ALCOHOL AND DRUG MISUSE

During recent years, the misuse of nicotine, alcohol, prescribed medications, over-the-counter drugs and illicit psychoactive substances has increased dramatically, resulting in health and socio-economic problems – to which every health care professional will need to recognise and respond.

Written by an experienced author and lecturer, this five-part text presents an introduction to alcohol and drug misuse and provides:

- an understanding of alcohol and drug misuse, and the nature and theories of addiction, as well as a historical overview and discussion of policy initiatives in contemporary society;
- an understanding of the problems associated with psychoactive substances and their impact on groups such as Black and ethnic minorities, young people, women, older people and the homeless;
- the generic role responses to substance misuse in a variety of different settings and contexts, including primary care, community and hospitals;
- a framework for assessment, care planning, harm reduction approach, dealing with overdose, intoxication and withdrawals, and psychological and pharmacological interventions;
- a skills-oriented approach to assist students and practitioners in dealing with drugs and alcohol misuse with accessible information about clinical issues, education and practice.

Alcohol and Drug Misuse takes into account current policy initiatives and practice for substance use and misuse and includes a range of pedagogical features to enhance learning. It is essential reading for nursing and health students taking substance misuse modules, as well as related CPD courses for health care professionals.

G. Hussein Rassool is Director of the Inter-Cultural Therapy Centre and Visiting Professor of Addiction and Mental Health at the University of São Paulo at Ribeirão Preto, Brazil.

ALCOHOL AND DRUG MISUSE

A HANDBOOK FOR STUDENTS AND HEALTH PROFESSIONALS

G. Hussein Rassool

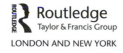

Routledge
Taylor & Francis Group

LONDON AND NEW YORK

First published 2009
by Routledge
2 Park Square, Milton Park, Abingdon, Oxon OX14 4RN

Simultaneously published in the USA and Canada
by Routledge
270 Madison Avenue, New York, NY 10016

Routledge is an imprint of the Taylor & Francis Group; an informa business

© 2009 G. Hussein Rassool

Typeset in Sabon and Futura by
Keystroke, 28 High Street, Tettenhall, Wolverhampton
Printed and bound in Great Britain by
TJ International Ltd, Padstow, Cornwall

British Library Cataloguing in Publication Data
A catalogue record for this book is available from the British Library

Library of Congress Cataloging in Publication Data
Rassool, G. Hussein.
Alcohol and drug misuse : a handbook for students and
health professionals/G. Hussein Rassool.
p. ; cm.
Includes bibliographical references.
1. Substance abuse–Handbooks. manuals, etc.
2. Alcoholism—Handbooks, manuals, etc.   I. Title.
[DNLM: 1. Substance-Related Disorders.   2. Harm Reduction.   3. Health Policy.
4. Substance-Related Disorders—prevention & control. WM 270 R228a 2008]
RC564.R33 2008
616.86—dc22   2008009169

ISBN 10: 0–415–40965–9 (hbk)
ISBN 10: 0–415–40967–5 (pbk)

ISBN 13: 978–0–415–40965–0 (hbk)
ISBN 13: 978–0–415–40967–4 (pbk)

Dedicated to Yasmin Soraya, Adam Ali Hussein, Reshad Hassan, Safian, Hassim, Mohamed Ally and Najmul Hussein.

Knowledge is of two kinds: that which is absorbed and that which is heard. And that which is heard does not profit if it is not absorbed.

Ali Ibn Abi Talib (RadiAllah Anhu)

CONTENTS

FIGURES AND TABLES

FIGURES

TABLES

PREFACE

Alcohol and drug misuse, their associated sequelae and their interventions strategies, are the subject of this book. The increase in the number of individuals with alcohol and drug problems has attracted considerable interest as one of the most important public health challenges. The book focuses on the approaches and intervention strategies that health and social care professionals can use to respond to this new challenge in specialist and non-specialist settings. The book underpins a number of current policy initiatives as applied to current practice and covers most aspects of alchol and drug misuse. An added dimension is the coverage of the special issues and needs of special populations, prevention and harm reduction, assessment, care planning, dealing with emergencies and psychological and pharmacological interventions.

The book provides a basic clinical and practical text on areas of clinical issues and practice, interventions, management and education. It will enable health and social care professionals and students to understand the extent and nature of substance use and misuse, and foster the knowledge and skills required in its management to provide effective care to patients they encounter in their daily practice. In addition, it provides a framework to assist practitioners in dealing with complex issues related to alcohol and drug misuse. It is envisaged that the book will act as a resource for health and social care practitioners who are unfamiliar with the substance misuse field. It will be of relevance to students in medicine, nursing, psychology, social work and criminal justice systems and those attending undergraduate and postgraduate courses in addiction and mental health studies. The book is practice-oriented and contains several activities related to the content of the chapters.

STRUCTURE OF THE BOOK

The book is presented in five parts. Part 1 provides an understanding of alcohol and drug misuse and the nature and theories of addiction, with a historical overview. It also includes the policy initiatives and strategies in alcohol and drug misuse that have shaped the provision and delivery of care. Part 2 presents the nature and problems associated with psychoactive substances from alcohol to eco-drugs. Part 3 deals with blood-borne viruses and special populations: Black and ethnic minority groups, young people, women, the elderly and homeless people. Part 4 deals with the generic role responses to substance misuse in a variety of different settings and contexts. These include engaging substance misusers in primary care, community and hospital settings. Subsequent chapters cover prevention and health education, strategies in helping people to change and working with diversity. Part 5 focuses on the framework for assessment, care planning, harm reduction approach, dealing with overdose, intoxication and withdrawals and psychological and pharmacological interventions.

The book contains a number of activities (True–False items, multiple-choice questions and questions requiring short answers) in most chapters. The reader is encouraged to undertake the activities found in each chapter to gain the added value of the contents. This book incorporates some of the knowledge and skills specification of DANOS (Drugs and Alcohol National Occupational Standards).

ACKNOWLEDGEMENTS

I would like to thank Eloise and Grace at Taylor & Francis for their support and patience throughout the process of writing and publication of this book.

I am also particularly grateful to Professor James P. Smith, Professor John Strang, Professor A. Hamid Ghodse, Dr Nek Oyefeso and the Florence Nightingale Research Foundation for their guidance in my professional development. Special thanks go to Professor Margarita Villar-Luis, Escola De Enfermagem de Ribeirao Preto, Universidade de São Paulo, Brazil, for collaboration and development in publishing, teaching and research activities in addiction and mental health.

Thanks go to my patients and students for teaching me about the practice in the addiction field. Thanks also go to all my brothers at Al-Furqan, Les Guibies for their friendships and support. I would like to acknowledge the contributions made by my teachers, who enabled me, through my own reflective practices, to follow the path.

My special thanks also to Mariam for all the help and support during the writing of the book. Finally, I owe my gratitude to my children, Yasmin, Adam and Reshad who keep me going and active in various endeavours and have taught me about life. Welcome to the family Leyla.

PART 1

OVERVIEW OF SUBSTANCE MISUSE AND POLICY INITIATIVES

CHAPTER 1

INTRODUCTION TO SUBSTANCE USE AND MISUSE

OBJECTIVES

- Have an understanding of the global drug scene.

- Explain the meaning of the following terms: drug, alcohol, substance misuse, addiction, problem-drug use and problem-alcohol use, hazardous drinker, harmful drinker, severely dependent drinkers and drinkers with complex problems.

- Examine the components of concept of dependence: tolerance, physical and psychological dependence.

In the twenty-first century, there is no lack of interest in the use of psychoactive substances and plants. Alcohol and drug use remain the social and psychological fabric of our society and are now regarded as a public health problem. Society has learned to co-exist with drugs and alcohol, and its views of which drugs should be legal or illicit change with time and economic and political considerations. For example, tea, coffee and tobacco have all been illegal in Britain at various points in history (Whitaker 1987), but with time, increasing availability and more widespread use opinions change, and the drug becomes 'normalized'. Alcohol and drug use cause a host of physical, social, psychological and economic harms not only to the individual but to the family and the community. The harms include higher risks of premature death; risk of acquiring blood-borne virus such as hepatitis B and C and HIV; overdose; respiratory failure; and mental health problems. It is stated that drug problems will not be beaten out of society by yet harsher laws, lectured out of society by yet more hours of 'health education', or treated out of society by yet more drug experts (Royal College of Psychiatrists 1987).

GLOBAL DRUG SCENES

The growing epidemic of drug misuse appeared to have slowed down with 'significant and positive changes' in world drugs markets according to a report of the United Nations Office on Drugs and Crime (UNODC 2007). The Report shows that global markets for illicit drugs remained largely stable in 2005–6. There are signs of overall stability in the production, trafficking or consumption of cocaine, heroin, cannabis and amphetamines. About 5 per cent of the world's population, about 200 million, between the ages of 15 and 64 uses illicit drugs each year but only a small share of these can be considered 'problem drug users' (0.6 per cent). The main problem of drugs at the global level continued to be the opiates (notably heroin), followed by cocaine. For most of Europe and Asia, opiates continued to be the main problem drug; in South America, drug-related treatment demand continued to be mainly linked to the misuse of cocaine; and in Africa, the bulk of all treatment demand is linked to cannabis. Countries experiencing an increase in heroin usage include those surrounding Afghanistan (Pakistan, Iran and Central Asia), as well as Russia, India and parts of Africa. Many of these areas have high levels of poverty and HIV, leaving them vulnerable to the worst effects of this drug.

Cocaine consumption has increased significantly in Europe, doubling or tripling in several countries over the last decade. In Africa, notably in the countries of western Africa, cocaine use has also increased. Overall cocaine consumption levels in Europe are still significantly lower than in North America. High and rising levels of cocaine use have also been reported from the UK, Spain and Italy. Cannabis is the largest illicit drug market by far, with roughly 160 million annual consumers. Although consumer demands for cannabis appear to have contracted somewhat, there has been a reported increase of cannabis use in Africa and in most countries of South America. The situation in Europe and Asia is mixed. Global demand for amphetamines (methamphetamine and amphetamine), which increased strongly in most parts of the world in the 1990s, is now showing signs of overall stabilisation.

The World Health Organization (WHO 2007) estimates that there are about two billion people worldwide who consume alcoholic beverages and 76.3 million with diagnosable alcohol use disorders. Alcohol is estimated to cause about 20–30 per cent of oesophageal cancer, liver cancer, cirrhosis of the liver, homicide, epileptic seizures, and motor vehicle accidents worldwide (WHO 2002). There are over one billion smokers across the world causing four million deaths a year (WHO 1998). There is an upward trend in tobacco smoking in Third World countries and in Eastern Europe.

WHAT IS A DRUG?

ACTIVITY 1.1

State by ticking yes or no what you think is/are the definition(s) of a drug

	Yes	No
A substance other than food intended to affect the structure or function of the body		
A substance intended for use in the diagnosis, cure, mitigation, treatment, or prevention of disease		
A substance used as a medication or in the preparation of medication		
A substance recognised in an official pharmacopoeia or formulary		
A substance intended for use as a component of a medicine but not a device or a component, part or accessory of a device		
A substance used in dyeing or chemical operations		
A commodity that is not salable or for which there is no demand		
Something, often an illegal substance that causes addiction, habituation, or a marked change in consciousness		
Any substance or chemical that alters the structure or functioning of a living being		
A psychoactive substance that affects the central nervous system and alters mood, perception and behaviour		

Source: 1–8 *Encyclopædia Britannica* (2007).
World Health Organization (1981)

In fact, the definitions in Activity 1.1 are all potential definitions of a drug. However, the language of 'addiction' is confusing but it is essential to have a common language for understanding the complexities of substance misuse. There are various elements in what constitute a drug (food or chocolate can be considered a drug) as the concept is heavily influenced by the socio-cultural context and purpose of its use. The therapeutic use of drugs refers to a pharmacological preparation used in the prevention, diagnosis and treatment of an abnormal or pathological condition whereas the non-therapeutic use of drugs commonly indicates the use of illegal or socially disapproved substances (Rassool 1998). However, drugs can be either therapeutic or non-therapeutic or both. According to the World Health Organization (1981), a drug is 'any substance or chemical that alters the structure or functioning of a living being'. Despite the broadness of the concept which limits its use for clinical and for certain practical purposes, it provides some perspective into its pervasive nature. A drug, in the broadest sense, is a chemical substance that has an effect on bodily systems and behaviour. This includes a wide range of prescribed drugs and illegal and socially accepted substances.

ACTIVITY 1.2

- What are drug misuse and abuse?
- What is meant by the terms problem drug user and problem drinker?
- Explain the following terms: substance abuse, dependence and addictive behaviour
- What is meant by tolerance?
- What is meant by physical and psychological dependence?
- Users of psychoactive substances are described as experimental, recreational or dependent. What do the terms experimental, recreational and experimental mean? What are their characteristics?

DRUG MISUSE AND ABUSE

The terms 'drug misuse' and 'drug abuse' are difficult to define precisely but the operational use of these concepts is heavily dependent on the particular culture, ideology, aetiology and clinical practice (Rassool 1998) and the effect of the substance on the individual. Drug use refers to the ingestion of a substance that is used for therapeutic purpose or as prescribed by medical practitioners. The term drug misuse may be seen as the use of a drug in a socially unacceptable way that is harmful or hazardous to the individual or others (Royal College of Psychiatrists and Royal College of Physicians 2000). Drug misuse is the result of a psychoactive substance being consumed in a way that it was not intended for and causes physical, social and psychological harm. Drug misuse also implies use outside the therapeutic use which harms health or functioning. It may take the form of physical or psychological dependence or be part of a wider spectrum of problematic or harmful behaviour. It is also used to represent the pattern of use: experimental, recreational and dependent. The generic term 'substance misuse' is often used to denote the misuse of alcohol and drugs.

The term 'drug abuse', often associated with addiction and dependence, is considered to be value-laden and has limited use in the addiction literature in the United Kingdom. In the United States, practitioners prefer the term 'abuse' for problems resulting from the use of alcohol or other mood-altering drugs and use the term 'addictive disorders' when the problems have escalated to dependency (Sullivan 1995). The World Health Organization recommends the use of the following terms:

- *Unsanctioned use*: A drug that is not approved by society
- *Hazardous use*: A drug leading to harm or dysfunction
- *Dysfunctional use*: A drug leading to impaired psychological or social functioning
- *Harmful use*: A drug that is known to have caused tissue damage or psychiatric disorders.

DRUG DEPENDENCE

The term 'drug dependence' refers to behavioural responses that always include a compulsion to take the drug in order to experience its physical or psychological effects, and sometimes to avoid the discomfort of its absence. Dependence is often described as either physical or psychological. Physical dependence is a common and often important, but not a necessary, element of drug dependence. This highlights the core features of dependence such as tolerance and psychological and physical dependence. These concepts need further explanations and are examined in the next section. Dependence, according to DSM-IV (APA 1994), requires three out of seven criteria to be occurring at any time in the same 12-month period. The DSM-IV criteria for dependence are briefly presented in Table 1.1. Dependence is also seen as comparable to addiction as 'the user has adapted physically and/or psychologically to the presence of the drug and would suffer if it is withdrawn' (Royal College of Psychiatrists and Royal College of Physicians 2000).

Table 1.1 DSM IV Diagnostic criteria for substance dependence

A maladaptive pattern of substance use leading to clinically significant impairment or distress is manifested by three or more of the following occurring during the same 12-month period:

1 Tolerance, as defined by either of the following:
   - need for markedly increased amounts of the substance to achieve intoxication or desired effect
   - markedly diminished effect of continued use of the same amount of the substance

2 Withdrawal, as manifested by either of the following:
   - the characteristic withdrawal syndrome for the substance
   - the same (or a closely related) substance is taken to relieve or avoid withdrawal symptoms

3 The substance is often taken in larger amounts or over a long period than was intended

4 A persistent desire or unsuccessful efforts to cut down or control substance use

5 A great deal of time is spent in activities necessary to obtain the substance (e g., visiting multiple doctors or driving long distances), in use of substance (e.g., chain-smoking), or recovering from its effects

6 Important social, occupational or recreational activities are given up or reduced because of substance use

7 The substance use is continued despite knowledge of having a persistent or recurrent physical or psychological problem that is likely to have been caused or exacerbated by the substance (e.g., current cocaine-induced depression, or continued drinking despite recognition that an ulcer was made worse by alcohol consumption)

ADDICTION AND ADDICTIVE BEHAVIOUR

The concept of addiction is synonymous with related terms such as dependence and misuse. Addictive behaviour includes the misuse of psychoactive substances and activities leading to excessive behavioural patterns. Individuals who have problems with excessive behaviours such as eating, drinking, drug use, gambling and sexuality present similar descriptions of the phenomenology of their disorders (Cummings, Gordon and Marlatt 1980, Orford 1985). This entails the classification of both pharmacological and non-pharmacological addictions under the more inclusive diagnostic category of addictive behaviour (Marks 1990, Ghodse 1995).

PROBLEM DRUG USERS AND PROBLEM DRINKERS

The terms 'problem drug user' and 'problem drinker' have been used to refer to those who are dependent on psychoactive substances. The problem drug user has been described as 'any person who experiences social, psychological, physical or legal problems related to intoxication and/or regular excessive consumption and/or dependence as a consequence of his own use of drugs or other chemical substances . . . and may involve or lead to sharing of injecting equipment' (ACMD 1982, 1988). This definition focuses on the needs and problems of the individual and places less emphasis on the substance-oriented approach. It is a holistic definition in acknowledging that the problem drug user has social, psychological, physical and legal needs, and the definition could be expanded to incorporate the spiritual needs of the individual of the problem drug user or problem drinker (Rassool 2001, Hammond and Rassool 2006).

HAZARDOUS DRINKERS

The World Health Organization (WHO 1994) defines hazardous use of a psychoactive substance, such as alcohol, as 'a pattern of substance use that increases the risk of harmful consequences for the user . . . hazardous use refers to patterns of use that are of public health significance despite the absence of any current disorder in the individual user'. Hazardous drinkers are drinking at levels over the sensible drinking limits, in terms of either regular excessive consumption or less frequent sessions of heavy drinking.

HARMFUL DRINKERS

The WHO International Classification of Diseases (ICD-10) (1992) defines harmful use of a psychoactive substance, such as alcohol, as 'a pattern of use which is already causing damage to health. The damage may be physical or mental'. This definition does not include those with alcohol dependence. Harmful drinkers are usually drinking at levels above those recommended for sensible drinking, typically at higher levels than most hazardous drinkers. Unlike hazardous drinkers, harmful drinkers show clear evidence of some alcohol-related harm.

MODERATELY DEPENDENT DRINKERS

Moderately dependent drinkers may recognise that they have a problem with drinking and they may not have reached the stage of 'relief drinking' – which is drinking to relieve or avoid physical discomfort from withdrawal symptoms (NTA 2006). In older terminology, drinkers in this category would probably not have been described as 'chronic alcoholics'. Treatment of moderately dependent drinkers can often be managed effectively in community settings, including medically assisted alcohol withdrawal in the community.

SEVERELY DEPENDENT DRINKERS

Individuals in this category may have serious and long-standing problems of 'chronic alcoholism', and may have been heavy users over prolonged periods. This habit of significant alcohol consumption may be due to stopping the withdrawal symptoms. Such individuals may have special needs, such as co-existing psychiatric problems, learning disabilities, polydrug use or complicated assisted alcohol withdrawal; others may need rehabilitation and strategies to address the level of their dependence, or to address other issues, such as homelessness or social dislocation. However, more severely dependent drinkers may be in need of inpatient assisted alcohol withdrawal and residential rehabilitation.

PSYCHOLOGICAL AND PHYSICAL DEPENDENCE

Tolerance

Tolerance refers to the way the body usually adapts to the repeated presence of a drug. Higher quantities or doses of the psychoactive substance are required to reproduce the desired or similar cognitive, affective or behavioural effects. Individuals can develop tolerance to a variety of psychoactive substances. Tolerance may develop rapidly in the case of LSD or slowly in the case of alcohol or opiates. The drug must be taken on a regular basis and in adequate quantities for tolerance to occur. For example, amphetamines can produce considerable tolerance and strong psychological dependence with little or no physical dependence, and cocaine can produce psychological dependence without tolerance or physical dependence. Furthermore, in certain medical applications, morphine has been reported to produce tolerance and physical dependence without a significant psychological component.

Psychological dependence

Psychological dependence can be described as a compulsion or a craving to continue to take the substance because of the need for stimulation, or because it relieves anxiety or depression. Psychological dependence is recognised as the most widespread and the most important. This kind of dependence is attributed not only to the use of psychoactive drugs but also to food, sex, gambling, relationships or physical activities.

Physical dependence

Physical dependence is characterised by the need to take a psychoactive substance to avoid physical disturbances or withdrawal symptoms following cessation of use. The withdrawal symptoms depend on the type or category of drugs. For example, for nicotine, the physiological withdrawal symptoms may be relatively slight. For other dependence-inducing psychoactive substances such as opiates and depressants, the withdrawal experience can range from mild to severe. The withdrawal from alcohol for instance can cause hallucinations or epileptic fits and may be life-threatening. Physical withdrawal syndromes are not, however, the essence of dependence. It is possible to have dependence without withdrawal and withdrawal without dependence (Royal College of Psychiatrists 1987). Many of the supposed signs of physical dependence are sometimes psychosomatic reactions triggered off not by the chemical properties of psychoactive drug but by the user's fears, beliefs and fantasies about what withdrawal entails (Plant 1987).

THE DEPENDENCE SYNDROME

The original framework of the dependence syndrome referred specifically to alcohol dependence but this has been expanded to include other psychoactive substances. The dependence syndrome, derived from the disease, biological and behavioural models, has provided a common language for academics and clinicians to talk about the same phenomena. According to Edwards and Gross (1976), there are seven components of the syndrome (See Table 1.2)

Table 1.2 The dependence syndrome

- Increased tolerance to the drug
- Repeated withdrawal symptoms
- Compulsion to use the drug (psychological state known as craving)
- Salience of drug-seeking behaviour (obtaining and using the drug become more important in the person's life)
- Relief or avoidance of withdrawal symptoms (the regular use of the drug to relieve withdrawal symptoms)
- Narrowing of the repertoire of drug taking (pattern of drinking may become an everyday activity
- Rapid reinstatement after abstinence

KEY POINTS

- Drug use includes a wide range of prescribed drugs and illegal and socially accepted substances.
- The terms 'problem drug user' and 'problem drinker' have been used to refer to those who are dependent on psychoactive substances.
- Individuals can develop tolerance to a variety of psychoactive substances.
- Dependence has two components: physical and psychological dependence.

- Drugs can produce considerable tolerance and strong psychological dependence with little or no physical dependence.
- The withdrawal symptoms depend on the type or category of drugs.

REFERENCES

Advisory Council on the Misuse of Drugs (1982) *Treatment and Rehabilitation*. London: HMSO.

Advisory Council on the Misuse of Drugs (1988) *Aids and Drug Misuse: Part 1*, London: HMSO.

American Psychiatric Association (1994) DSM-IV: *Diagnostic and Statistic Manual of Mental Disorders*, 4th edition. Washington DC: American Psychiatric Association, 75–90.

Cummings, C., Gordon, J.R. and Marlatt, G.A. (1980) Relapse: prevention and prediction. In W.R. Miller (ed.) *The Addictive Behaviours: Treatment of Alcoholism, Drug Abuse, Smoking and Obesity*. New York: Pergamon Press.

Edwards, G. and Gross, M. (1976) Alcohol dependence: provisional description of a clinical syndrome. *British Journal of Addiction*, 81: 171–3.

Encyclopædia Britannica (2007), from Encyclopædia Britannica Ultimate Reference Suite 2005 DVD. Copyright © 1994–2004 Encyclopædia Britannica, Inc. Encyclopædia Britannica www.britannica.com/dictionary (accessed 15 March 2007).

Ghodse, A.H. (1995) *Drugs and Addictive Behaviour*. Oxford: Blackwell Science.

Hamond, A. and Rassool, G. Hussein (2006) Spiritual and cultural needs: integration in dual diagnosis care. In G. Hussein Rassool (ed.), *Dual Diagnosis Nursing*, Oxford: Blackwell Publishing.

Marks, I. (1990) Behavioural (non-chemical) addictions. *British Journal of Addiction*, 85: 1389–94.

Merriam-Webster's Collegiate Dictionary, from Encyclopædia Britannica Ultimate Reference Suite 2005 DVD. Copyright © 1994–2004 Merriam-Webster, Inc. (accessed 15 March 2007).

NTA (2006) *Models of Care for Alcohol Misusers* (MoCAM). London: National Treatment Agency.

Orford, J. (1985) *Excessive Appetites: A Psychological View of Addictions*. Chichester: John Wiley & Sons.

Plant, M. (1987) *Drugs in Perspective*. London: Hodder and Stoughton.

Rassool, G. Hussein (1998) *Substance Use and Misuse: Nature, Context and Clinical Interventions*. Oxford: Blackwell Science.

Rassool, G. Hussein (2001) *Substance Use and Dual Diagnosis: Concepts, Theories and Models*. In G. Hussein Rassool (ed.), *Dual Diagnosis: Substance Misuse and Psychiatric Disorders*. Oxford: Blackwell Science.

Royal College of Psychiatrists (1987) *Drug Scenes: A Report on Drugs and Drug Dependence*. The Royal College of Psychiatrists. London: Gaskell.

Royal College of Psychiatrists and Royal College of Physicians Working Party (2000) *Drugs: Dilemmas and Choices*. London: Gaskell.

Sullivan, E.J. (1995) *Nursing Care of Clients with Substance Abuse*. St Louis, Missouri: Mosby-Year Book, Inc.

United Nations Office of Drugs and Crime (2007) *World Drug Report 2007* http://www.unodc.org/unodc/en/world_drug_report.html (accessed 15 March 2007).

Whitaker, B. (1987) *The Global Connection: The Crisis of Drug Addiction*. London: Jonathan Cape.

WHO (1981) Nomenclature and classification of drug- and alcohol-related problems: A WHO Memorandum. *Bulletin of the World Health Organization*, 59: 225–42.

WHO (1992) *International Classification of Diseases: The ICD-10 Classification of Mental and Behavioural Disorders (ICD-10)*. Geneva: World Health Organization.

WHO (1994) *Lexicon of Alcohol and Drug Terms*. Geneva: World Health Organization.

WHO (1998) *Health for All*. Data Base: European Region, Geneva: World Health Organization.

WHO (2002) *Alcohol in Developing Societies: A Public Health Approach*, Geneva: WHO.

WHO (2007) *WHO Expert Committee on Problems Related to Alcohol Consumption, Second Report*, Technical Series No. 944. Geneva: World Health Organization.

CHAPTER 2

SELF-AWARENESS AND ATTITUDE

OBJECTIVES

- Have developed greater sensitivity regarding substance misusers.

- Be more accepting of individuals with alcohol or drug problems.

- Describe briefly the stigmatisation and stereotypes of alcohol and drug users.

- List some of the harmful substances.

- Be more aware and confident around drug/alcohol issues.

In this chapter, we will consider your own use of alcohol and drugs. In order to understand the nature and reasons behind the use of alcohol and drugs, you will need first to understand your own 'dependence' on psychoactive substances and other things. You need also to be more aware of your own attitude towards substance misusers. Understanding why individuals become dependent on alcohol or drugs may enable you to have a more positive attitude (feeling, thinking and behaviour) about substance misusers and help them to change their behaviour.

ACTIVITY 2.1

1   List your dependencies
    (a) Substances
    (b) Activities
    (c) People or things
2   (a) Why do you think you may be dependent on them?
2   (b) Why do you need them?
2   (c) What do they do for you?
3   (a) How would you feel if you had to give up your preferred choice of dependence?
3   (b) Would it be easy or difficult?
3   (c) Would you have physical or psychological withdrawal symptoms or both?

Source: Scottish Drugs Training Project, University of Stirling

---

This activity explores one's own 'dependency' on substances (alcohol and drugs), things, people or activities (Scottish Drugs Training Project, University of Stirling). For example, people may be dependent on coffee, tea, chocolate, alcohol at the end of the working day, first cigarette on waking up, jogging, horse racing, the internet and soap opera – in fact, anything, any substances, things or activities that would cause a void in your daily life if taken away from you.

The reasons why people use drugs and continue to use drugs are two different propositions. The reasons may or may not be the same. Physical and psychological withdrawals of psychoactive substances are discussed in Part 2.

ATTITUDE

An attitude is the way we feel, think and behave towards an individual or things. For example, people can have a good (or positive) attitude towards their working with alcohol and drug misusers, usually meaning that they feel good about their work and their roles in working with this client group. Others may think or feel differently about substance misusers – for example, that most alcohol or drug misusers are unpleasant to work with or the penalties for drinking and driving are too lenient.

Attitudes are influenced by a variety of factors, including past experiences (positive and negative), knowledge, education, context of the situation, and cultural and religious factors. Changing attitudes are a complex problem as an individual's attitudes may be closely tied to their personal values, belief system or important aspects of their self-identity (Wood 2000). Many factors impact on nurses and other health care professionals' willingness to intervene with individuals who use drug and alcohol. These factors include knowledge, training, organisational structure and policies and previous positive or negative experiences. Attitudes towards drug users represent one factor within this wider set that may impact on health professionals' responses to individuals with problematic drug use.

Acceptance of new attitudes 'depends on who is presenting the knowledge, how it is presented, how the person is perceived, the credibility of the communicator, and the conditions by which the knowledge was received' (Halloran 1967: 60–1). Attitude cannot be changed solely by simple education. It is important to recognise, however, that work colleagues, supervisors and the organisational culture may also influence workers' attitudes towards individuals who use alcohol and drug (Pidd *et al*. 2004)

Attitudes towards individuals who use alcohol or drug can be broadly categorised as professional or personal views. Professional attitudes refer to beliefs concerning professional practice such as role legitimacy (i.e., is it appropriate for me to respond to drug use within my professional role?), confidence (perceived level of skill and ability) and perceived efficacy of available treatments and interventions. Personal attitudes refer to feelings and beliefs that stem from the stigmatised nature of drug use, for example blame and anger.

ATTITUDE AND STIGMATISATION

Attitudes towards substance abusers remain a perennial problem. Despite the magnitude of the problem, and even when alcohol and drug problems are identified, health care professionals may be reluctant to respond appropriately because of negative attitudes towards substance misusers. Social prejudice, negative attitudes and stereotyped perceptions of substance misusers and dual-diagnosis patients are held widely amongst health care professionals and this may lead to minimal care being given to this population (Rassool 1998, Selleck and Redding 1998, Williams 1999, Richmond and Foster 2003). Gafoor and Rassool (1998) stated that overtly self-abusive behaviour, particularly when it involves illicit drugs, can be dealt with in a suppressive and moralist way by many health care workers not least nurses, probably out of a sense of frustration or inadequacy about an ability to effect any change.

There is some evidence that health professionals' attitudes towards substance abusers exert a significant influence on their willingness to intervene and the quality of such interventions (Karam-Hage *et al*. 2001). Subsequently, negative attitudes towards substance misusers are likely to make nurses less reluctant to work with alcohol and drug abusers or to cause them to provide minimal care to this group of patients. Negative attitudes have been associated with the application of alcohol and drug training into clinical practice by nurses, reduced likelihood that clients will pursue referrals and reluctance to engage in management and treatment with substance abusers (Ask *et al*. 1998, Abouyanni *et al*. 2000, Mistral and Velleman, 2001). There is also evidence to suggest that substance misusers are reluctant to utilise health services for drug-related or other health problems because of the negative attitudes and behaviours of staff. (McLaughlin *et al*. 2000).

Complete the Rassool Attitude Towards Substance Misusers Questionnaire (© G. Hussein Rassool 2004. Permission should be obtained from the author for the use of the questionnaire) in Activity 2.2. Reflect on your attitudes towards alcohol and drug misusers. Write in your reflective journal about your own substance use and your attitude towards substance misusers.

ACTIVITY 2.2

Rassool Attitude Towards Substance Misusers Questionnaire (RATSMQ-10)

The following statements reflect several different opinions, beliefs and viewpoints about substance use and misuse. Indicate how strongly you agree or disagree with each statement. To complete the questionnaire, place a tick in the box that best reflects how strongly you agree or disagree with each statement.

1. Personal use of illicit drug should be legal in the confines of one's home.

    ❑   ❑   ❑   ❑   ❑
    Strongly agree   Agree   Uncertain   Disagree   Strongly disagree

2. Drug addicts suffer from feelings of inferiority.

    ❑   ❑   ❑   ❑   ❑
    Strongly agree   Agree   Uncertain   Disagree   Strongly disagree

3. People who use illicit drug do not respect authority.

    ❑   ❑   ❑   ❑   ❑
    Strongly agree   Agree   Uncertain   Disagree   Strongly disagree

4. Heroin is so addictive that no one can really recover once he or she becomes an addict.

    ❑   ❑   ❑   ❑   ❑
    Strongly agree   Agree   Uncertain   Disagree   Strongly disagree

5. Rehabilitation of drug misusers always fails.

    ❑   ❑   ❑   ❑   ❑
    Strongly agree   Agree   Uncertain   Disagree   Strongly disagree

6. Illicit drug users are a financial and social drain on the community.

    ❑   ❑   ❑   ❑   ❑
    Strongly agree   Agree   Uncertain   Disagree   Strongly disagree

7. Compulsory treatment is necessary for those who are addicted to drug and/or alcohol.

    ❑   ❑   ❑   ❑   ❑
    Strongly agree   Agree   Uncertain   Disagree   Strongly disagree

8. Alcohol misusers should be referred to a specialist once health problems are identified.

    ❑   ❑   ❑   ❑   ❑
    Strongly agree   Agree   Uncertain   Disagree   Strongly disagree

9.   Those who are addicted to drugs are unpleasant to work with.

❑   ❑   ❑   ❑   ❑
Strongly agree   Agree   Uncertain   Disagree   Strongly disagree

10.   Drug addicts are stigmatised by health care professionals.

❑   ❑   ❑   ❑   ❑
Strongly agree   Agree   Uncertain   Disagree   Strongly disagree

---

It is clear that, unless nursing education addresses the attitudes that underpin the stigmatisation of substance abusing patients, and supports the acquisition of the necessary skills and knowledge, a significant proportion of patients will be denied due response and intervention (Rassool 2007).

HARM

Public health policy regarding drug and alcohol misuse is primarily aimed at reducing the harm caused to individual users, their families and society. Some drugs are more harmful than others. Harm caused by substance misuse includes physical harms, social harms, psychological harms and economic harms. Currently, harmful substances are currently regulated according to classification systems (Misuse of Drugs Act) that purport to relate to the harms and risks of each drug.

ACTIVITY 2.3

List of substances

Alcohol	Ecstasy
Alkyl nitrates	GHB
Amphetamines	Heroin
Anabolic steroids	Ketamine
Barbiturates	Khat
Benzodiazepines	LSD
Buprenorphine	Methadone (street)
Cocaine	Solvents
Cannabis	Tobacco

Classify each substance listed in the table above according to the relative degree of harm you think it causes. For example, if you think that ecstasy is the most harmful substance in the list, you should write it in the number 1 ranking overleaf.

1	10
2	11
3	12
4	13
5	14
6	15
7	16
8	17
9	18

Activity 2.3 examines an individual's notion of a 'harmful' drug. You should classify and write each substance according to the relative degree of harm you think it causes.

A new 'matrix of harm' for drugs of abuse has been proposed by Nutt *et al*. (2007). The study proposes that drugs should be classified by the amount of harm that they do, rather than the sharp A, B and C divisions in the UK Misuse of Drugs Act. Nutt *et al*. (2007) identified three main factors that together determine the harm associated with any drug of potential abuse:

- the physical harm to the individual user caused by the drug
- the tendency of the drug to induce dependence
- the effect of drug use on families, communities, and society.

The new ranking places alcohol and tobacco in the upper half of the league table. These socially accepted drugs were judged more harmful than cannabis, and substantially more dangerous than the class A drugs LSD, 4-methylthioamphetamine and ecstasy (see Figure 2.1 for new ranking). Heroin and cocaine were ranked most dangerous, followed by barbiturates and street methadone. Alcohol was the fifth most harmful drug and tobacco the ninth most harmful. Cannabis came in eleventh, and near the bottom of the list was ecstasy.

Now compare your own classification with those of Nutt *et al*. (2007) as shown in Figure 2.1. What are the similarities or differences in comparison? Are your ideas of harm of substances based on the media, your personal experience or experiences of others? Is the notion of harm based on medical, moral, social or legal criteria?

CONFIDENCE SKILLS

In order to work with alcohol and drug misusers, there is a need to have confidence in our own abilities. Confidence is a psychological quality that arises from considering if a person or thing is capable of something. Confidence can be a self-fulfilling prophecy, as those without it may fail or not try because they lack it, and those with it may succeed because they have it, rather than because of an innate ability (wikipedia.org/wiki/Confidence 2007). Nurses and other health care professionals will have some areas of their nursing or health activity where they feel quite confident, while at the same time they do not feel at all confident in other areas. Confidence is something which comes naturally with experience and practice but for some individuals could be an attitude or a habit of thought. Taking a positive attitude may help the development of confidence skills in working with alcohol and drug misusers.

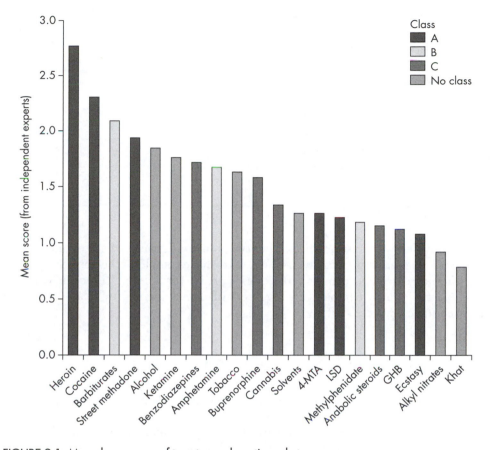

FIGURE 2.1 Mean harm score of twenty psychoactive substances

Source: Nutt *et al.* (2007)

ACTIVITY 2.4

Addiction intervention skills questionnaire (© Rassool 2004)

To complete the questionnaire, please tick the box that best reflects your confidence level

	Low confidence	Moderate confidence	High confidence
Providing alcohol use education and prevention information			
Recognising signs and symptoms of alcohol problems			
Talking to patients about risks of alcohol misuse			
Taking an alcohol history			
Referring patients for alcohol treatment			
Providing care for patients with alcohol problems			

Providing drug use education and prevention information

Recognising signs and symptoms of drug problems

Talking to patients about risks of drug misuse

Taking a drug history

Referring patients for drug treatment

Providing care for patients with drug problems

Giving health risk information on prescribed medication

Informing smokers about health risks of tobacco smoking

Providing tobacco education and prevention information

Knowledge of drug and alcohol services

Complete the questionnaire of intervention confidence skills in working with substance misusers now (Activity 2.4). When you have completed the book or a course, you should return and complete the questionnaire for a second time. It would be valuable for you to compare the two sets of questionnaires in relation to your intervention confidence skills.

KEY POINTS

- There is a need to be self-aware about own dependence on substances, things, activities or people.
- Reflect on our own attitude towards those with alcohol and drug problems.
- It is important to develop a positive attitude in order to enhance the quality of care given to those with alcohol or drug problems.
- Public health policy regarding drug and alcohol misuse is primarily aimed at reducing the harm caused to individual users, their families and society.
- Harm caused by substance misuse includes physical harms, social harms, psychological harms and economic harms.
- Working with substance misusers requires confidence, which comes with experience and practice.
- Taking a positive attitude may help the development of confidence skills in working with alcohol and drug misusers.

REFERENCES

Abouyanni, G., Stevens, L., Harris, M., Wickes, W., Ramakrishna, S., Ta, E. *et al*. (2000) GP attitudes to managing drug- and alcohol-dependent patients: a reluctant role. *Drug and Alcohol Review*, 19: 165–70.

Ask, A., Ashenden, R., Allsop, S., Cormack, S., Addy, D. and Beel, A. (1998) *Education and Training Programs for Frontline Professionals Responding to Drug Problems in Australia: A Literature Review*. Adelaide, South Australia: National Centre for Education and Training on Addiction (NCETA).

Gafoor, M. and Rassool, G. Hussein (1998) The co-existence of psychiatric disorders and substance misuse: working with dual diagnosis patients. *Journal of Advanced Nursing*, 27: 497–502.

Halloran, J.D. (1967) *Attitude Formation and Change*. Leicester: Leicester University Press.

Karam-Hage, M., Nerenberg, L. and Brower, K.J. (2001) Modifying residents' attitudes about substance abuse treatment and training. *American Journal on Addictions*, 10: 40–7.

McLaughlin, D., McKenna, H. and Leslie, J.C. (2000) The perceptions and aspirations of illicit drug users hold towards health care staff and the care they receive. *Journal of Psychiatric and Mental Health Nursing*, 7: 435–41.

Mistral, W. and Velleman, R. (2001). Substance-misusing patients in primary care: incidence, services provided and problems. A survey of general practitioners in Wiltshire. *Drugs: Education, Prevention and Policy*, 8: 61–71.

Nutt, D., King, L.A., Saulsbury, W. and Blakemore, C. (2007) Development of a rational scale to assess the harm of drugs of potential misuse. *The Lancet*, 369, 9566: 1047–53.

Pidd, K., Freemen, T., Skinner, N., Addy, D., Shoobridge, J. and Roche, A.M. (2004) *From Training to Work Practice Change: An Examination of Factors Influencing Training Transfer in the Alcohol and Other Drugs Field*. Adelaide: National Centre for Education and Training on Addiction, Flinders University.

Rassool, G. Hussein (1998) Contemporary issues in addiction nursing. In G. Hussein Rassool (ed.) *Substance Use and Misuse: Nature, Context and Clinical Interventions*. Oxford: Blackwell Science.

Rassool G. Hussein (2007) Some considerations on attitude to addictions: waiting for the tide to change. Guest Editorial. *Journal of Addictions Nursing*, 18, 2: 61–3.

Richmond, I.C. and Foster, J.H. (2003) Negative attitudes towards people with co-morbid mental health and substance misuse problems: an investigation of mental health professionals. *Journal of Mental Health*, 12, 4: 393–403.

Selleck, C. and Redding, B. (1998) Knowledge and attitudes of registered nurses toward perinatal substance abuse. *Journal of Obstetric, Gynecologic & Neonatal Nursing*, 27, 1: 70–7.

wikipedia.org/wiki/Confidence 2007 (accessed 30 June 2007).

Williams, K. (1999) Attitudes of mental health professionals to co-morbidity between mental health problems and substance misuse. *Journal of Mental Health*, 8, 6: 606–13.

Wood, I. (1998) Effects of continuing professional education on the clinical practice of nurses: a review of the literature. *International Journal of Nursing Studies*, 35, 3: 125–31.

Wood, W. (2000) Attitude change: persuasion and social influence. *Annual Review of Psychology*, 51, 2: 539–70.

HISTORICAL OVERVIEW

Substance use dates back thousand of years, and records of ancient civilisations provide evidence of the use of alcohol and plants with psychoactive properties. From the earliest times, alcohol and drugs have been used for medicinal, religious, cultural and recreational purposes and as a social lubricant. The use of alcohol and drugs throughout history helps us to understand the distinctive nature of psychoactive substances in today's society and the changes in the use and misuse of alcohol and drug.

ACTIVITY 3.1

Are the following statements true or false?

	True	False
Throughout history, alcohol has been used for medicinal purposes		
The term alcohol is derived from the Arabic language 'Al-Kuhl'		
Habitual drunkness was uncommon in ancient Greece		
Beer or ale has been used as a payment for rent		

Opium contains morphine and codeine

In nineteenth-century England, you could buy opium products from the grocery store

Opium-based products have been given to young children

Cocaine has been used for the treatment of alcohol and drug addiction

Cocaine has been sold in cigarettes and chewing gum

Amphetamine has been used in the treatment of hyperactive children

LSD has been used in the treatment of addiction and mental health problems

Tobacco would be considered as an illicit substance if it was found today

Drinking coffee has been seen as a deviant behaviour

ALCOHOL

The word 'alcohol' comes from the Arabic language, and may be derived from the *al-kuhl*, the name of an early distilled substance, or perhaps from *al-gawl*, meaning 'spirit' or 'demon' and akin to liquors being called 'spirits' in English. The discovery of late Stone Age beer jugs has established the fact that intentionally fermented beverages existed at least as early as the Neolithic period (c. 10,000 BC), and it has been suggested that beer may have preceded bread as a staple; wine clearly appeared as a finished product in Egyptian pictographs around 4000 BC (Hanson 1995). The earliest reference to the misuse of alcohol appears in the Old Testament referring to Noah's plantation of a vineyard and his drunkenness. In ancient Egypt alcoholic beverages were considered a necessity of life, and Osiris, the god of wine, was worshipped throughout the country. Alcohol was used for pleasure, nutrition, medicine, ritual, remuneration and funerary purposes. Drinking bouts and excessive drinking were common in ancient Egypt and Assyria for religious rituals and festive occasions.

The first alcoholic drink to obtain widespread popularity in what is now Greece was mead, a fermented beverage made from honey and water. Wine drinking was used in religious rituals, in social encounter and hospitality and for medicinal purposes, and it became an integral part of daily meals. In ancient Greece, habitual drunkenness was uncommon because of the social etiquette attached to drinking and drinking behaviour. Contemporary writers observed that the Greeks were among the most temperate of ancient peoples. This appears to result from their rules stressing moderate drinking, their praise of temperance and their avoidance of excess in general (Hanson 1995).

A variety of alcoholic beverages were used in China from prehistoric times. Alcohol, known in Chinese as *Jiu*, was considered a spiritual food rather than a material (physical) food. Alcoholic drinks were widely used in all segments of Chinese society as a source of inspiration, were important for hospitality, were considered an antidote for fatigue and throughout the 'rite of passage' from birth to death and were sometimes misused. A Chinese imperial edict of about 1116 BC makes it clear that the use of alcohol in moderation was believed to be prescribed by heaven (Hanson 1995). In India, alcoholic beverages were already in use between 3000 BC and 2000 BC. *Sura*, a beverage distilled from rice meal, was popular among the warriors and the peasant population.

The use of these beverages was well defined within specific social contexts (Peele and Grant 1999)

At the height of the Roman Empire, the shift from ceremonial drinking – confined to banquets and special occasions – to casual, everyday drinking was accompanied by an increase in chronic drunkenness, which today would be labelled alcoholism (Babor 1986). Roman abuse of alcohol appears to have peaked around the mid first century (Jellinek 1976). Wine had become the most popular beverage, and, as Rome attracted a large influx of displaced persons, it was distributed free or at cost (Babor 1986). This led to occasional excesses at festivals, victory triumphs and other celebrations, as described by contemporaries. Although there continued to be some criticisms of abusive drinking over the next several hundred years, most evidence indicates a decline of such behaviour (Austin 1985). With the collapse of the Roman Empire, religious institutions, particularly the monasteries, became the repositories of the brewing and wine-making techniques developed in the ancient world (Babor 1986). It is argued that the early ritualisation of alcohol in Christian Europe and the revulsion for mind-altering psychoactive substances spread by the Church added to alcohol achieving dominance in European nations (Gossop 1989). By the millennium, the most popular form of festivities in England was known as 'ales', and both ale (brewed without hops) and beer were at the top of lists of products to be given to lords for rent.

The most important development regarding alcohol throughout the Middle Ages was probably that of distillation. The isolation of ethanol (alcohol) as a pure compound was first achieved by Muslim chemists who developed the art of distillation during the Abbasid caliphate (AD 750–1258), the most notable of whom were Jabir ibn Hayyan (Geber), Al-Kindi (Alkindus) and Al-Razi (Rhazes) (Al-Hassan and Hill 1986, Al-Hassan 2001). Pure distilled alcohol was first produced by Muslim chemists in the Islamic world during the eighth and ninth centuries. Geber (Jabir Ibn Hayyan, AD 721–815) invented the alembic still; he observed that heated wine from this still released a flammable vapour, which he described as 'of little use, but of great importance to science'. Not much later, Al-Razi (AD 864–930) described the distillation of alcohol and its use in medicine (Al-Hassan and Hill 1986). The word was introduced into Europe, together with the art of distillation and the resulting substance itself, around the twelfth century by various European authors who translated and popularised the discoveries of Islamic and Persian alchemists (Hassan 2001)

In summary, alcohol throughout history has been valued by various cultures and societies. From the earliest times alcohol has played an important role in religious worship, as a source of nutrients and calories, as a substitute for polluted water, for medicinal and therapeutic purposes and as a social lubricant. However, the harm of purified drugs seems even more apparent when the psychoactive substance is consumed outside their historical and cultural contexts. Whitaker (1987) suggested that distilled alcohol inflicted more havoc on North American Indians and Australians Aborigines than any other drug throughout history.

OPIUM

Opium is an extract of the exudates derived from seedpods of the opium poppy. The opium plant produces lots of small black seeds called poppy-seeds. Poppy-seeds can be ground into flour; used in salad dressings; added to sauces as flavouring or thickening-agents; and the oil can be expressed and used in cooking. Poppy-heads are infused to make a traditional sedative drink. Opium is a complex chemical mixture containing sugars, proteins, fats, water, meconic acid, plant wax, latex, gums, ammonia, sulphuric and lactic acids, and numerous alkaloids, most notably morphine (10–15%), codeine (1–3%), noscapine (4–8%), papaverine (1–3%), and thebaine (1–2%).

The poppy plant was cultivated in the ancient civilisations of Persia, Egypt and Mesopotamia. Fossil remains of poppy-seed cake and poppy-pods have been found in Neolithic Swiss lake-dwellings dating from over four thousand years ago. Plants such as the opium poppy were used by Middle Eastern and Asian cultures, and were brought to Europe through the opening of trade, hostilities and expeditions. Hippocrates, 'the father of medicine', dismisses the magical attributes of opium but acknowledges its usefulness as a narcotic and styptic in treating internal diseases, diseases of women and epidemics. References to the juice of the poppy occur in the Assyrian medical tablets of the seventh century BC, and in Sumerian ideograms of about 4000 BC the poppy is called 'plant of joy' (Berridge and Edwards 1987).

Throughout Egyptian civilisation, priest-physicians promoted the household use of opium preparations and the pharaohs were entombed with opium artefacts by their side. Opium could also readily be bought on the street markets of Rome. By the eighth century AD, opium use had spread to Arabia, India and China. The Arab physicians such as Ibn-sina (or Avicenna 980–1037) used opium extensively, writing special treatises on its preparations, and recommended the plant especially for diarrhoea and diseases of the eye.

In Britain, opium was chiefly used as a narcotic and a hypnotic. The drug's soporific and narcotic qualities appeared in Chaucer's *Canterbury Tales* and Shakespeare's *Othello*. Opium was variously called the Sacred Anchor of Life, Milk of Paradise, the Hand of God, and Destroyer of Grief. Thomas Sydenham, the seventeenth-century pioneer of English medicine, introduced the use of opium in medicine. Sydenham, however, went on to standardise laudanum in the now classic formulation – 2 ounces of opium; 1 ounce of saffron; a drachm of cinnamon and cloves – all dissolved in a pint of Canary wine. In the nineteenth century, laudanum, a mixture of alcohol solution and tincture of opium, could be bought over the counter at any grocer's shop and for decades it was every family's favourite remedy for minor aches and pains (Royal College of Psychiatrists 1989). Substances with opium-based preparations such as Godfrey's Cordial, a soothing syrup of opium tincture, effective against colic, Street's Infants' Quietness, Atkinson's Infants' Preservative, and Mrs Winslow's Soothing Syrup were used for babies and young children for sedation. In effect, opium was used in preference to alcohol and in various forms for endemic conditions such as malaria. Opium was most popular among the rural peasantry of the Fens (Lincolnshire, Norfolk, Cambridgeshire, Huntingdonshire, Northamptonshire and Suffolk). The British Medical Association estimated that sparsely populated Cambridgeshire and its environs consumed around half of Britain's annual opium imports. This consumption was topped up by generous use of poppy tea brewed from homegrown poppies.

By the late 1700s, the British East India Company controlled the Asian opium trade. Opium was already heavily used in China as a recreational drug. In 1839, the Qing Emperor ordered his minister to take action and instructed the confiscation of twenty thousand barrels of opium and detained some foreign traders. The British retaliated by attacking the port-city of Canton. Thus began the First Opium War, launched by Britain. The Chinese were defeated and were forced to sign the Treaty of Nanjing in 1842. The British required that the opium trade be allowed to continue; that the Chinese pay a large settlement and open five new ports to foreign trade; and that China cede Hong Kong to Britain. A Second Opium War began and ended in 1856 over western demands that opium markets be expanded. The Chinese were again defeated and opium importation to China was formally legalised. By the end of the nineteenth century, it has been estimated that over a quarter of the adult male Chinese population were addicted.

Morphine was first isolated from opium in 1805 by a German pharmacist, Wilhelm Sertürner, who named it morphium – after Morpheus, the Greek god of dreams. In the late nineteenth century, morphine became the drug of choice for high society and middle-class professionals. The development of the hypodermic syringe in the mid nineteenth century allowed the injection of pure morphine. It was believed that injecting morphine was not addictive and would be effective treating those with opium dependence. However, the search began for a powerful non-addictive alternative to opium and morphine. Subsequently, the identification of the active alkaloids of opium and the development of the process of acetylation by which morphine is converted to heroin changed the whole pattern of opiate use, not only in the West where the discovery was made but also in the East, where the parent drug originated (Ghodse 1995). In 1874, the English pharmacist C.R. Alder Wright had boiled morphine and acetic acid to produce diacetylmorphine, $C_{17}H_{17}NO (C_2H_3O_2)_2$. Diacetylmorphine was synthesised and marketed commercially by the German pharmaceutical giant, Bayer. In 1898, Bayer launched the best-selling drug brand of all time, heroin (http://opioids.com/.)

CANNABIS

Cannabis sativa (or Indian hemp), more commonly known as cannabis or marijuana, was one of the first plants to be cultivated for its non-food properties, and was primarily harvested for its fibre. It is thought to have originated in Asia, around 2700 BC in China. It was recommended for its pharmacological properties by the Emperor Shen Nung to his citizens for the treatment of pain, gout, absentmindedness and other ailments (Maisto *et al.* 1995). In addition, it has been speculated that cannabis was also used for countering of evil spirits and for its psychoactive properties (Abel 1980). With the spread of cannabis to neighbouring countries, in India, this psychoactive substance was regarded as a sacred plant and used for religious function and ritual. Whereas marijuana is the leafy top portion of the plant, hashish, made from the resin, was identified amongst the Arabs around the tenth century (Abel 1980). The use of the drug for its recreational and intoxicating effects appears to be associated with the Middle East and North Africa. The drug most probably first reached European countries in the nineteenth century following the Arab invasion of Spain.

The exposure of cannabis to Europe was also influenced by the printed literature describing the personal experiences in the use of hashish. The medical profession began to show an interest in the use of cannabis by the middle of the nineteenth century. An Irish physician, William O'Shaughnessy, who described the medical application of cannabis whilst in India, introduced cannabis in Great Britain (Bloomquist 1971). In France, the use and effects of hashish were described by a small group of writers, intellectuals and artists. In the 1840s, Le Club des Hachishins (The Hashish Club) was founded in an exclusive hotel in Paris. French authors such as Charles Baudelaire and Théophile Gautier described the splendours of their hallucinatory experiences in the use of hashish. The elements of mystery, joy, ecstasy, fear and paranoia were described by Gautier. For a description of the experiences see Gautier 1844/1966. Despite its attraction as a recreational or intoxicating drug, it did not immediately spread in Europe. However, the widespread use of cannabis or hashish for its psychoactive properties in Europe in the 1960s seems to have occurred as a result of the cultural movement of the young generation imported from the United States. During the last four decades, cannabis has remained the most frequently used illicit drug in the United Kingdom. The plant grows freely throughout the world but is indigenous to Central Asia and the Himalayan region and is cultivated widely in Africa, India, North America and the Caribbean region. Today, cannabis is grown in at least 172 countries, often in small plots by the users themselves (UNDOC 2007).

COCAINE

The use of the coca leaf dates back to the Inca civilisations and their descendants. The Inca people apparently learned the practice of chewing the coca leaf from the Aymara people of Bolivia whose use dates back to around 300 BC (Grinspoon and Bakalar 1976). For centuries the coca leaf has been chewed by the Andean Indians of Peru and other South American countries. The coca plant was used for medicinal, religious significance, rituals and burials and for special occasions. The Peruvian Indians use coca to increase their physical strength, to lessen fatigue and for the prevention of hunger. After the Spanish conquistadores conquered the Incas, they encouraged the use of the coca leaf in the beliefs that it helped the Inca to work longer and harder. In fact, because of its social importance, the Spanish eventually took over coca production and distribution and used coca as a tool to control the conquered population (Petersen 1977).

It was not until the early 1800s that Europeans started to experiment with the use of coca. In the 1850s European chemists were able to isolate the far more potent ingredient in the leaf which they called cocaine. 'The extraction of cocaine from the leaf led to a whole new era in the history of stimulant drug use and misuse.' Freud, in his first major publication, 'On Coca', advocated the therapeutic and recreational use of cocaine. Freud also thought that cocaine was an aphrodisiac (Byck 1974). He recommended the use of cocaine as a local anaesthetic and as a treatment for drug addiction, alcoholism, depression, various neuroses, indigestion, asthma and syphilis. By the 1880s cocaine was widely available in patent medicines that could be obtained without prescription. These include Mariani's Coca Wine, a best-seller in Europe, and Coca-Cola. (Despite the name, Coca-Cola no longer contains coca or cola.) Cocaine became very popular and was also sold in cigarettes, in nose sprays and in chewing gum (Gossop 1989).

It was not until the 1980s that the United States of America experienced a 'cocaine epidemic'. However, the acceptance of cocaine has been fostered by an association with glamorous imagery and compounded with the idea of the 'non-addictive' nature of the drug. Consumption of cocaine has increased significantly in Europe, doubling or tripling in several countries over the last decade (UNDOC 2007). Coca leaves and other psychoactive substances such as coffee, tea and tobacco were introduced to Europe from South America. The coca plant is indigenous in the Andean Highlands of Bolivia, Columbia and Peru.

AMPHETAMINE

Another psychoactive substance that was synthesised in 1887 was amphetamine. It was marketed in the form of a benzedrine inhaler for use in the treatment of nasal congestion, mild depression, schizophrenia, alcoholism and obesity. During the Second World War, amphetamines were widely used by the armed forces to keep the troops functioning under stressful and physically demanding conditions. More recently, amphetamines have also been used in the treatment of narcolepsy and hyperactivity in children. The use of the stimulant was also widespread amongst athletes and sports men and women to enhance their exploits and performances. During the 1950s, there was over-prescription of amphetamines by doctors for use in the treatment of common conditions. It was not until the 1960s that amphetamine misuse erupted in the UK among young people and subsequently resulted in an epidemic of injection of methamphetamine. It is argued that in the UK the largest positive influence limiting amphetamine misuse has been the slow growth in medical awareness of the danger of these drugs, leading to changes in medical prescribing as well as a growing realisation among the general population that 'pep-pills' are none-too-wise a prop (Royal College of Psychiatrists 1987).

HALLUCINOGENIC DRUGS

Hallucinogenic drugs are among the categories of psychoactive substances which in the past caused and still cause intense controversy in their use. Originally called 'phantastica' (Lewin 1964), during the 1960s the drugs were referred to as 'psychedelics' (Stevens 1987). The Indian peoples of Central and South America used the naturally occurring psychoactive plant as part of religious rituals and practices and for predicting the future. The medicine man or shaman also used the substances in the healing of the sick. It has been suggested that the psilocybin mushroom, regarded as a sacred mushroom, was used by the Mayan civilisation dating back to more than 1000 BC (Schultes 1976). Mexico has been the source of hallucinogenic mushrooms and the cactus plant (peyote) and both have played an important role in the cultural and religious traditions. The use of sacred mushrooms and morning glory seeds (ergine and isoergine) still persists in parts of Mexico with rituals for healing and divination (Schultes 1976).

These hallucinogenic psychoactive plants had very little impact on European culture, despite its long history of drug use, until the 1960s. It was the synthetic hallucinogens such as LSD (lysergic acid diethylamide) that came under scientific and medical scrutiny. In 1943, Albert Hofmann, a chemist working at Sandoz Laboratories in Switzerland, discovered LSD. Initially, LSD was primarily used as an adjunct to psychotherapy and later in the treatment of alcoholism, drug dependence, sexual problems and psychotic and neurotic disorders. By the early 1960s the drug was used by the emerging 'hippy subculture' for spiritual enlightenment and for mystical peak experiences. Throughout the 1980s in the UK there was a decline in the use of LSD but it resurfaced in the late 1980s together with other hallucinogens in the 'Rave' subculture. Ecstasy (MDMA), although not a new drug, appeared on the scene in 1985 and since then there has been an increase in the consumption of both ecstasy and LSD by young people. The drug was first synthesised in Germany to be used as an appetite suppressant.

CAFFEINE

Since ancient times plants that contain caffeine and other methylxanthines have been used to make beverages. Caffeine is the world's favourite and most popular psychoactive substance. Coffee was known to the Arab travellers in the sixth century and was used medicinally and for religious purposes particularly by the Dervishes to keep themselves awake during long religious practices and rituals (Ghodse 1995). During the seventeenth century, coffee drinking spread from the Arab world and Persia to Britain and other European countries, and in eighteenth-century England coffee was seen as an alternative to sex and as a cure for alcohol intoxication. In the 1840s the 'Bohemians' of Paris took drugs as part of their lifestyle, and the taking of the drugs shocked public opinion at that time. The drug was coffee. According to Ghodse (1995: xi), attempts were made in different countries 'to close down the coffee houses which were seen as centres of sedition and dissent and to ban the use of coffee altogether'.

Coffee is the major source of caffeine; other familiar psychoactive substances such as tea, cocoa and chocolate also contain caffeine. During the last four decades, soft drinks have risen dramatically as a significant source of caffeine. Brazil is the world's major leading producer of coffee, and the major producers of tea are China and the Indian subcontinent. Cocoa is primarily produced in Africa, and Switzerland has the highest per capita consumption of cocoa (James 1991).

TOBACCO

Although small amounts of nicotine may be found in some Old World plants, including belladonna and Nicotiana africana, and nicotine metabolites have been found in human remains and pipes in the Near East and Africa, there is no indication of habitual tobacco use in the ancient world, on any continent save the Americas (Borio 2007). Tobacco is a plant that grows natively in North and South America. It is in the same family as the potato, pepper and the poisonous nightshade. Tobacco was believed to be a cure-all, and was used to dress wounds, as well as a pain killer for toothache. In South and Central America, a complex system of religious and political rites was developed around tobacco use (www.imperialtobaccocanada.com 2007).

On 15 October 1492, Christopher Columbus was offered dried tobacco leaves as a gift from the American Indians whom he encountered. The growing popularity of tobacco in Europe was due to its supposed healing properties. In 1571, a Spanish doctor named Nicolas Monardes wrote a book about the history of medicinal plants of the new world. In this book, he claimed that tobacco could cure 36 health problems. During the 1600s, tobacco was frequently used as a currency for exchange of goods. The health concerns of the dangerous effects of smoking tobacco were being noticed, and in 1610 Sir Francis Bacon noted that trying to quit nicotine smoking was really hard. In 1632, it was illegal to smoke publicly in Massachusetts. The moral belief prevails at this period of time with the new settlers in America.

In 1826, the pure form of nicotine was finally discovered. Scientists began to understand the chemicals in tobacco and the dangerous health effects smoking produces. In 1847, the famous British company Phillip Morris was established, selling hand-rolled Turkish cigarettes. In 1902, Phillip Morris set up a New York headquarters to market its cigarettes, including the famous Marlboro brand. Cigarettes in the US were mainly made from scraps left over after the production of other tobacco products, especially chewing tobacco. Chewing tobacco became quite popular at this time with the 'cowboys' of the American west. In Britain, the habit of tobacco smoking in pipes was introduced by Sir Walter Raleigh in the seventeenth century.

During the Crimean War (1854–6), soldiers were offered cigarettes to overcome the misery of food deprivations. Cigarettes became popular around this time when soldiers brought them back to England from the Russian and Turkish soldiers. The use of cigarettes exploded during the first World War (1914–18), when cigarettes were called the 'soldier's smoke'. During the Second World War (1939–45), cigarettes were included in a soldier's rations. The tobacco companies sent millions of cigarettes to the soldiers for free, thus developing potential customers when these soldiers came home.

During the 1950s, important epidemiological studies provided the first powerful links between smoking and lung cancer. In Britain, Richard Doll and A. Braford Hill published the first report on smoking and carcinoma of the lung in the *British Medical Journal*, finding that heavy smokers were fifty times as likely as non-smokers to contract lung cancer. Although the tobacco industry denied such health hazards, they promoted new products which were 'safer', such as those with lower tar and filtered cigarettes. In 1954, Doll and Hill published 'The mortality of doctors and their smoking habits' in the *British Medical Journal* resulting from most doctors giving up smoking, confirming the link between lung cancer and smoking. As a result of Doll and Hill's studies and the government-approved scientific committee's findings, the British government officially acknowledged the smoking/lung cancer link. It was in 1971 that tobacco manufacturers in the UK voluntarily put health warnings on cigarette packs.

During the 1980s and 1990s, the tobacco industry started marketing heavily in areas outside the US, especially developing countries in Asia and Africa. In recent years, there is growing evidence that the tobacco industry has known all along that cigarettes are harmful, but continued to market and sell them. During the late 1990s smoking became prohibited in bars and restaurants in many countries and subsequently this was followed by total ban in public places.

CONCLUSIONS

This brief overview has covered only a few drugs that have been used over the years and in different cultures for their psychoactive products. There seems to be a parallel development in the therapeutic uses of psychoactive substances and the non-medical or recreational use of these drugs. Most of the 'old' drugs such as cannabis, tobacco and alcohol have been used for religious or medicinal purposes. In modern times, these drugs have been primarily used as part of recreational and social activities. It is argued that England's emergence as a colonial power in the seventeenth century was based chiefly upon tobacco, and the development of the European market for tobacco was seen as being essential to England's economic future (Harrison 1993).

However, in the 1920s Britain had its first notable drugs panic. The detection of a drug underground of cocaine and heroin provided a way of speaking simultaneously about women, race, sex and the nation's place in the world. In the past, the outlawing of drugs was the consequence not of their pharmacology but of their association with social groups that were perceived as potentially dangerous (Kohn 1992). In reality, it was the British who promoted the use of psychoactive substances such as opium to the Chinese, and the Opium Wars safeguarded the opium trade. In addition, the remnants of this belief still remain in the public consciousness. Contrary to popular mythology, most of the biggest drug importers and criminal gang in Britain are led not by Blacks but by white businessmen or criminals who have the necessary capital (Clutterbuck 1995).

The anti-drug stance and the 'war on drugs' have consolidated little gain in the proliferation of psychoactive substances. When the UN General Assembly Special Session on drugs convened in 1998, it committed to 'eliminating or significantly reducing the illicit cultivation of the coca bush, the cannabis plant and the opium poppy by the year 2008' and to 'achieving significant and measurable results in the field of demand reduction'. In 2007, there were signs of overall stability in the production, trafficking or consumption of cocaine, heroin, cannabis and amphetamines. Whether, a 'drug-free world', which the United Nations describes as a realistic goal, is attainable remains to be seen.

KEY POINTS

- From the earliest time, alcohol and drugs have been used for medicinal, religious, cultural and recreational purposes and as a social lubricant.
- Alcohol has been used for pleasure, nutrition, medicine, ritual, remuneration and funerary purposes.
- Opium is an extract of the exudates derived from seed-pods of the opium poppy.
- During the last four decades, cannabis has remained the most frequently used illicit drug in the United Kingdom.
- Amphetamines were widely used by the armed forces to keep the troops functioning under stressful and physically demanding conditions and in the treatment of narcolepsy and hyperactivity in children.
- In the late nineteenth century, cocaine became very popular and was also sold in cigarettes, in nose sprays and in chewing gum.
- Morphine was used for the treatment of opium addiction.
- LSD was primarily used as an adjunct to psychotherapy, in the treatment of alcoholism, drug dependence, sexual problems and psychotic and neurotic disorders.
- Caffeine is the world's favourite and most popular psychoactive substance.

- Tobacco was believed to be a cure-all, and was used to dress wounds, as well as a pain killer for toothache.
- The anti-drug stance and the 'war on drugs' have consolidated little gain in the proliferation of psychoactive substances.

REFERENCES

Abel E.L. (1980) *Marijuana: The First Twelve Thousand Years*. New York: Plenum Press.

Al-Hassan, A.Y. (2001) *The Different Aspects of Islamic Culture, Science and Technology in Islam*, Vol. 4, Part II, UNESCO. Cambridge: Cambridge University Press.

Al-Hassan, A.Y. and Hill, D. (1986) *Islamic Technology: An Illustrated History*, UNESCO. Cambridge: Cambridge University Press.

Austin, G.A. (1985) *Alcohol in Western Society from Antiquity to 1800: A Chronological History*. Santa Barbara, CA: ABC – Clio.

Babor, T. (1989) *Alcohol – Customs and Rituals*. London: Burke Publishing Company Limited.

Berridge, V. and Edwards, G. (1987) *Opium and the People. Opiate Use in Nineteenth-Century England*. London: Yale University Press.

Bloomquist, E.R. (1971) *Marijuana: The Second Trip* (revised edn). Beverly Hills, CA: Glencoe Press.

Borio, G. (2007) Tobacco BBS (212-982-4645). http://www.tobacco.org) (accessed 15 June 2006).

Byck, R. (ed.) (1974) *Cocaine Papers by Sigmund Freud*. New York: Stonehill Publishing Company.

Clutterbuck, R. (1995) *Drugs, Crime and Corruption*. Basingstoke: Macmillan Press.

Edwards, G. (1971) *Unreason in an Age of Reason*. Edwin Stevens Lecture for the Laity, London: Royal Society of Medicine.

Gautier, T. (1844/1966) *Le club de hasishins*. In D. Solomon (ed.), *The Marijuana Papers*, pp. 121–35. New York: Bobbs-Merrill.

Ghodse, A.H. (1995) *Drugs and Addictive Behaviour: A Guide to Treatment*. Oxford: Blackwell Science.

Gossop, M. (1989) *Living with Drugs*. Aldershot: Wilwood publications.

Grinspoon, L. and Bakalar, J.B. (1976) *Cocaine: A drug and Its Social Evolutions*. New York: Basic Books Inc.

Hanson, David J. (1995) *History of Alcohol and Drinking around the World*. Wesport, CT: Praeger.

Harrison, L. (ed.) (1993) *Race, Culture and Substance Problems*. Hull: Department of Social Policy and Professional Studies, University of Hull.

http//info.opiate (accessed 15 June 2007).

Institute for the Study of Drug Dependence (1993) *National Audit of Drug Misuse in Britain*. London: ISDD.

James, J.E (1991) *Caffeine and Health*. New York: Academic Press.

Jellinek, E.M. (1976) Drinkers and alcoholics in ancient Rome. *Journal of Studies on Alcohol*, 37: 1718–41.

Kohn, M. (1992) *Dope Girls: The Birth of the British Drug Underground*. London: Lawrence & Wishart.

Lewin, L. (1964) *Phantastica-narcotic and Stimulating Drugs: Their Use and Abuse*. London: Routledge and Kegan Paul.

Maisto, S.A., Galizio, M. and Connors, G.J. (1995) *Drug Use and Abuse*, 2nd edition. London: The Harcourt Press.

Peele, S. and Grant, M. (eds) (1999) *Alcohol and Pleasure: A Health Perspective*. Philadelphia: Brunner/Mazel.

Petersen, R.C. (1977) History of cocaine. In R.C. Petersen and R.C. Stillman (eds), Cocaine, Research Monograph 13, 17–34. Washington DC: National Institute of Drug Abuse.

Royal College of Psychiatrists (1987) *Drug Scenes: A Report on Drugs and Drug Dependence.* London: Gaskell.

Schultes, R.E. (1976) *Hallucinogenic Plants.* New York: Golden Press.

Stevens, J. (1987) *Storming Heaven: LSD and the American Dream.* New York: Atlantic Monthly Press.

United Nations Drugs office and Crime (2007) *World Drug Report 2007.* http://www.unodc. org/pdf/research/wdr07/WDR_2007_executive_summary.pdf (accessed 17 June 2007).

Whitaker, B. (1987) *The Global Connection: The Crisis of Drug Addiction.* London: Jonathan Cape Ltd.

www.imperialtobaccocanada.com/ *Tobacco History 2007* (accessed 16 June 2007).

CHAPTER 4

THEORIES OF ADDICTION

OBJECTIVES

■ Gain a greater knowledge of the broad range of theories of addiction.

■ Develop one's own working theory of addiction.

Many models and theories have proposed to explain the use or misuse of alcohol and drugs and the causes of substance use. The theories range from those which stress the genetic or biological causes and those which stress social or psychological causes. Some theories attempt to view addiction as both a physiological and a psycho-social phenomenon. That is a bio-psychosocial theory of addiction.

The models or theories provide explanations for the initiation into substance misuse or for why individuals begin to use drugs and the process of addiction. Some theories explain both initial and continuing use of drugs (Addiction Research Foundation 1986). However, the reason why people start using drugs may not be the same reason why they continue to use drugs. It will become apparent that no single theory is sufficient to explain substance use and misuse per se, and that a range of 'risk factors' has to be considered. Most of the studies are retrospective in design, and more research has been conducted in relation to alcohol rather than any other substances. There are a number of theories but none should be considered to be the definitive account nor is any one theory mutually exclusive of any other.

MORAL THEORY

The moral theory or model is based on the belief that using alcohol or drug is a sign of moral weakness, bad character or sinful people. The individual has deviated from the acceptable religious and social norms. The proponents of this model do not accept that there is any biological basis for addiction. According to the moral theory, individuals are responsible for their behavioural choices and their own recovery. Much of the stigma faced by individuals with an alcohol or drug problem is based on this underlying moral notion that labels anyone with an alcohol or drug habit as a 'bad person'. This is where the 'victim-blaming' approach is evident. This model contributes little to our understanding of why people are dependent on drug and alcohol and has limited therapeutic value. The focus of intervention under this model is the control of behaviour through social disapproval, spiritual guidance, moral persuasion or imprisonment.

DISEASE THEORY

In contrast with the moral model of 'victim-blaming' for the development of addiction, the disease theory of addiction maintains that addiction is a disease due to the impairment of either behavioural or neurochemical processes, or of some combination of the two. This theory views substance misuse as a progressive, incurable disorder and the cause of the disease is firmly attributed to the genetic or biological make up of the individual (Jellinek 1960, Valliant 1983). The theory holds that alcohol and drug addiction is a unique, irreversible, and progressive disease and its primary symptom is the inability to control consumption. According to the disease theory of alcoholism, once a drink is taken, craving is increased and the physical demand for alcohol overrides any cognitive or voluntary control (Jellinek 1960). The proponents of this model hold that, while alcohol or drug addiction cannot be cured, abstinence is the only option. Defining alcohol or drug addiction as a physical or biological disease enables those with alcohol or drug addiction to have access to health care and treatment instead of punitive action or imprisonment.

   This disease approach implies the adoption of the sick role by the alcohol and drug misusers, and the individuals are expected to be treated as having a 'disease'. Spontaneous recovery is unlikely and, even with treatment, the potential for relapse is always present. This approach also implies that recovery from drug or alcohol misuse can be sustained only through the goal of total abstinence within support from self-help group movements such as AA, NA and GA (Alcoholics Anonymous, Narcotics Anonymous, Gamblers Anonymous). The disease concept of addictive behaviour is incorporated in the philosophy underpinning the approaches of NA or AA in the adoption of the 'Minnesota Model' (Cook 1988). However, the disease model of addiction reduces the scope of analysis to features that are physiological in origin and isolates the importance of the interrelationship of both psychological and socio-cultural factors in the maintenance of substance use behaviour.

GENETIC THEORY

The genetic model posits a genetic predisposition to alcohol or drug addiction. A number of studies have suggested that alcohol or drug addiction is the result of genetic or induced biological abnormality of a physiological, structural or chemical nature. There is strong evidence that early-onset alcoholism is genetically determined (Cloninger 1987, Blum *et al.* 1990, Pickens *et al.* 1991). Problem drinkers have a 50 per cent chance of having at least one member of their family becoming dependent on alcohol, and there is a 90 per cent chance of two or more family members being dependent on alcohol (Miller 1991).

In adoption studies, children whose adopted parents were dependent on alcohol were more likely themselves to develop a problem with alcohol, though their biological parents were not dependent on alcohol (Miller 1991). However, the findings of the Copenhagen study (Goodwin *et al.* 1977), the best study to date on methodological grounds, showed that there was a fourfold increase in the incidence of alcoholism among male adoptees who were removed from their alcoholic parents soon after birth. In a study of pairs of twins by Tsuang *et al.* (1996), the findings suggest that the likelihood of developing a dependence to opiates or stimulants is more influenced by genetic factors than by shared environmental factors. Some people may experience a less intense reaction to alcoholic beverages, and such vulnerable individuals drink more before feeling intoxicated. It also appears that a genetic predisposition may also protect some individuals who have a genetically based metabolic sensitivity to indulging in psychoactive substances such as alcohol (Wolf 1972).

The available data to date indicate that dependency on alcohol is a genetically influenced disorder with a rate of heritability similar to that expected for diabetes or peptic ulcer (Schuckit 1995). Adyitanjee and Murray's (1991) review of twin studies of alcoholism and normal drinking looks at a number of studies in a similar culture and racial group: they indicate that alcoholism tends to run in families but acknowledge that no one is clear about what it is that may or may not be transmitted through genetic inheritance. However, when evaluating the pattern of inheritance, all studies showed that it is sons and not daughters who are more at risk of developing alcohol disorder.

One aspect of inheritance is understood amongst members of particular races. Eskimos, American Indians and Asians, for example, are all genetically predisposed to have a deficiency in the production of acetaldehyde, an enzyme important for alcohol degradation. These groups are hypersensitive to the effects of alcohol and, once higher levels of alcohol are reached in their bodily system, they develop a flushing known as 'Asian Flushing'. The lack of these enzymes (alcohol dehydrogenase and aldehyde dehydrogenase) makes it more difficult to metabolise alcohol, causing it to accumulate faster in a person's system, and does not allow the alcohol to break down as quickly.

Many of the studies have been based on alcohol rather than on drugs. The different methodologies used in several studies (mainly alcohol studies), such as face-to-face interviews, records such as those of hospitalisation and arrests, and the use of different operational definitions of 'alcoholism', may have implications in comparing and confirming the different findings, especially in adoption and twin studies. The degree to which genetic factors play a role in addictive behaviour is still unclear and remains to be further investigated.

PSYCHOLOGICAL THEORIES

There are a number of psychological theories that attempt to explain the causation of drug- and alcohol-dependent behaviour. The theories view heavy alcohol and drug use as problem behaviours. A brief overview of selected theories is presented here.

Psychoanalytic theory

Psychoanalytic theory is derived from the work of Freud based on the components of the self and their functioning during the stages of psychosexual development. Early psychoanalytical explanations stem from the belief that addiction stems from the unconscious death wishes as a form of 'slow suicide' (Khantzian 1980). Other schools of thought include the notions of conflict between a repressed idea and the defence against it and a deficient ego (Leeds and Morgenstern 1996, Murphy and Khantzian 1995).

Freud made little reference to alcohol disorder in his published works but did suggest that the consumption of alcohol provided relief from the conflict generated by oral fixation, or repressed homosexuality. According to the psychoanalytic theory, adaptive behaviour requires the harmonious functioning of the id, ego and superego (the self). These components change during the stages of psychosexual development. Alcoholism and other pathological conditions are attributed to the conflicts in these stages of development, resulting in the destructive interactions among the three components of the self. The aetiology of alcohol or drug dependence is assumed to develop from sensual satisfaction (avoidance of pain or anxiety), conflict among the id, ego and superego and fixation in the infantile past (Allen 1996). In order to avoid pain or anxiety, alcohol intoxication is assumed to provide this relief.

Mental defence mechanisms seem to operate in the case of conflicts among the components of the self. Denial, repression, projection and displacement can be seen as part of the behavioural repertoires. The use of alcohol or drugs (smoking) is related to the 'fixation' at the oral stage of development. According to Treece and Khantzian (1986), there are certain pychodynamic characteristics observed in substance-dependent individuals. These include problems in affect management, narcissism, object relations, judgement and self-care. These problems may predispose individuals to drug dependence because they are the basis of anxieties or distresses that are relieved by taking psycho-active substance. Dependency involves the gradual incorporation of the drug effects and their experienced need into the defensive structure building activity of the ego itself (Treece and Khantzian 1986). There are major methodological problems with psychoanalytic studies, and limited empirical evidence has been found to support this theory.

Behavioural theories

In behavioural theories, the use of psychoactive substances is viewed as an acquired behaviour, a response that is learned through the process of classical conditioning (Pavlovian's conditioning), operant conditioning (Skinner) and social learning. In classical conditioning, dependence is in part acquired through the process of associative learning. That is, the desire to use drugs may be the result of specific factors associated with the use of a particular substance. The maintenance of drug-taking behaviour is the result of past associations with a drug-taking environment or situation.

Wickler (1948, 1961) first suggested the significant role played by classical conditioning in the development of the motivation to use drugs. However, the theory of classical conditioning does not make provision for individual differences (genetic factors), social factors or the expectations of drug effects. In operant conditioning learning occurs when the response or behaviour is followed by reinforcement. Reinforcements strengthen behaviour and may be positive (rewarding behaviour) or negative (avoidance of an unpleasant experience). The role of positive reinforcement in the use of psychoactive substances can be explained by the fact that drugs can cause pleasurable sensations. The more pleasure or in some cases fear of withdrawal reinforces the continued use of the substance.

Social learning theory

Social learning theory (or cognitive social learning) provides an explanation of how behaviour (adaptive or maladaptive) is formed and maintained through the process of positive and negative reinforcement. Behaviour is assumed to be also influenced by role modelling and the need to conform (Becker 1966, Bandura 1977, Barnes 1990). Collins and Marlatt (1981) have demonstrated that modelling affects drinking behaviour – for example, how an individual's consumption of alcohol will vary to match that of a drinking partner. Their findings indicate that heavy-drinking males seem to exhibit the strongest response to a heavy-drinking model of the same sex. In effect, patterns of behaviour and attitudes can also be acquired through observation of social models without any reinforcement of overt behaviour. In the cognitive social learning theory, in order to understand the effects of alcohol or drug, cognitive processes must be considered in relation to other factors. In addition, there is also an interrelationship between personal (expectations, beliefs, cognitions) and environmental factors (context, social setting). That is, an individual's prior experience with alcohol or drug and the social setting in which drinking or drug-taking occurs must be considered.

Other cognitive theories or models include the tension-reduction theory, self-awareness model and the expectancy theory. The tension-reduction theory is based on the notion that individuals drink in order to reduce tension or anxiety. The drinking of alcohol or drug-taking becomes the reinforcer because it produces a reduction in tension (Cappell and Greeley 1987). The self-awareness model (Hull 1981) attempts to understand the cause and effects of psychoactive substances in terms of disinhibiting social behaviour by reducing an individual's level of self-awareness. The expectancy theory seeks to explain the role of cognitive factors in the initiation of substance use and the maintenance of drug-taking behaviour despite the consequences (Stacy et al. 1990). This theory focuses on beliefs about psychoactive substance that develop at an early age. 'Outcome expectancy' may link drug or alcohol use with a specific incoming situation. Studies amongst adolescents show that expectations predicted drinking behaviour more accurately than social background and demographic variables (ethnicity, religious affiliation, parental attitudes) and that alcohol would improve their cognitive and motor functioning (Christiansen and Goldman 1983). Orford (1985) proposes a theory of 'excessive appetites' within the context of social learning paradigm. He develops a theory of addiction and maintains that the degree of an individual's involvement with 'appetitive activities' has multiple interacting determinants. These include biological, personality, social and ecological determinants.

Personality theory

Within the framework of psychological theories, personality theory stresses the importance of personal traits and characteristics in the formation and maintenance of dependence. Traits such as hyperactivity, sensation-seeking, antisocial behaviour and impulsivity have been found to be associated with substance misuse (Sher *et al.* 1991). According to Ghodse (1995: 20), while 'there is an epidemiological association between drug misuse and personality disorder, no deductions can be made about causality as most studies have compared drug-dependent with non-dependent individuals'. He asserted that there might be personality traits which change the likelihood of an individual becoming dependent on drugs.

SOCIO-CULTURAL THEORIES

Socio-cultural theories include a number of sub-theories such as systems theory, family interaction theory, anthropological theory, economic theory, gateway theory and availability theory. In the systems theory, behaviour is determined and maintained by the ongoing demands of interpersonal systems in which an individual interacts. The aetiology is based on behaviour observed in family contexts such as behaviour resulting from the interactions between relevant significant others. Steinglass's (1987) work supports the idea of alcoholism as a 'family disease' or 'family disorder'. In the family interaction theory, the most significant aetiological factor is probably parental deficits that occur as a product of parental alcoholism. These deficits may include parental absence, family tension, rejection, emotional distancing and parental alienation. There is also some evidence to suggest that alcohol may serve as an adaptive function in a marital relationship by facilitation of interaction (Jacob and Leonard 1988).

The availability theory suggests that, the greater the availability of alcohol or other psychoactive substances, the greater the prevalence and severity of substance use problems in society. According to Ghodse (1995) the availability of the drug is a prerequisite for misuse and dependence and the rapid transport system of the modern world ensure that drugs or alcohol are obtainable everywhere. Influences such as availability of drugs, relative cost, social pressures, legal sanctions and marketing practices are the best predictors of the development of dependence (Henningfield *et al.* 1991).

The cultural model recognizes that the influence of culture is a strong determinant of whether or not individuals fall prey to certain addictions. Cultural and religious attitudes have been considered to be a defensive shield against alcohol and drug addiction. For example, the uses of moderate or controlled drinking within the family setup have an influence on the drinking behaviour of their children. This perception tends to encourage individuals to view alcohol as a social lubricant with clearly defined social rules and etiquette. Both ethnicity and religious values have a strong influence on the nature and pattern of drug-taking and drinking behaviour. However, drug-taking and drinking patterns may alter as a result of immigration and social and economic constraints. The psychoactive substances misused by Black and ethnic minority groups are not clearly different from those used by the white population. Nevertheless there seem to be preferences for a certain class or classes of substances and mode of consumption by different ethnic groups which are linked with the historical and cultural characteristics of each ethnic group (Oyefeso *et al*. 2000, Sangster *et al*. 2002).

Other socio-cultural factors that may have an influence on the choice of drug and alcohol use and misuse include gender, age, occupation, social class, ethno-cultural background, subcultures, alienated groups, family dysfunction and religious affiliation.

Bio-psychosocial theory

Many models of addiction could be criticised for failing to attend sufficiently to social and environmental factors (Copello and Orford 2002). There have been several attempts to amalgamate the biological, psychological and sociological theories of drug and alcohol addiction into a megatheory – the bio-psychosocial perspectives (Galizio and Maisto 1985, Kumpter *et al*. 1990, Wallace 1990). Even though the focus here is on biological and psychological processes, social factors are also included in this model through learning, perceiving and interpreting the world about us as well as through the person's social relationships and larger cultural environment.

The bio-psychosocial model takes into consideration a broad range of factors which interact resulting in addiction. Thus, drug and alcohol addiction are viewed as the result of multi-factorial causation rather than having uni-dimensional cause. Kumpter *et al*.'s (1990) bio-psychosocial 'vulnerability model' includes biological factors (genetic inheritance, physiological differences), psychosocial factors and environmental factors (family, community, peer or social pressure). In addition, another component may be added to the bio-psychosocial theory, that is the spiritual dimension. The model views these factors 'as temporarily ordered in its interactions' that lead to addiction. Whether the goal is prevention, treatment or research, the health care professionals can understand the individuals from a holistic perspective. By adopting a multi-dimensional approach, the bio-psychosocial theory has provided a new conception of alcohol and drug misuse that focuses attention towards a new set of questions about the nature and process of addiction. A summary of the advantages of the bio-psychosocial model is presented in Table 4.1.

ACTIVITY 4.1

There is only one correct answer to the following multiple-choice questions

Which of the following is not a major theory of addiction?
a.   Genetic
b.   Adaptation
c.   Moral
d.   Psychological

Table 4.1 Characteristics and focus of the bio-psychosocial theory

Characteristics	Focus
The bio-psychosocial theory unifies prior biological, psychological and social theories of addiction	Multidimensional and multi-professional approach to addiction
This theory postulates a role for social and spiritual factors in the development of and recovery from substance misuse and allows for future analysis of these elements	
A conceptual framework that allows attention to be focused on all problems related on a continuum, from experimental users to those who are dependent on psychoactive substances	Provision of a comprehensive range of services
Characterises the population of substance misusers as heterogeneous	Meeting individual or holistic needs
Supports the concept of a hierarchy of harm reduction outcome goals including abstinence-related goals	Allows for the delivery of harm reduction services
Congruent with other modern theories of health and education	Diversity of health needs within a population or community. Matching needs to services or treatment. Measuring treatment outcomes on all dimensions

Source: Adapted from Adult Addictions Services Branch, Alcohol and Drug Services (1996) British Columbia Ministry for Children and Families, Victoria

Which statement is incorrect?
a. The moral theory is based on the belief that using alcohol or drug is a sign of moral weakness
b. The moral theory accepts that there is any biological basis for addiction
c. According to the moral theory, individuals are responsible for their behavioural choices and their own recovery
d. 'Victim-blaming' approach is evident in the moral theory

Which statement is incorrect? The disease theory of addiction
a. Maintains that addiction is a disease due to either the impairment of behavioural and/or neurochemical processes
b. Claims that the cause of the disease is not attributed to the genetic or biological make up of the individual
c. Holds that alcohol and drug addiction are unique, irreversible, and progressive diseases
d. Holds that while alcohol or drug addiction cannot be cured, abstinence is the only option

Which statement is incorrect? The genetic theory of addiction
a. Put forward a genetic predisposition to alcohol or drug addiction
b. Maintains that early-onset alcoholism is genetically determined

c.   Is based on evidence mainly from drug research studies

d.   Incorporates the psychosocial factors in the development of addiction

Which statement is incorrect?

a.   Asians encompass the only race that exhibits Asian flushing

b.   Acetaldehyde is an important enzyme for alcohol metabolism

c.   American Indians and Eskimos are genetically identical

d.   Flushing is common amongst white Europeans

Regarding genetic studies of addiction, which statement is incorrect?

a.   Twin studies are the most powerful

b.   Twins reared apart studies are the most powerful

c.   Family studies are scientifically sound

d.   Adoption studies are easy to do because good records are kept

Which statement is false?

a.   Family studies have shown an increased incidence of alcoholism in families

b.   Adoption studies have not shown any correlation between addiction and genetics

c.   Twins reared apart studies are the most powerful

d.   Monozygotic twins and diszygotic twin studies show slightly different outcomes

Which one of the following factors is not considered to be a component in psychological theories?

a.   Psychoanalytical

b.   Genetic

c.   Personality

d.   Social learning

Which statement is incorrect? The psychoanalytic theory of addiction

a.   Stems from the belief that addiction stems from the unconscious death wishes

b.   Includes the notions of conflict between a repressed idea and the defence against it

c.   Proposes that aetiology of alcohol or drug dependence is assumed to develop from the avoidance of pain or anxiety

d.   States that use of alcohol or drug (smoking) is related to the 'fixation' at the anal stage of development

Which one of the following is not considered in behavioural theories?

a.   The theory makes provision for individual differences (genetic factors)

b.   The use of psychoactive substances is viewed as an acquired behaviour

c.   Behaviour is learned through the process of classical conditioning and operant conditioning

d.   The theory of classical conditioning does not include social factors or the expectations of drug effects

Which one of the following is not considered in social learning theories?

a. The theory is formed and maintained through the process of positive and negative reinforcement
b. Behaviour is through role-modelling and need to conform
c. In order to understand the effects of alcohol or drug, cognitive processes must be considered in relation to other factors
d. An individual's prior experience with alcohol or drug and the social setting in which drinking or drug taking occurs are least important in the theory

Which one of the following is not considered in socio-cultural theories?

a. In the systems theory, behaviour is determined and maintained by the ongoing demands of interpersonal systems in which an individual interacts
b. In the cultural theory, behaviour is through role-modelling and the satisfaction of a hierarchy of needs
c. The availability theory suggests that the greater the availability the greater the prevalence and severity of substance use problems in society
d. Cultural and religious attitudes have been considered to be a defensive shield against alcohol and drug addiction

Which one of the following is not considered in bio-psychosocial theories?

a. In the bio-psychosocial theory, behaviour is mainly determined and maintained by the genetic factors
b. The theory includes genetic inheritance, physiological differences, family, community, peer or social pressure
c. This theory postulates a role for social and spiritual factors in the development of and recovery from addiction
d. The theory supports the concept of a hierarchy of harm reduction outcome goals including abstinence related goals.

KEY POINTS

- The moral theory is based on the belief that using alcohol or drug is a sign of moral weakness.
- The disease theory of addiction maintains that addiction is a disease caused by the impairment of either behavioural or neurochemical processes or both.
- The genetic theory of addiction puts forward a genetic predisposition to alcohol or drug addiction.
- Family studies have shown an increased incidence of alcoholism in families.
- The psychoanalytic theory of addiction stems from the belief that addiction stems from the unconscious death wishes.
- Behaviour is learned through the process of classical conditioning and operant conditioning.
- In social learning theory, in order to understand the effects of alcohol or drugs, cognitive processes must be considered in relation to other factors.
- In the socio-cultural theories, behaviour is determined and maintained by the ongoing demands of interpersonal systems in which an individual interacts.

- In the bio-psychosocial theory genetic inheritance, physiological differences, family, community, peer or social pressure are all considered.

REFERENCES

Addiction Foundation Research (1986) *Essential Concepts and Strategies*, Toronto, Canada: Canadian Government Publishing Centre, Supply and Services.

Adyitanjee, Murray, R.M. (1991) The role of genetic predisposition in alcoholism. In I.B. Glass (ed.), *The International Handbook of Addiction Behaviour*. London: Tavistock/ Routledge.

Allen, K.M. (1996) Theoretical perspectives for addictions nursing practice. In K.M. Allen (ed.), *Nursing Care of the Addicted Client*. Philadelphia: Lippincott.

Bandura, A. (1977) *Social Learning Theory*. Englewood Cliffs: Prentice-Hall.

Barnes, G. (1990) Impact of the family on adolescent drinking patterns. In R. Collins, K. Leonard and J. Searles (eds), *Alcohol and the Family: Research and Clinical Perspectives*. New York: Guilford Press.

Becker, H. (1966) *Outsiders: Studies in the Sociology of Deviance*. New York: The Free Press.

Blum, K., Noble, E.P., Sheridan, P.J. *et al.* (1990) Allelic association of human dopamine D2 receptor gene in alcoholism. *Journal of American Medical Association*, 263: 2055–60.

Cappell, H. and Greeley J. (1987) Alcohol and tension reduction: an update on research and theory. In H.T. Blane and K.E. Leonard (eds), *Psychological Theories of Drinking and Alcoholism*. New York: Guilford Press.

Christiansen, B. and Goldman, M. (1983) Alcohol related expectancies versus demographic background variables in the prediction of adolescent drinking. *Journal of Consulting and Clinical Psychology*, 51: 249–57.

Cloninger, C.R. (1987) Neurogenetic adaptive mechanisms in alcoholism. *Science*, 236: 410–15.

Collins, R. and Marlatt, G. (1981) Social modelling as a determinant of drinking behaviour: implications for prevention and treatment. *Addictive Behaviours*, 6: 233–40.

Copello, A. and Orford, J. (2002). Alcohol and the family: is it time for services to take notice of the evidence? *Addiction*, 97: 1361–3.

Cook, C. (1988) The Minnesota Model in the management of drug and alcohol dependency: miracle, method or myth? Part 1. The philosophy and the programme. *British Journal of Addiction*, 83: 625–34.

Galizio, M. and Maisto, S.A. (1985) Towards a biopsychosocial theory of substance abuse. In M. Galizio and S.S. Maisto (eds), *Determinants of Substance Abuse: Biological, Psychological and Environmental*. New York: Plenum.

Ghodse, A.H. (1995) *Drugs and Addictive Behaviour*. Oxford: Blackwell Science.

Goodwin, D.W., Schulsinger, F., Knop, J., Mednick, S. and Guze, S.B. (1977) Alcoholism and depression in adopted-out daughters of alcoholics. *Archives of General Psychiatry*, 34: 751–5.

Henningfield, J.E., Cohen, C. and Slade, J.D. (1991) Is nicotine more addictive than cocaine? *British Journal of Addiction*, 86, 5: 565.

Hull, J. (1981) A self-awareness model of the causes and effects of alcohol consumption. *Journal of Abnormal Psychology*, 90: 586–600.

Jacob, T. and Leonard, K. (1988) Alcohol-spouse interaction as a function of alcoholism subtype and alcohol consumption interaction. *Journal of Abnormal Psychology*, 97: 231–7.

Jellinek, E.M. (1960) *The Disease Concept of Alcoholism*. New Haven: Hillhouse Press.

Khantzian, E.J. (1980) An ego/self theory of substance dependence: a contemporary psychoanalytical perspective. In D.J. Littieri, M. Sayers and H.W. Pearson (eds), *Theories on Drug Abuse: Selected Contemporary Perspectives*, Washington: DHSS adm84–967.

Khantzian, E.J. (1985) The self-medication hypothesis of addictive disorders: focus on heroin and cocaine dependence. *American Journal of Psychiatry*, 142, 11: 1259–64.

Khantzian, E.J. (1997) The self-medication hypothesis of addictive disorders: A reconsideration and recent applications. *Harvard Review of Psychiatry*, 4: 231–44.

Khantzian, E.J. and Treece, C. (1985) DSM-III psychiatric diagnosis of narcotic addicts. Recent findings. *Archives of General Psychiatry*, 42, 11: 1067–71.

Kumpter, K.L., Trunnell, E.P. and Whiteside, H.O (1990) The biopsychosocial model: Applications to the addictions field. In R.C. Eng (ed.), *Controversies in the Addictions Field*, vol. 1, Dubuque, Iowa: Kendall/Hunt Publishing Company.

Leeds, J. and Morgenstern, J. (1996) Psychoanalytic theories of substance abuse. In F. Rotgers, D.S. Keller and J. Morgenstern (eds), *Treating Substance Abuse: Theory and Technique*. New York: Guilford Press.

Miller, N.S. (1991) *The Pharmacology of Alcohol and Drugs of Abuse and Addiction*. New York: Springer-Verlag.

Murphy, S.L. and Khantzian, E.J. (1995) Addiction as a 'self-medication' disorder: application of ego psychology to the treatment of substance abuse. In A.M. Washton (ed.), *Psychotherapy and Substance Abuse: A Practitioner's Handbook*. New York: Guilford Press.

Orford, J. (1985) *Excessive Appetites: A Psychological View of Addictions*. Chichester: John Wiley & Sons.

Oyefeso, A., Ghodse, H., Keating, A., Annan, J., Phillips, T., Pollard. M. and Nash, P. (2000) *Drug Treatment Needs of Black and Minority Ethnic Residents of the London Borough of Merton*. Addictions Resource Agency for Commissioners (ARAC) Monograph Series on Ethnic Minority Issues. London: ARAC.

Pickens, R., Svikis, D., McGue, M., Lykken, D., Hesten, L. and Clayton P. (1991) Heterogeneity in the inheritance of alcoholism. *Archives of General Psychiatry*, 48, 1: 19–28.

Sangster, D., Shiner. M., Sheikh. N. and Patel, K. (2002) *Delivering Drug Services to Black and Minority Ethnic Communities*. DPAS/P16. London: Home Office Drug Prevention and Advisory Service (DPAS). Also available on thttp://www.drugs.gov.uk tp://www.drugs.gov.uk.

Schuckit, M.A. (1995) *Drug and Alcohol Abuse. A Clinical Guide to Diagnosis and Treatment*, 4th edition. New York: Plenum Medical Book Company.

Sher, K., Walitzer, K., Wood, P. and Brent, E. (1991) Characteristics of children of alcoholics: putative risk factors, substance use and abuse, and psychopathology. *Journal of Abnormal Psychology*. 100, 4: 427–48.

Stacy, A., Widaman, K. and Marlatt, G. (1990) Expectancy models of alcohol use. *Journal of Personal and Social Psychology*, 58, 5: 418–28.

Steinglass, P. (1987). A systems view of family interaction and psychopathology. In T. Jacob (ed.), *Family Interaction and Psychopathology: Theories, Methods, and Findings*, pp. 25–65. New York: Plenum.

Treece, C. and Khantzian, E.J. (1986) Psychodynamic factors in the development of drug dependence. *Psychiatric Clinics of North America*, 9, 3: 399–412.

Tsuang, M.T., Lyons, M.J., Eisen, S.A., Goldberg, J. *et al.* (1996) Genetic influences on DSM III-R. Drug abuse and dependence. A study of 3372 pairs of twins. *American Journal of Medical Genetic*, 67: 473.

Valliant, G.E. (1983) *The Natural History of Alcoholism*. Cambridge, MA: Harvard University Press.

Wallace, J. (1990) The new disease model of alcoholism. *Western Journal of Medicine*, 152, 5: 502.

Wikler, A. (1948) Recent progress in research on the neurophysiological basis of morphine addiction. *American Journal of Psychiatry*, 105: 329–38.

Wikler, A. (1961) On the nature of addiction and habituation. *British Journal of Addiction*, 57: 73–9.

Wolf, P.H. (1972) Ethnic differences in alcohol sensitivity. *Science*, 175: 449–50.

CHAPTER 5

NATURE OF ADDICTION

OBJECTIVES

- Discuss the drug experience in relation to the 'drug' 'set' and 'setting'.

- State the reasons why people take drugs.

- Describe the pattern of alcohol or drug misuse.

- Describe the various routes of drug administration.

- Identify the risks of injecting behaviour.

ACTIVITY 5.1

Please circle or tick the correct answer. There is only one correct answer for each statement

The drug experience depends on
a. The pharmacological properties of the drug and the environment
b. The physical environment where the drug is used and the laws related to drug use
c. The social context of alcohol and drug use
d. The pharmacological properties, social context and the personality of the individual

Experimental users are characterised by
a.   Choice of drug is discriminate; conforms to pattern of use and depends on availability and subculture
b.   Choice of drug is indiscriminate; does not conform to pattern of use and does not depend on availability and subculture
c.   Choice of drug is indiscriminate; choice of substance depends on availability and subculture but does not conform to any pattern of use
d.   Choice of drug is discriminate and conforms to a pattern of use and at an early stage of contact with drug

Recreational users are characterised by
a.   Having a strict adherence to the pattern of use
b.   Having no preference for a particular drug (drug of choice)
c.   Estimating the main risks and benefits of their drug of choice
d.   Their tendency to use drugs or alcohol to complement their social and recreational activities

Dependent users are characterised by
a.   Physical dependence; little or no control over drug use; injecting is not common; polydrug user
b.   Psychological dependence; no control over drug use; injecting is common; polydrug user
c.   Psychological dependence; less frequent in the use of drug; drug of choice and social activities very important
d.   Physical and psychological dependence; no control over drug use; injecting is common; polydrug user

The complications of injecting drug misuse are
a.   Abscess; arterial puncture; headache and vomiting
b.   Hepatitis; abscess; arterial puncture and deep vein thrombosis
c.   Deep vein thrombosis; headache; nausea and abscess
d.   Cellulitis; headache; nausea; abscess

In Chapter 4, many models and theories were put forward to explain why people use or misuse psychoactive substances and about the causes of substance. The theories provide explanations for the initiation into substance misuse or for why individuals begin to use drugs and the process of addiction. It is apparent that no single theory is sufficient to explain substance use and misuse per se, and that a range of 'risk factors' has to be considered. This chapter examines the drug experience, why people take drugs, the pattern of use and misuse and the routes of drug administration.

THE DRUG EXPERIENCE

It is acknowledged that the effect of a psychoactive substance or 'drug experience' will have on a given individual will depend on several other factors beside the pharmacological properties of the drug. The gamut of 'drug experience' involves interrelated sets of non-pharmacological and pharmacological factors. These include pharmacological factors, the personality of the individual and the context or setting (Ghodse 1995). The pharmacological factors include the chemical properties or type of drug used. Different drugs have different mode of action on the body owing to their pharmacological properties, the drug dosage and the route of administration.

In addition, the effects or actions of a psychoactive drug are influenced by the personal characteristics of the drug user. These characteristics include factors such as the person's biological make up, personality, gender, age and drug tolerance (Rassool 1998). For instance, some individuals may develop a toxic reaction to a single cup of coffee or the normally insignificant elevation of heart rate caused by cannabis can be painful for those suffering from angina pectoris, whereas glaucoma patients may find cannabis beneficial but a few cups of coffee may aggravate their conditions (ISDD 1996). The psychological state of drug users is very important as this has a significant influence on the effects and dangers of alcohol and drug use. For example, if they have low mood or are anxious or depressed they are more liable to have disturbing experiences when using psychoactive substances. Their psychological state may be more pronounced and they are likely to become more anxious, disorientated and potentially aggressive. Individuals with psychological disorders such as anorexia nervosa or bulimia can also deteriorate as a result of the use of psychoactive substances. Health problems such as cardiovascular disease, hypertension, asthma, epilepsy, diabetes mellitus or liver disease can exacerbate the use of psychoactive substances and make them more unsafe.

The knowledge, attitude and expectations (psychological set) about a drug will have an influence on the 'drug experience'. For example, if an individual believes or expects, as a self-fulfilling prophecy, that a particular substance will produce a certain effect, the desired effect may be experienced. There is a need to look beyond the immediate intoxicating effects of drugs, and consider drug taking within the wider social context. The last set of factors is the setting or context in which a drug is used. This includes the physical environment where the drug is used, the cultural influences of the community where the drug is consumed, the laws related to drug use and the context in which a drug is used.

All the three interrelated factors, pharmacological properties, individual differences and context of use influence the individual experiences of drug taking. It is stated that 'it is necessary to see the drug–brain interaction not as a simple chemical event but as a matter of considerable complexity involving the drug, the particular person, and the messages and teachings which come from the environment and which powerfully influence the nature and meaning of the drug experience' (Royal College of Psychiatrists 1987).

ACTIVITY 5.2

1   List the reasons why people start taking alcohol or drugs
2   List the reasons why people continue to use alcohol or drugs

WHY DO PEOPLE USE DRUGS?

Psychoactive substances cause a series of temporary changes in the nervous system that produce a feeling of 'high'. One of these changes is the rise in available levels of certain neurotransmitters associated with feelings of pleasure. Key among these is dopamine, a naturally occurring neurotransmitter that some scientists now think is implicated in most of the basic human experiences of pleasure (Palfai and Jankiewicz 1997). In fact, there is evidence to suggest that the mere display of food causes a significant elevation in brain dopamine, a neurotransmitter associated with feelings of pleasure and reward (Volkow *et al.* 2002). In that study, healthy subjects were allowed to observe and smell their favourite foods, but not eat them; the more the subjects desired the foods, the higher their dopamine levels went. This activation of the brain's dopamine may be similar to what addicts experience when craving drugs. When an individual takes a psychoactive substance such as cocaine or smokes tobacco, the substance causes an increase in dopamine levels in the brain resulting in a rush of euphoria or pleasure. There are other chemicals (neurotransmitters) such as serotonin, norepinephrine and gamma amino butyric acid (GABA) that may be involved in process of addiction to psychoactive substances, but dopamine seems to be the essential one.

There is a myth that individuals use illicit psychoactive substances because they are having problems. This is usually not true. They may be attracted to illicit drugs for similar reasons as they are to alcohol. In fact, the subjective initial experiences of taking psychoactive substances is often pleasurable. Furthermore, the use of drugs for pleasure is readily identifiable throughout history and across most cultures (Siegel 2005).

Environmental risk factors are a major influence on an individual's surroundings that increase their likelihood of using psychoactive substances. Drug and alcohol misuse tend to thrive in areas of multiple deprivation, with high unemployment and low-quality housing, and where the surrounding infrastructure of local services is fractured and poorly resourced. In fact, having a less stressful, more privileged environment may provide a degree of protection from addiction or relapse during recovery, according to a recent review of the role of environment in addiction (Nader and Czoty 2005). However, substance misuse is certainly not restricted to areas of urban deprivation. Curiosity, subset of youth culture and music, social acceptability, peer pressure and the media can also promote drug use. Research funded by Cancer Research UK has shown that cigarette advertising encourages young people to start smoking. Teenagers aged 15 and 16 are aware of and participate in many forms of tobacco marketing, and this is consistently associated with becoming a smoker (MacFadyen *et al.* 2001). A list of the reasons why people use drugs is presented in Table 5.1

However, the reason why people start using drugs may not be the same reason why they continue to use drugs. Continued substance use among alcohol and drug users is driven more by physiological and psychological dependence rather than by rational decisions. The reasons why people continue to use drugs may be related to a combination of factors such as dependence, chaotic use, fear of withdrawal symptoms, social exclusions, mental health problems and other psychosocial and environmental conditions. What is common to many alcohol and drug misusers is that they may in fact be able to stop for short periods of time without withdrawal but could not remain abstinent.

Table 5.1 Why people use drugs

- To enjoy the experience
- To get the same experience as alcohol
- To enjoy the short-term effects
- To feel confident
- To 'break the rules'
- To be part of the subculture
- To be curious about the effects
- The drugs are easily accessible and available
- Friends use them
- To avoid unpleasant feelings
- To enhance work performances

- To counter the unpleasant effects of prescribed medications.
- To continue the habit
- It is part of one's home or social life
- To relieve boredom
- To alleviate pain
- To satisfy cravings
- To avoid withdrawal symptoms
- To counter the withdrawal effects of other drugs (use of benzodiazepines after stimulants)
- To lose weight
- To escape from stress

PATTERNS OF SUBSTANCE USE AND MISUSE

The progression of an addiction reflects a broad spectrum, ranging from no use to dependence. The patterns of drug or alcohol use and misuse for some individuals sometimes vary over a period of time. Individuals may move back and forth within this continuum, but generally they advance from no use, to use, misuse and finally to dependence. The patterns of substance misuse are often described as no use, experimental, recreational and problematic users. Other patterns of substance misuse include binge drinking or drug-taking and chaotic use.

No use

In this stage there is no use of alcohol or other drug. People have their own reasons not to be involved, including religious beliefs, age, the criminal justice system, etc.

Experimental users

Experimental users can be described as those who have used drugs, legal or illicit, on a few occasions. By definition, anyone's initial use of a drug, alcohol or tobacco smoking is experimental (Rassool 1998). At this stage, using alcohol or drugs feels good because there is no consequence or minimal consequences at this point or having a low tolerance to the drug. There is no 'pattern' in the use of psychoactive substances but the choice of the drug misused is indiscriminate. The use of psychoactive substances is usually unplanned. The choice of drug depends on factors such as availability, social marketing and reputation of the drug, subculture, fashion and peer-group influence.

The motivating factors include curiosity, desire to share a social experience, anticipation of effects, availability and value for money (cost of drug). This stage usually forms part of the desire among adolescents to experiment and try new risky experiences and can be seen as a normal developmental pattern. There is usually no change in behaviour and the experimental user is practically identical to the non-user in terms of lifestyle, activities, social integration and school performance. Experimental use of illicit psychoactive substance is usually a short-lived experience, and the majority of people may confine the consumption to drugs that are socially acceptable. Experimental users, however, are in the highest category of risk for infections (if injecting), medical complications or overdose owing to the indiscriminate use of adulterated psychoactive substances. What is unclear is the likelihood of further engagement with, or disengagement from, further alcohol and drug use.

Recreational users

The most common drugs used by recreational users are alcohol, caffeine, nicotine, cannabis, LSD and ecstasy. Experimental users may or may not become recreational users of illicit psychoactive substances and come from all strata of society. The term 'recreational' refers to a form of substance use in which pleasure and relaxation are the prime motivations. There is a strict adherence to the pattern of use so that the drug is used only on certain occasions such as weekends and less likely on consecutive days. There is usually a preference for a particular drug (drug of choice); the user has learnt how to use it and appreciate its effects. Drug or alcohol use is one aspect of the user's life and tends to complement social and recreational activities. There are usually no adverse medical or social consequences as a result of the recreational use as in the case of controlled drinking.

A study by Parker *et al.* (1998) found that taking recreational drugs is best understood as a matter of the complex calculation of risks and benefits. Recreational users estimate the main hazards as damage to their health, or legal risks (getting caught), and the main benefits as gaining 'time-out' from stress as leading to leisure and relaxation. On the whole, recreational users refrain from using hard drugs as a result of their personal calculations of risks and pleasures. Recreational users, however, are also in the highest category of risk for infections. Some recreational drugs act as sexual stimulants, lowering inhibition and increasing sexual drive which often leads to risky sexual behaviour and increased likelihood of HIV infection.

Dependent users

By definition, a dependent user has progressed to regular and problematic use of a psychoactive drug or becoming a polydrug user (multiple drug use). Tolerance is very high and there is the presence of psychological and/or physical dependence; it is distinguished from experimental and recreational use. The pattern of use is more frequent and regular but less controlled. However, use continues despite the negative consequences. The process in obtaining the drug is more important to the user than the quality of experience. This tends to displace rather than complement social activities. Injecting drugs is common, and the frequent use creates problems of intoxication, infections if sharing needle and syringe, and other medical complications. Personal, social, psychological and legal problems may be present in this group.

CHAOTIC USE

Chaotic use is referred to when an individual is regarded as taking a drug or drugs in a spontaneous way that tends not to follow any typical drug-using pattern. It is generally associated with problematic bouts of heavy use that may cause the user harm (Drugscope 2007). This is often the excessive use of multiple drugs or polydrug use over a prolonged period of time. The individual's life is circumscribed by their drug use in completely unordered and unpredictable ways and is combined with other significant health issues such as HIV, liver damage and mental health problems.

BINGE DRINKING

In recent years the term 'binge drinking' has gained currency as referring to a high intake of alcohol in a single drinking occasion. Binge drinking is often defined as the consumption of more than a certain number of drinks over a short period of time – a single drinking session or at least a single day (men consuming at least eight, and women at least six standard units of alcohol) (Institute of Alcohol Studies 2004). The features of binge drinking (MCM Research 2004):

- drinking with the intention of getting drunk, often mixing drinks
- drinking to the point at which you lose control
- drinking as much as possible in a short space of time
- occasional, heavy drinking.

A much simpler definition of binge drinking is drinking too much alcohol over a short period of time and is usually the type of drinking that leads to drunkenness (Alcohol Concern 2007). Binge drinking and severe intoxication can cause muscular incoordination, blurred vision, stupor, hypothermia, convulsions, depressed reflexes, respiratory depression, hypotension and coma. Death can occur from respiratory or circulatory failure or if binge drinkers inhale their own vomit (Institute of Alcohol Studies 2004). It is well known that binge drinkers are at increased risk of accidents, alcohol poisoning, unsafe sex and having poor social behaviour. These patterns of behaviour are also relevant to the episodic use of a psychoactive drug other than alcohol, in large quantities over a period of time, followed by limited use or abstinence.

ROUTES OF DRUG ADMINISTRATION (HOW PEOPLE TAKE DRUGS)

The absorption of a drug is in part dependent upon its route of administration. Since psychoactive drugs must enter the bloodstream to reach their site of action, the route of administration is very important in the speed of influencing the physical and psychological effects of the drug. The routes of taking drug are oral, smoking, inhalation and by injection. The most common route of administration is oral, in either liquid or tablet form. When a drug is required to act more rapidly the preferred route of administration is by injection. Drugs of misuse, such as heroin, are often administered intravenously, for example directly into a vein. Certain drugs are smoked, for example cannabis, crack cocaine, heroin. Some psychoactive drugs, for example cocaine and amphetamine, are also taken by the intranasal route. Identical drugs can produce different results depending on the route of administration. For example, naloxone, an antagonist of opiates, is given intravenously and is therefore used in the treatment of opiate overdose: the same drug, given orally, acts differently and is used in the treatment of constipation.

Oral

The oral route (swallowing) is the most popular method of drug administration although effectively the slowest route because of the slow absorption of the drug into the blood stream. There is no stigma attached, compared to smoking and injecting, to take a psychoactive substance orally either in tablet form or in the form of beverages containing alcohol or caffeine

Smoking

Smoking is also a very effective route where the drug is inhaled as in the case of tobacco or heroin smoking ('chasing the dragon'). Cannabis or marijuana is also smoked in the form of a 'joint' which is usually mixed with tobacco.

Inhalation

The inhalation route (sniffing) is also used to self-administer drugs. Absorption of the drug is through the mucous membrane of the nose and mouth. The types of drugs that are inhaled include cocaine, tobacco snuff and volatile substances and solvents. Inhalation may also produce rapid absorption and response as in the case of crack cocaine.

Injecting

The methods of drug injecting include intramuscularly or subcutaneously and/or intravenously. Injection of drugs is less widespread than other routes of drug administration but also the most hazardous. The major dangers of injecting are risk of overdose because of the concentrated effect of this method. There is also the risk of infection from non-sterile injection methods including hepatitis B and HIV infections, abscesses, gangrene and thromboses. The onset of the effects of the drug is rapid when it is administered intravenously: this is a major reason why drugs are often self-administered by injecting. Drugs that are mainly injected include heroin, cocaine, amphetamines and some hypnosedatives. Table 5.2 summarises the complications of injecting.

Table 5.2 Complications of injecting

Equipment	Agent	Site of injection	Effects
Environment	Drug	Trauma and Infection	Overdose
Cooker	Drug interactions	Skin abscess	Poisoning
Water	Allergy	Fat necrosis	Infection
Filter	Contaminants	'Simple' miss	Thrombosis
Syringe	Infectious agents	Connective tissue	Embolism
Needle		Arterial injection	
		Nerves	
		Lungs, breasts, penises, necks	

Adapted from Pates, R., McBride, A. and Arnold, K. (2005) *Injecting Illicit Drugs*, p. xiii. Oxford: Blackwell Publishing.

KEY POINTS

- All the three interrelated factors, pharmacological properties, individual differences and context of use influence the individual experiences of drug taking.
- Continued substance use among alcohol and drug users is driven more by physiological and psychological dependence than by rational decisions.
- The patterns of drug or alcohol use and misuse for some individuals sometimes vary over a period of time.
- Experimental use of illicit psychoactive substance is usually a short-lived experience and the majority of people may confine their consumption to drugs that are socially acceptable.
- The most common drugs used by recreational users are alcohol, caffeine, nicotine, cannabis, LSD and ecstasy.
- A dependent user has progressed to regular and problematic use of a psychoactive drug or becoming a multiple drug user.
- Binge drinking is drinking with the intention of getting drunk.
- Chaotic use is referred to when an individual is regarded as taking a drug or drugs in a spontaneous way that tends not to follow any typical drug-using pattern.
- The routes of administration are oral, smoking, inhalation and injection.
- Injecting drugs is less widespread than other routes of drug administration but also the most hazardous.

REFERENCES

Alcohol Concern (2007) *Binge Drinking Factsheet Summary*. London: Alcohol Concern.

Drugscope (1997) *Media Guide Glossary*. London: Drugscope. http://www.drugscope.org.uk/resources/mediaguide/glossary.

Ghodse, A.H. (1995) *Drugs and Addictive Behaviour*. Oxford: Blackwell Science.

Institute of Alcohol Studies (2004) *Binge Drinking: Nature, Prevalence and Causes*. St Ives: Institute of Alcohol Studies.

Institute for the Study of Drug Dependence (1996) *Drug Abuse Briefings*, 6th edition. London: ISDD.

MacFadyen, L., Hastings, G. and MacKintosh A.M (2001) Cross sectional study of young people's awareness of and involvement with tobacco marketing. *British Medical Journal*, 322: 513–17.

MCM Research Limited (2004) *WTAG Binge-drinking Research*. Oxford: MCM Research Limited.

Nader, P.W. and Czoty, M.A (2005) PET imaging of dopamine D2 receptors in monkey models of cocaine abuse: genetic predisposition versus environmental modulation. *American Journal of Psychiatry*, 162: 1473–82.

Palfai, T. and Jankiewicz H. (1997) *Drugs and Human Behaviour*, 2nd edition. Madison: Brown & Benchmark.

Parker, H., Aldridge, J. and Measham F. (1998) *Illegal Leisure: The Normalization of Adolescent Recreational Drug Use*. London: Routledge.

Rassool, G. Hussein (1998) *Substance Use and Misuse: Nature, Context and Clinical Interventions*. Oxford: Blackwell Science.

Royal College of Psychiatrists (1987) *Drug Scenes: A Report on Drugs and Drug Dependence*. London: Gaskell.

Siegel, R. (2005) *Intoxication: The Universal Drive for Mind-Altering Substances*. Vermont: Park Street Press.

Volkow, N.D., Wang, G.J., Fowler, J.S. *et al.* (2002) Nonhedonic food motivation in humans involves dopamine in the dorsal striatum and methylphenidate amplifies this effect, *Synapse*, 44, 3: 175–80.

CHAPTER 6

POLICY INITIATIVES AND STRATEGY IN ALCOHOL AND DRUG USE

OBJECTIVES

■ Understand the laws concerning psychoactive substances.

■ Be familiar with policy issues and initiatives in takling alcohol and drug misuse.

■ Be aware of the implications of the 'models of care' in the management of and treatment for alcohol and drug misusers.

This chapter focuses on selected policy issues which are important in the understanding of the larger context of alcohol and drugs. Despite the long-standing political prominence of the problem, relatively coherent strategies and substantial investment, the United Kingdom remains at the top of the European ladder with the highest level of dependent and recreational drug use (UKDCP 2007). Since the 1990s, the UK government has responded to high-profile alcohol and drug problems with various policies and initiatives in dealing with this public health problem. At international level, various conventions have attempted to control the manufacturing, distribution and use of psychoactive substances. The Single Convention on Narcotic Drugs (1961, 1972) placed strict controls on the cultivation of opium poppy, coca bush and cannabis plants. The Convention on Psychotropic Substances (1971) widened the international drug control system to cover stimulants, hypnosedatives and hallucinogens. The 1988 Convention against Illicit Traffic in Narcotic Drugs and Psychotropic substances covers areas of drug-trafficking activities including money laundering. In the UK, the Misuse of Drugs Act 1971 continued a process of increasing legal control of psychoactive substances.

THE MISUSE OF DRUGS ACT 1971

The Misuse of Drugs Act 1971 deals with nearly all drugs and defines a series of offences, including unlawful supply, intent to supply, import or export (all these are collectively known as 'trafficking' offences), unlawful production and cultivation. It also lays down specific requirements for their prescriptions, safe custody and record-keeping. The Misuse of Drugs Act regulates what are termed controlled drugs. The main difference from the Medicines Act is that the Misuse of Drugs Act also prohibits unlawful possession. The legislation also lays down the prescribing responsibilities of the medical practitioner. The Act divides drugs into three classes as follows: class A, B and C (see Table 6.1). Class A drugs are those considered to be the most harmful.

The possession of a controlled drug such as amphetamines, barbiturates, methadone, minor tranquillisers and occasionally heroin is not illegal and the drugs can be obtained through a legitimate doctor's prescription. However, allowing your home to be used for the consumption of certain controlled drugs (smoking of cannabis or opium) or for the supply or production of any controlled drug is a criminal offence. Professionals could be prosecuted if they knowingly allowed any of these things to occur on work premises. The Drugs Act 2005 came into force on 1 January 2006. Key points of the Act are presented in Table 6.2 (Drugscope 2007).

Table 6.1 The Misuse of Drugs Act 1971

Class	Drug	Penalties for possession	Penalties for dealing
A	Cocaine and crack, ecstasy, heroin, LSD, morphine, opium, pethidine, methadone, methamphetamine (crystal meth), magic mushrooms and any class B drug which is injected. Class A drugs are treated by the law as the most dangerous	Up to seven years in prison or an unlimited fine. Or both	Up to life in prison or an unlimited fine. Or both
B	These include oral preparations of amphetamine (not methamphetamine), barbiturates, and codeine	Up to five years in prison or an unlimited fine. Or both	Up to 14 years in prison or an unlimited fine. Or both
C	These include cannabis (in resin, oil or herbal form), amphetamines, anabolic steroids and minor tranquillisers	Up to two years in prison or an unlimited fine. Or both	Up to 14 years in prison or an unlimited fine. Or both

Table 6.2 The Drugs Act 2005

- The Act allows compulsory drug testing of arrested people where police have 'reasonable grounds' for believing that class A drugs were involved in the commission of an offence. Failure to comply with this testing is itself an offence and positive tests can lead to compulsory drug treatment assessment
- The Act allows a reversal of the burden of proof in cases where suspects are found in possession of a quantity of drugs greater than that which would be required for personal use. In other words, it is up to the defendant to prove that there was no intent to supply. The actual amount has yet to be defined
- The Act includes fresh liberty cap or 'magic' mushrooms in class A of the Misuse of Drugs Act. Before this Bill, only dried or prepared mushrooms were considered illegal
- The Act has also linked drug legislation with measures to deal with antisocial behaviour so that anyone given an Anti Social Behaviour Order must undergo compulsory testing and drug treatment

In May 2008, cannabis was recommended to be reclassified from class C to class B. The reclassification of cannabis to class B would take effect from early 2009, if approved by parliament.

TACKLING DRUGS TO BUILD A BETTER BRITAIN: POLICY DEVELOPMENT

The Advisory Council of the Misuse of Drugs' report on 'Treatment and Rehabilitation' (ACMD 1982) highlighted the need for a comprehensive approach and multi-professional response to substance misuse, calling for the active involvement of a wide range of both specialist and non-specialist service provision. In England, the most significant health policy document, *The Health of the Nation* (Department of Health 1992), signalled a shift of emphasis towards the prevention of alcohol-related problems and HIV/AIDS and sexual health. In addition, the aim of the British government's strategy, as set out in the White Paper *Tackling Drugs Together* (Home Office 1995), is 'to take effective action by vigorous law enforcement, accessible treatment and a new emphasis on education and prevention'. It introduced Drug Action Teams to implement the strategy depending on local need and set up local multi-agency reference groups. The government has built on this policy with the publication of *Tackling Drugs to Build a Better Britain* in 1998; it updated this in 2002 and again in 2004 with the publication of *Tackling Drugs: Changing Lives* (Home Office 2004)

The updated drug strategy (Home Office 2002) builds on the foundations laid and lessons learned from previous drug strategies. This updated strategy sets out a range of policies and interventions which concentrate on the most dangerous drugs, the most damaged communities and the individuals whose addiction and chaotic lifestyles are most harmful, both to themselves and to others. Implicit in the strategy is that the government has no intention to legalise any illicit drug. The focus of the strategy is

- to help young people resist drugs misuse to achieve their full potential
- to protect communities from antisocial and criminal behaviour
- to enable people with drug problems to overcome them and live healthy and crime-free lives
- to stifle availability of illegal drugs on our streets.

One of the main focuses of the ten-year strategy is the provision of access to treatment and rehabilitation services for substance misusers and the Drug Interventions Programme (DIP). The DIP is a critical part of the government's strategy. Service provision has been expanded to interface with the criminal justice system to provide a tailored solution for adults who commit crime to fund their drug misuse. Its principal focus is to reduce drug-related crime. Its aim is to break the cycle of drug misuse and offending behaviour by intervening at every stage of the criminal justice system to engage offenders in drug treatment.

The government's wider national drugs strategy is to reduce drug-related death due to overdose and blood-borne viruses. Blood-borne virus infections can cause chronic poor health and can lead to serious disease and to premature death. In 2005, 1,506 drug users died in England from 'overdose' or poisoning due to drug misuse. A report on Reducing Drug-related Harm: An Action Plan (Department of Health/NTA 2007) sets out a harm reduction approach aimed at reducing the number of drug-related deaths and blood-borne virus infections. Its wider goals are to prevent drug misuse and of encouraging stabilisation in treatment and support for abstinence. The aims of the strategy are to provide effective substitution treatments and effective support for abstinence.

A ten-year strategy (2008–2018) (Home Office 2008), unveiled in 2008, aims to restrict the supply of illegal drugs and focuses on protecting families and strengthening communities.

THE ALCOHOL HARM REDUCTION STRATEGY FOR ENGLAND

The *Alcohol Harm Reduction Strategy for England* (Prime Minister's Strategy Unit 2004, 2007) is a coherent strategy that sets out the government's aims for reducing alcohol-related harm and costs of alcohol misuse. The strategy recognises the need for co-ordination of services and commits to working within the *Models of Care* framework on integrated care pathways. It also has a series of measures which aim to tackle alcohol-related disorder in town and city centres, improve treatment and support for people with alcohol problems, clamp down on irresponsible promotions by the industry and provide better information to consumers about the dangers of alcohol misuse.

The strategy includes a series of measures aimed at achieving a long-term change in attitudes to irresponsible drinking and behaviour and proposes a number of measures to improve early identification and treatment of alcohol problems. The strategy will build on the good practice of some existing initiatives and involve the alcohol industry in new initiatives both at national level (drinks producers) and at local level (retailers, pubs and clubs). The strategy sets out:

- to improve the information available to individuals and to start the process of change in the culture of drinking to get drunk
- to better identify and treat alcohol misuse
- to prevent and tackle alcohol-related crime and disorder and deliver improved services to victims and witnesses
- to work with the industry in tackling the harms caused by alcohol.

The report *Safe. Sensible. Social: The Next Steps in the National Alcohol Strategy* (Department of Health, Home Office, Department for Education and Skills and Department for Culture, Media and Sport 2007) reviews progress since the publication of the *Alcohol Harm Reduction Strategy for England* (2004) The document outlines further sharpening of criminal justice for drunken behaviour; a review of NHS alcohol spending; more help for people who want to drink less; toughened enforcement of underage sales; trusted guidance for parents and young people; public information campaigns to promote a new 'sensible drinking' culture; public consultation on alcohol pricing and promotion; and local alcohol strategies and actions to achieve long-term reductions in alcohol-related ill health and crime.

In *Choosing Health: Making Healthy Choices Easier* (Department of Health 2004), the report places alcohol firmly in the realm of public health practice and highlights action on reducing alcohol-related harm and encouraging sensible drinking as one of its six priorities. *Choosing Health* emphasises and builds on the recommendations in the alcohol harm reduction strategy for England (Department of Health 2002). It proposes:

- a national information campaign to tackle the problems of binge drinking
- a social responsibility scheme
- training for professionals
- piloting screening and brief interventions in primary and secondary health settings, including accident and emergency
- similar pilots in criminal justice settings
- a programme of improvements for treatment services
- additional funding.

In addition, the report highlighted the need for a public health approach and set out a number of priorities for action including action on smoking and sexual health. For tobacco smoking, the strategy aims to reduce the numbers of people who smoke by implementing a campaign to reduce smoking rates and motivate smokers in different groups to quit. This will be supported by clear information about health risks, reasons not to smoke and access to NHS support to quit, including Stop Smoking Services and nicotine replacement therapy. In the areas of sexual health the report proposes a new national campaign targeted particularly at younger men and women. This is to ensure that they understand the real risk of unprotected sex and to persuade them of the benefits of using condoms to avoid the risk of sexually transmitted infections or unplanned pregnancies.

NATIONAL TREATMENT AGENCY

The National Treatment Agency (NTA), created by the government in 2001, is a special health authority with a remit to increase the availability, capacity and effectiveness of treatment for drug misuse in England, thus ensuring that there is more access to treatment modalities, better or effective treatment and fairer treatment available to all those who need it. This is the first time an organisation has been established to oversee the development of drug treatment services at a national level. Parallel structures have been established with the Scottish Executive and the Welsh and Northern Ireland Assemblies. The NTA focuses on the following priority areas: treatment capacity; retention of individuals in treatment systems; ensuring that offenders can access treatment at every stage of their passage through the criminal justice system; access to treatment facilities within three weeks and that those already in treatment will wait no longer than three weeks between treatment modalities; treatment effectiveness and diversity.

The NTA works closely with Department of Health with the sexual health and substance misuse team; with the Home Office; with the Drug Strategy Directorate, criminal justice agencies (probation, police, prison services and youth justice board); Healthcare Commission in developing standards and inspection procedures for drug treatment services; with the royal colleges and training organisations to increase the level of training on drug misuse available in their courses; with academic institutions and researchers to identify best practice in drug treatment; and with government office drug teams whose responsibility is to implement the national drugs strategy at regional level. In addition the Drug Alcohol Action Teams (DAATs) implement the national drug treatment policies and strategies on a regional and local level. The DAATs are multi-agency government-funded teams responsible for the effective management and commissioning of drug treatment services. Representatives from the police, the county councils, probation, Customs and Excise, local NHS services and voluntary groups make up the partnership board of the DAATs. Other partnerships are formed with the NHS regional directors of public health to reduce drug-related deaths and the spread of blood-borne diseases; with drug treatment providers; and with service user and carer groups.

THE 2007 CLINICAL GUIDELINES

The *Drug Misuse and Dependence: UK Guidelines on Clinical Management* (Department of Health 2007), referred to as the 2007 Clinical Guidelines, provide guidance on the treatment of drug misuse in the UK, based on current evidence and professional consensus. The report places its emphasis on the rights of individual drug users to receive appropriate treatment and on the responsibility of all doctors to address drug-related problems. It is intended for all clinicians, non-medical prescribers (nurses and pharmacists) and those providing pharmacological interventions for drug misusers as a component of drug misuse treatment. The 2007 Clinical Guidelines focus on drug treatment effectiveness, principles of clinical governance, essential elements of treatment provision, psychosocial components of treatment, health considerations and specific treatment situations and populations

MODELS OF CARE: DRUGS

Models of Care for Treatment of Adult Drug Misusers (MoCDM) (NTA 2002) sets out a national framework, in England, for the commissioning of adult treatment for drug misuse to meet the needs of diverse local populations. The MoCDM has the same status, in terms of local planning and delivery, as a national service framework for drug treatment. The framework has also 'great relevance' for alcohol service provision and provides specific guidance to support the co-ordination of drug and alcohol treatment and effective management of care across drug misuse treatment services and general health, social and other care. The MoCDM advocates a whole system approach to meeting the multiple needs of drug and alcohol misusers through the development of local systems that integrate drug and alcohol treatment services with other generic health, social and criminal justice services including throughcare and aftercare.

The MoCDM was updated in 2006. The *Update 2006* (NTA 2006) is intended to build on the framework and concepts in *Models of Care 2002* rather than replace them. It requires drug treatment commissioners and providers to have implemented the key tenets previously described in Models of Care 2002, including:

- the four-tiered model of commissioning
- local screening and assessment systems

- the care planning and co-ordination of care at the heart of structured drug treatment
- the development of integrated care pathways.

Models of Care: Update 2006 also incorporates the new strategy to improve the quality and effectiveness of drug treatment. The key differences between *Models of Care 2002* and *Models of Care: Update 2006* are: the context of improving treatment effectiveness and improving clients' journeys; a reiteration of the four tiers system (see below) updated information on assessment, care planning and integrated care pathways; definitions of the full range of treatment interventions in the context of local treatment systems; and quality requirements which are in line with the NHS policy and performance management structures. In addition, *Models of Care: Update 2006* advocates the commissioning and provision of a wide range of interventions to reduce the adverse effects of drug misuse on drug users, with particular focus on reducing the risk of immediate death due to overdose and risks of morbidity and mortality due to blood-borne virus and other infections. This may include interventions to reduce drug-related harm by increasing the availability of clean injecting equipment; encouraging drug injectors not to share injecting equipment, to use ingestion methods as an alternative to injecting; and to attracting drug users into oral substitute treatment when appropriate.

Models of Care (NTA 2002) introduced a four tiers system of models of care. A summary of the key points is presented in Table 6.3.

Tier 1 services are generic (non-substance-misuse-specific) services requiring interface with drug and alcohol treatment but their sole purpose is not drug or alcohol treatment. The role of Tier 1 services, in this context, includes the provision of generic services plus, as a minimum, screening and referral to local drug and alcohol treatment services in Tiers 2 and 3. There may be a need for a specialised drug treatment or 'addiction' liaison service to provide a co-coordinated response with Tier 1 where there is a high prevalence rate of substance misuse.

The aim of the treatment in Tier 2 is to engage substance abusers in drug treatment and reduce drug-related harm. This tier is defined by having a low threshold to access services, and includes needle exchange, drug and alcohol advice and information services, and ad hoc support not delivered in the context of a care plan. Specialist social workers can provide services within this tier, including the provision of access to social work advice, childcare or parenting assessment, and assessment of social care needs. Tier 2 can also include low-threshold prescribing programmes aimed at engaging opioid users to reduce drug-related harm.

Tier 3 services are provided solely for drug and alcohol misusers in structured programmes of care. Tier 3 services require the drug and alcohol abusers to receive a drug assessment and to have a care plan, which is agreed between the service provider and the client. For clients whose needs cross several domains, there should be a care co-coordinator, responsible for co-ordination of that individual's care on behalf of all the agencies and services involved. Tier 3 services and mental health services should work closely together to meet the needs of drug abusers with dual diagnosis. Tier 3 structured services include a whole gamut of pharmacotherapy and psychosocial interventions.

Tier 4 services are aimed at individuals with multiple needs. Services in this tier include inpatient drug and alcohol units, residential rehabilitation units and crisis intervention centres. Referral is usually from Tiers 2 or 3 services or via community care

Table 6.3 Models of Care four tiers system: drugs

Tier	Settings	Professionals	Intervention strategies
1	• Primary healthcare services • Acute hospitals, e.g. A&E departments • Psychiatric services • Social services departments • Homelessness services • Antenatal clinics • General hospital wards • Police settings, e.g. custody cells • Probation services • Prison service • Education and vocational services • Occupational health services • Hepathology services	• Primary care • General medical services • Social workers • Community pharmacists • Probation officers • Housing officers • Homeless persons units	• Drug and alcohol screening • Referral to alcohol and drug services • Assessment • Information to reduce drug-related harm • Liaison with drug and alcohol services • General medical care • Housing support • Hepatitis B vaccination
2	• Drug advice and information centres • Drop-in services • Pharmacy • Outreach services • Self-Referrals • Referral from variety of other sources	• Specialist drug and alcohol workers • Specialist social workers	• Drug and alcohol screening and assessment. • Care planning and management • Criminal justice screening and referral • Motivation and brief interventions • Drug and alcohol information services • Needle exchange • Ad hoc support (no care planning) • Social work advice • Childcare or parenting assessment • Assessment of social care needs • Low-threshold prescribing programme • Outreach work

Table 6.3 Continued

Tier	Settings	Professionals	Intervention strategies
3	• Community-based specialist drug and alcohol services • Structured community-based services for stimulant users, young people, Black and ethnic minority groups, women, HIV and AIDs, dual diagnosis • Self-referrals • Referral from variety of sources	• Specialist drug and alcohol workers • Dual diagnosis workers • Specialist social workers	• Drug assessment • Care plan • Care-co-ordinator • Shared-care prescribing • Testing order drug treatment • Cognitive behaviour therapy • Motivational interventions • Counselling • Methadone maintenance programmes • Community detoxification • Day care • After-care programme
4a	• Inpatient drug and alcohol detoxification services • Drug and alcohol residential rehabilitation units • Residential drug crisis intervention centres • Referral from Tiers 2 or 3 services	• Drug and alcohol specialist workers • Counsellors or therapists • Specialist liaison services to Tiers 1–4a services	• Provision of holistic care: physical, psychological, social and spiritual care • Pharmacotherapy • Psychological interventions • Social interventions • Educational interventions
4b	• Non-substance-misuse-specific	• Specialist liver disease units • HIV clinics and genito-urinary clinics • Eating disorder units • Forensic services • Personality disorder units • Terminal care services	

Source: Adapted from Models of Care for Adult Misusers (NTA 2002, 2006)

assessment. Tier 4a services may be abstinence-oriented programmes, detoxification services or services which stabilise clients (e.g. on substitute drugs). Access to Tier 4a requires careful assessment, detoxification prior to placement in a drug- and alcohol-free residential programme and preparation of the client in order to maximise readiness, compliance and programmes effectiveness. Drug and alcohol abusers receiving Tier 4 services require a designated care co-coordinator, allocated before entry to this tier. Tier 4b services are non-substance-misuse-specific and have close links with services in other tiers. Some highly specialist Tier 4b services also provide specialist liaison services to Tiers 1–4a services, for example HIV liaison clinics, forensic services and genito-urinary medicine.

MODELS OF CARE: ALCOHOL

Model of Care for Alcohol Misusers (MoCAM) (Department of Health/NTA 2006) is based on all the key foundations laid down in the document *Models of Care for the Treatment of Adult Drug Misusers* (MoCDM) (NTA 2002). MoCAM develops the notion of integrated local treatment ' systems', the tiered framework of provision, effective use of screening and assessment, a central role of care planning in structured treatment and the development of integrated care pathways to enhance pathways of care ('alcohol treatment pathways'). The document describes key quality criteria for the commissioning and provision of services and interventions strategies. MoCAM identifies four main categories of alcohol misusers who may benefit from some kind of intervention or treatment: hazardous drinkers; harmful drinkers; moderately dependent drinkers and severely dependent drinkers (see Chapter 3).

MoCAM outlined the four-tiered framework of provision for commissioning evidence-based alcohol treatment in England. Tier 1 interventions include provision of identification of hazardous, harmful and dependent drinkers; information on sensible drinking; simple brief interventions to reduce alcohol-related harm; and referral of those with alcohol dependence or harm for more intensive interventions. Tier 2 interventions include provision of open access facilities and outreach that provide alcohol-specific advice, information and support; extended brief interventions to help alcohol misusers reduce alcohol-related harm; and assessment and referral of those with more serious alcohol-related problems for care-planned treatment. Tier 3 interventions include provision of community-based specialised alcohol-misuse assessment, and alcohol treatment that is care-co-ordinated and care-planned. Tier 4 interventions include provision of residential, specialised alcohol treatments which are care-planned and co-ordinated to ensure continuity of care and after-care. Key points of the four-tiered framework are presented in Table 6.4

DEVELOPMENT OF SERVICES FOR SPECIAL POPULATIONS

There has been a notable absence from recent national drug policies in the UK of attempts to address the health status and health care needs of Black and ethnic minority

Table 6.4 Models of Care four tiers system: alcohol

Tier	Settings	Specialist settings	Intervention strategies
1	• Primary healthcare services • Acute hospitals, e.g. A&E departments • Psychiatric services • Social services departments • Homelessness services • Antenatal clinics • General hospital wards • Police settings, e.g. custody cells • Probation services • Prison services • Education and vocational services • Occupational health services	• Specialist liver disease units • Specialist psychiatric wards • Forensic units • Residential provision for the homeless • Domestic abuse services	• Interventions include provision of: identification of hazardous, harmful and dependent drinkers • Information on sensible drinking; simple brief interventions to reduce alcohol-related harm • Referral of those with alcohol dependence or harm for more intensive interventions
2	• Primary healthcare services • Acute hospitals, e.g. A&E departments • Psychiatric services • Social services departments • Homelessness services • Antenatal clinics • General hospital wards • Police settings, e.g. custody cells • Probation services. Prison service • Education and vocational services • Occupational health services	• Alcohol services	• Alcohol-specific information, advice and support • Extended brief interventions and brief treatment to reduce alcohol-related harm • Alcohol-specific assessment and referral of those requiring more structured alcohol treatment • Partnership or 'shared care' with staff from Tier 3 and Tier 4 • Provision, or joint care of individuals attending other services providing Tier 1 interventions • Mutual aid groups, e.g. Alcoholics Anonymous • Triage assessment, which may be provided as part of locally agreed arrangements

| 3 | Primary care settings (shared care schemes)
• GP-led prescribing services
• The work in community settings can be delivered by statutory, voluntary or independent services providing care-planned, structured alcohol treatment | • Community-based, structured, care-planned alcohol treatment | • Comprehensive substance misuse assessment
• Care planning
• Case management
• Community detoxification
• Prescribing interventions to reduce risk of relapse
• Psychosocial therapies and support
• Interventions to address co-existing conditions
• Day programmes
• Liaison services, e.g. for acute medical and psychiatric health services(such as pregnancy, mental health or hepatitis services)
• Social care services (such as child care and housing services and other generic services) |
| 4 | • Inpatient provision in the context of general psychiatric wards
• Hospital services for pregnancy, liver problems, etc. with specialised alcohol liaison support | • Alcohol specialist inpatient treatment and residential rehabilitation | • Comprehensive substance misuse assessment
• Care planning and review
• Prescribing interventions
• Alcohol detoxification
• Prescribing interventions to reduce risk of relapse
• Psychosocial therapies and support
• Provision of information, advice and training and 'shared care' to others |

Source: Adapted from *Models of Care for Alcohol Misusers* (NTA 2006)

people, young people and women. This section focuses only on Black and ethnic minority substance abusers. According to the Advisory Council on the Misuse of Drugs (ACMD 1998: 52), 'Ethnic differences in patterns of drug misuse suggest that the needs of some minority ethnic groups are marginalized by existing services, which tend to focus on injecting rather than smoking'. The current UK drug policy, *Tackling Drugs to Build a Better Britain* (Home Office 1998) and the updated drug strategy (Home Office 2002) recognised the failure of Black and ethnic minority drug abusers to utilise the range of available treatment services and provided guidance for those involved in the purchasing and provision of drug services to tackle race equality, accessibility and practice. In addition, the strategy encouraged drug action teams (DATs) to undertake health care needs assessment and consider cultural diversity in service provision and delivery. The National Treatment Agency for Substance Misuse (NTA) has identified diversity as one of its key strategic objectives, recognising the need to ensure equal access to service provision regardless of age, gender, sexuality, disability and ethnicity.

In *Models of Care for Adult Drug Misusers* (NTA 2002), the treatment needs of Black and ethnic minority substance misusers are recognised throughout the document. In addition, there is a specific section on Black and ethnic minority communities (pp. 130–8) focusing on service accessibility and service utilisation, the barriers to drug treatment services, service appropriateness, professional guidance and legal framework, care pathways, needs assessment and treatment. The document also reiterates that service provisions need to be sensitive to the needs of these groups, to be aware of legislation relating to race and racial discrimination, and to employ approaches in order to maximise treatment engagement and retention of these groups.

EFFECTIVENESS OF UK DRUG POLICY

An Analysis of UK Drug Policy was commissioned by the UK Drug Policy Commission (2007) to provide an independent overview of UK drug policy. The key findings of the report suggest that:

- Britain has an unusually severe drug problem compared with its European neighbours – it has the highest prevalence rates of problem drug use and the highest levels of recreational drug use in Europe
- the government has successfully increased the number of dependent drug users entering treatment resulting to substantial reductions in drug use, crime and health problems at the individual level
- UK policy of harm reduction has scored some significant successes, including a level of HIV among injecting drug users lower than in most of Europe
- general drug education and prevention efforts in schools and through campaigns appear to make little difference to risk behaviour among the young
- the international evidence suggests however that drug policy appears to have very limited impact on the overall level of drug use. The authors argue that this is more influenced by wider social, economic and cultural factors
- the arena where government drug policy needs to focus further effort and where it can make an impact is in reducing the levels of drug-related harms (crime, death and disease and other associated problems) through the expansion of and innovation in treatment and harm reduction services.

KEY POINTS

- The UK government has adopted a comprehensive demand reduction strategy to tackle alcohol and drug misuse through various policies and guidelines and has scored some significant successes.
- With the introduction of the National Treatment Agency for Substance Misusers, the purpose is to double the number of people in effective, well-managed treatment; and to increase the proportion of people completing or appropriately continuing treatment, year on year.
- The government's wider national drugs strategy sets out a harm reduction approach at reducing the number of drug-related deaths and blood-borne virus infections.
- The 2007 Clinical Guidelines focus on drug treatment effectiveness, principles of clinical governance essential elements of treatment provision, psychosocial components of treatment, health considerations and specific treatment situations and populations
- *Models of Care for Treatment of Adult Drug Misusers* (MoCDM) sets out a national framework, in England, for the commissioning of adult treatment for drug misuse to meet the needs of diverse local populations and to improve the quality and effectiveness of drug treatment.
- *Model of Care for Alcohol Misusers* (MoCAM) sets out a framework for the development of structured treatment and of integrated care pathways for those who misuse alcohol.

REFERENCES

Advisory Council for the Misuse of Drugs (1982) *Treatment and Rehabilitation*. London: HMSO.

Advisory Council for the Misuse of Drugs (ACMD) (1998) *Drug Misuse and the Environment*. London: The Stationery Office.

Department of Health (2004) *Choosing Health: Making Healthy Choices Easier*. London: Department of Health.

Department of Health / National Treatment Agency for Substance Misuse (2007) *Reducing Drug-related Harm: An Action Plan*. London: Department of Health.

Department of Health (2007) *Drug Misuse and Dependence: Guidelines on Clinical Management*. London: HMSO.

Department of Health, Home Office, Department for Education and Skills, Department for Culture, Media and Sport (2007) *Safe. Sensible. Social. The Next Steps in the National Alcohol Strategy*. London: Department of Health / Home Office.

Drugscope (1997) *Media Guide Glossary*. London: Drugscope. http://www.drugscope.org.uk/resources/mediaguide/glossary.

Home Office (1995) *Tackling Drugs Together*. London: HMSO. www.homeoffice.gov.uk.

Home Office (1998) *Tackling Drugs to Build a Better Britain*. London: HMSO. www.homeoffice.gov.uk.

Home Office (2002) *Tackling Drugs to Build a Better Britain: Updated Strategy*. London: HMSO. www.homeoffice.gov.uk.

Home Office (2004) *Tackling Drugs. Changing Lives*. London: HMSO. www.homeoffice.gov.uk.

Home Office (2008) Drugs: protecting families and communities 2008–2018 Strategy, London: HMSO.

NTA (2002) *Models of Care for Adult Drug Misusers*. Parts 1 and 2 London: National Treatment Agency Publications.

NTA (2006) *Models of Care for Adult Drug Misusers Updated*. London: National Treatment Agency Publications.

NTA (2007) *Models of Care for Alcohol Misusers*. London: National Treatment Agency Publications.

Prime Minister's Strategy Unit (2004) *Alcohol Harm Reduction Strategy for England*. London: Cabinet Office. http://www.huntsdc.gov.uk/NR/rdonlyres/05CA6CC6-4DDE-40B7-98FE-6EB3704DFB19/0/AlcoholHarmStrategy.pdf.

Prime Minister's Strategy Unit (2007) *Alcohol Harm Reduction Strategy for England*. London: Cabinet Office. http://www.cabinetoffice.gov.uk/strategy/work_areas/alcohol_misuse.aspx (accessed 20 June 2007).

UK Drug Policy Commission (2007) *An Analysis of UK Drug Policy*. London: UK Drug Policy Commission. www.ukdpc.org.uk.

PART 2

PSYCHOACTIVE SUBSTANCES

CHAPTER 7

ALCOHOL

OBJECTIVES

- Describe the pattern and extent of alcohol use.

- Discuss the harms caused by alcohol misuse.

- Have an understanding of the law regulating alcohol.

- Describe briefly the metabolism of alcohol.

- Describe effects of alcohol on the human body and how these changes affect behaviour.

- Calculate the strengths of a range of alcoholic drinks.

- Use the unit measuring system to assess how much a client is drinking.

ACTIVITY 7.1

Tick true or false for each of the statements listed below and provide some reasons why you chose that answer

	True	False

Alcohol is a central nervous system depressant

Alcoholism is one of the four most serious public health problems

It is illegal to give an alcoholic drink to a child under five years of age

Cannabis causes more problems than other drugs among young people in the UK

Men and women can drink the same amount of alcohol to have the same effect

Carbonated drinks cause the body to absorb alcohol more quickly

Everyone eliminates alcohol from their body at the same rate

Food in the stomach slows down the rate at which alcohol has its effects

Different kinds of alcoholic drinks contain different types of alcohol

It is dangerous to drink alcohol when taking drugs

Drinking water with alcohol prevents a hangover

Black coffee will help you to sober up after drinking too much

Alcohol firstly affects our sense of moral judgement, then our physical co-ordination

Alcohol can have a negative impact on sleep pattern and stress levels

A large quantity of alcohol affects respiration and heart rate

If a little alcohol may be good for your heart, more is probably even better

An average mixed drink contains nearly twice as much alcohol as a pint of beer

A pint of beer has the same alcohol content as a double whisky

Alcopops can contain as much alcohol as beer

Drinkers are more likely to have casual sex that leads to unwanted pregnancies and sexually transmitted diseases

Pregnant women have to worry about harming their baby only if they drink alcohol heavily

The legal breath/alcohol limit for driving in the UK is 35 mg per 100 ml of breath

---

Alcohol is part of the social and cultural fabric of Judeo-Christian societies and is enjoyed by the majority of the UK adult population. It is actively promoted in many cultural, social and religious circumstances, and assists in supporting national economies through taxation (Prime Minister's Strategy Unit 2004). However, alcohol is not generally perceived as a psychoactive substance with addictive potential resulting in physical, psychological, social, economic and legal consequences. Public-health problems associated with alcohol consumption have reached alarming proportions, and alcohol has become one of the most important risks to health globally (WHO 2004).

The World Health Organization (WHO 2004) estimates that there are about two billion people worldwide who consume alcoholic beverages and 76.3 million with diagnosable alcohol use disorders. From a public health perspective, the global burden related to alcohol consumption, both in terms of morbidity and mortality, is considerable in most parts of the world. Alcohol is estimated to cause about 20–30% of oesophageal cancer, liver cancer, cirrhosis of the liver, homicide, epileptic seizures, and motor vehicle accidents worldwide (WHO 2002). Alcohol causes 1.8 million deaths (3.2% of total) and a loss of 58.3 million (4% of total) of disability-adjusted life years (DALYs) (WHO 2002). Unintentional injuries alone account for about one-third of the 1.8 million deaths, while neuro-psychiatric conditions account for close to 40% of the 58.3 million DALYs. Alcohol consumption is the leading risk factor for disease burden in low-mortality developing countries and the third largest risk factor in developed countries.

In Europe, alcohol is public health enemy number 3, behind only tobacco and high blood pressure, and ahead of obesity, lack of exercise or illicit drugs. The European Union is the heaviest drinking region of the world, with each adult drinking 11 litres of pure alcohol each year, a level two and a half times the rest of the world's average (Anderson and Baumberg 2007). The UK is one of the top bingeing nations in western Europe, binge-drinking 28 times per year on average – about once every 13 days. UK adolescents are also the third-worst binge drinkers in the EU, with more than a quarter of 15–16-year-olds binge drinking three or more times in the last month (Anderson and Baumberg 2007).

PATTERN AND EXTENT OF USE

Alcohol misuse is associated with a wide range of problems, including cancer, heart disease, offending behaviours, social exclusion, domestic violence, suicide and deliberate self-harm, child abuse, child neglect and mental health problems which co-exist with alcohol misuse and homelessness. In England, around 90 % of adults consume alcohol and the majority do not experience problems. Over three-quarters of the adult population are either non-drinkers (4.7 million people) or drink less than the government's previously recommended weekly guidelines (Office for National Statistics 2001).

In England in 2005, 73% of men and 58% of women reported drinking an alcoholic drink on at least one day a week. Eighteen per cent of men and 8% of women had drunk more than twice the recommended daily intake. Among men, 24% reported drinking on average more than 21 units in a week. For women, 13% reported drinking more than 14 units in an average week (Information Centre 2007). Older people were more likely to drink regularly: 28% of men and 18% of women aged 45–64 drank on five or more days in a week. Younger people were more likely to drink heavily, with 42% of men and 36% of women aged 16–24 drinking above the daily recommendations, compared to 16% of men and 4% of women aged 65 and over (Information Centre 2007). In England in 2005, 45 per cent of pregnant women did not drink during pregnancy, while 39 per cent reported drinking on average less than 1 unit a week and only 8 per cent drank 1 to 2 units. In Great Britain in 2006, 69% of adults reported that they had heard of the government guidelines on alcohol consumption. And 32% of adults had seen units of alcohol displayed on labels of alcoholic drinks. In 2006, men were more likely to drink normal-strength beer, lager and cider and less likely to drink strong beer, lager and cider, and women were more likely to drink wine and less likely to drink strong beer, lager and cider and Alco pops (National Statistics 2007)

Binge drinking is a normal mode of consumption among 18–24-year-old men and women, bingeing here being defined subjectively in terms of experience of being drunk (Richardson and Budd 2003). UK adults and adolescents are among the worst binge drinkers in Europe, says an Institute of Alcohol Studies report (Anderson 2007). The average rate of binge drinking in the UK is about once every 13 days – the third highest rate in Europe and four times higher than in Italy. Over the last ten years, binge drinking in UK girls has increased to the second highest level in Europe. A Home Office Survey (Matthews and Richardson 2005) found 44% of 18–24-year-olds (49% men, 39% women) to be binge drinkers (using in this case an intoxication-based definition). General Household Survey 2003 (Office of National Statistics 2005) data show that 23% of men and 9% of women had engaged in 'binge drinking' at least once in the last week. This is based on the ONS definition of 'heavy drinking' (men drinking more than eight units on at least one day in the last week, and women drinking at least six units on at least one day in the last week). For both sexes, the prevalence of binge drinking is highest in the 16 to 24 age group and decreases with age. Thirty-seven per cent of men and 26% of women aged 16 to 24 drank heavily in the week before the survey.

A study by Jefferis *et al.* (2005) found that young binge drinkers are more likely to still be drinking to excess well into adulthood. Binge drinking was defined as consuming ten or more units of alcohol at a sitting for men, and seven or more units for women. The study found that young men who drank seven units of alcohol or more weekly at age 16 were one and a half times more likely to be binge drinkers in their 30s and 40s. Those men who binged at age 23 were found to be twice as likely to still be doing so 26 years later; women were one and a half times more likely to be bingers in their 40s if they binged in their 20s. Several factors are contributing to a rise in binge drinking in Britain, among them cheaper and more accessible alcohol, changing drinking patterns and a jump in drinking among young women. The Alcohol Needs Assessment Research Project (Department of Health 2005) found that 23% of the population (aged 16–64) drink hazardously or harmfully, which equates to approximately 7.1 million people in England. The prevalence of alcohol dependence overall was 3.6%, with 6% of men and 2% of women meeting these criteria nationally. This equates to 1.1 million people with alcohol dependence nationally. Twenty-one per cent of men and 9% of women are binge drinkers.

USE OF HEALTH SERVICES

In 2005/6, there were 187,640 NHS hospital admissions among adults aged 16 and over with either a primary or secondary diagnosis specifically related to alcohol (Information Centre 2007). Among children under 16, there were 5,280 NHS hospital admissions in 2005/6 with either a primary or secondary diagnosis specifically related to alcohol.

Alcohol consumption seems to be a significant factor for those presenting to accident and emergency departments, and around 70% of attendances between midnight and 5 am on weekend nights are alcohol-related (Department of Health 2004). In a study (Sharkey *et al.* 1996) of 464 people attending a general hospital in Northern Ireland, it was found that 15% of outpatients, 16% of inpatients and 38.5% of those attending the accident and emergency department scored as misusers of alcohol according to the AUDIT questionnaire. Males were three times more likely to misuse alcohol than females. An unexpectedly large number of those attending the gynaecological clinic reported alcohol misuse (Sharkey *et al.* 1996). Alcoholic liver disease was a much less common alcohol-related diagnosis than mental or behavioural disorders, but more than doubled between 1995/6 (14,350) and 2004/5 (35,393). Men were more likely to be admitted with alcoholic liver disease than women and twice as many men as women were admitted with this diagnosis. A diagnosis of toxic effects of alcohol was much less common, with only 1,646 admissions in 2004/5 (Information Centre 2007). The number of hospital admissions with a primary diagnosis of mental and behavioural disorders due to alcohol was 35,600 in 2004/5. Around two-thirds (68%) of those admitted with this primary diagnosis were men (Information Centre 2007). About one male drinker in seven (14%) had discussed drinking in the last year with his general practitioner (GP) or someone else at the surgery, or a doctor or other medical person elsewhere. Women were less likely to have had discussions (only 8% had done so) (National Statistics 2006).

ALCOHOL AND MORTALITY

The alcohol-related death rate in the UK increased from 6.9 per 100,000 population in 1991 to 12.9 in 2005. The number of alcohol-related deaths has more than doubled from 4,144 in 1991 to 8,386 in 2005 (Office of National Statistics 2005). Most of the alcohol-related deaths were caused by cirrhosis and chronic liver disease, but many also resulted from accidental alcohol poisoning or other problems. In England and Wales 4,037 people died from alcohol liver disease in 2004. More men than women died from each of the alcohol-related causes except for chronic hepatitis, where the reverse was true. The rise in deaths from cirrhosis amongst younger people is of particular concern where binge drinking patterns appear to be common. From 1970 to 2000, deaths from chronic liver disease have increased among men in the age group 25–44 years from 49 per annum to 470 (959%) and among women aged 25–44 years from 29 to 268 (924%) (Information Centre 2007).

In a Northern Ireland suicide study (case-control psychological autopsy), it was found that the prevalence of alcohol use disorders among people who committed suicide was 43% (Foster *et al.* 1997). A study looking at deaths from injury and poisoning among young men aged 15–39 years in England and Wales found that the most common cause of death was poisoning by alcohol and drugs (Stanistreet and Jeffrey 2003).

Provisional estimates in the Road Casualties Great Britain (2004) report suggest that 6% of road traffic accidents involved illegal alcohol levels. Drink-driving-related deaths have been increasing steadily since 1999 (460), rising to 590 in 2004. Fifteen per cent of road deaths occurred when someone was driving over the legal limit for alcohol.

SOCIAL AND ECONOMIC COSTS

As well as health risks and death, alcohol misuse also has an impact on social and economic factors. It is estimated that 360,000 incidents of domestic violence are linked to alcohol misuse, around a third of all domestic violence. Half of all violent crimes are alcohol-related. Up to 17 million days absent from work are alcohol-related. The cost to the National Health Service of alcohol misuse was £1.4 to £1.7 billion a year, including 1 in 26 NHS bed days (about £2 million), 1 in 80 NHS day cases, and up to 35% of all accident and emergency attendance costs (Department of Health 2004). The loss to the economy of premature death from alcohol misuse is around £2.4 billion each year. Alcohol misuse imposes a greater burden on the criminal justice system than on both the health service and social work services.

DRUGS AND THE LAW

In the United Kingdom, there are strict laws on the sale of alcohol, on who and when people can enter a pub or bar where it is sold and on buying alcohol. These restrictions apply in particular to young people. In England and Wales from late 2005, drinking establishments can apply for licences to stay open and serve alcohol for 24 hours. Police have powers to confiscate alcohol from you if you are drinking in public and can contact your parents. You can get a criminal record for offences of drunkenness. It is an offence to drive with more than the following amounts of alcohol in your body:

*   80 milligrams of alcohol in 100 millilitres of blood, or
*   35 micrograms of alcohol in 100 millilitres of breath if a breath test is used.

A summary of the Licensing law, applicable to England and Wales only, is presented in Table 7.1

Table 7.1 Licensing Act 2003 (England and Wales)

Age	Law
Under 5	It is illegal to give alcohol to a child under five except under medical supervision
Under 16	A 14-year-old can now go into licensed premises only when accompanied by someone aged 18 or over. Can drink only non-alcoholic drinks
Aged 16 or 17	16- and 17-year-olds can now drink, but not buy, beer, cider and wine when having a substantial table meal provided that they are accompanied by someone aged 18 or over who buys the alcohol for them
Under 18	Cannot be given alcohol or drink alcohol in a pub except with a table meal (see above). Cannot buy or attempt to buy alcohol anywhere

METABOLISM OF ALCOHOL

Ethyl alcohol or ethanol (C_2H_5OH) is a colourless, inflammable liquid with a characteristic smell and a burning taste. Alcohol is a psychoactive substance that depresses the central nervous system and provides calories. Unlike other foods, alcohol does not have to be digested in order for absorption to occur. Alcoholic beverages with a higher concentration of alcohol such as whisky or brandy, and carbonated drinks such as champagnes, are absorbed more quickly.

Alcohol is absorbed in the mouth, oesophagus and stomach. For the most part absorption of alcohol takes place in the initial part of the small intestine. The rate of alcohol absorption varies widely among people, depending on individual differences in physiology, contents of the stomach and situational factors. Once absorbed into the circulatory system, alcohol is carried to the liver where it is metabolised. The enzyme acetaldehyde dehydrogenase is active in the breakdown of alcohol into acetaldehyde which is then changed to acetic acid. On average, the liver is able to metabolise one drink equivalent per hour. The product acetic acid is rapidly converted to carbon dioxide and water. It is worth pointing out that alcohol, although fattening, affects the body's ability to absorb and use nutrients effectively. This adds to the problem of poor malnutrition or vitamin deficiencies in heavy alcohol drinkers.

There are considerable gender differences in the way alcohol affects the bodily system. Women can become more intoxicated than men on the same amount of alcohol intake, even if they weigh the same. This is because women have different fat distribution and less water in their bodies than men, so alcohol is less diluted and has greater potency. Pre-menstrual status, birth control pills and hormone replacement therapy (oestrogen) have an impact on the absorption rate of alcohol in women. As women do not metabolise alcohol as effectively as men, they are more vulnerable to the consequences of alcohol drinking. This level of alcohol consumption in women has implications for clinicians.

EFFECTS OF ALCOHOL

Initially small amounts of alcohol produce a feeling of relaxation and euphoria, and the individuals experience less inhibition. Both thinking process and motor functions are slightly impaired. At a higher level of consumption, there is cognitive, perceptual and behavioural impairment and these changes are proportional to the amount of alcohol consumed. This may include slurred speech, poor co-ordination, unsteady gait, uncontrolled movement of the pupils (nystagmus), poor judgement, insomnia, hangover and blackouts. Blackout is a memory impairment that occurs in anyone who drinks large amount of alcohol in one session. The lethal dose of alcohol is generally related to body size and physiology. Death can occur from high consumption of alcohol or withdrawal from alcohol. Chronic alcohol use may result in significant memory problems and cognitive impairment.

In women, menstrual disorders and fertility problems have been associated with harmful drinking. Women seem to be more susceptible to the influence of alcohol just prior to or during their menstrual cycle. A study by Epstein *et al.* (2006) found that drinking frequency was higher in the premenstrual than the 'other' phase and endorsed the premenstrual phase of the menstrual cycle as a drinking cue. Foetal alcohol syndrome is the biggest cause of non-genetic mental handicap in the western world and the only one that is entirely preventable. Foetal alcohol syndrome is caused by prenatal alcohol exposure and can cause permanent damage to the baby's brain, resulting in neurological impairment of the executive functions. It is unknown whether amount, frequency or timing of alcohol consumption during pregnancy causes a difference in amount of damage done to the foetus. The syndrome is characterised by underweight and small babies, facial abnormality, speech impairments, heart and eye disorders, genital deformities and behavioural problems. There is no safe level of drinking during pregnancy.

A summary of the problems associated with alcohol intoxication and harmful drinking is presented in Table 7.2 and 7.3.

WERNICKE'S ENCEPHALOPATHY AND KORSAKOFF'S PSYCHOSIS

Wernicke's encephalopathy is caused by alcohol and thiamine deficiency (Vitamin B_1). Thiamine is essential for normal growth and development and helps to maintain proper functioning of the heart and the nervous and digestive systems. Many heavy drinkers have poor eating habits and their nutrition is inadequate and will not contain essential vitamins. In addition, alcohol can inflame the stomach lining and impede the body's ability to absorb the key vitamins it receives. Wernicke's encephalopathy is characterised by unsteady gait (ataxia); involuntary, jerky eye movements or paralysis of muscles moving the eyes; drowsiness and confusion. The symptoms may not always present, so diagnosis may be difficult. However, if Wernicke's is left untreated, or is not treated in time, brain damage may result. In some cases the person may die. If treatment, with high

Table 7.2 Problems associated with alcohol intoxication

Physical	Psychological	Social
Accidents	Anger	Absenteeism
Acute alcohol poisoning	Anxiety	Aggression
Cardiac arrhythmia	Amnesia	Assault
Failure to take prescribed medications	Attempted suicide	Burglary
Foetal damage	Depression	Child neglect or abuse
Gastritis	Impaired relationships	Domestic violence
Gout	Insomnia	Drinking and driving
Hepatitis	Suicide	Family arguments
HIV (through sexual behaviour)		Football hooliganism
Impotence		Homicide
Pancreatitis		Public drunkenness
Stroke		Theft
		Unsafe sex
		Unwanted pregnancy

Source: Adapted from the Royal College of Psychiatrists (1986) *Alcohol: Our Favourite Drug.* London: Tavistock Publications

Table 7.3 Problems associated with harmful drinking

Physical	Psychological	Social
Brain damage	Attempted suicide	Divorce
Breast cancer	Amnesia	Family problems
Cirrhosis	Anxiety	Financial liability
Cancer of mouth, larynx, oesophagus	Delirium tremens	Fraud
Cardiomyopathy	Dementia	Habitual conviction for drunkenness
Diabetes	Depression	Homelessness
Fatty liver	Gambling	Poor social behaviour
Gastritis	Hallucinosis	Unemployment
Hepatitis	Misuse of other drugs	Vagrancy
Hypertension	Personality changes	Work difficulties
Infertility	Suicide	
Neuropathy	Withdrawal fits	
Nutritional deficiencies		
Obesity		
Pancreatitis		
Reactions to other drugs		
Sexual dysfunction		
Stroke		

Source: Adapted from the Royal College of Psychiatrists (1986) *Alcohol: Our Favourite Drug.* London: Tavistock Publications

doses of thiamine, is carried out in time most symptoms should be reversed in a few hours.

If Wernicke's encephalopathy is untreated or is not treated soon enough, Korsakoff's psychosis may follow. Korsakoff's psychosis may develop gradually, resulting in severe memory impairment. However, many other abilities may remain intact. Korsakoff's differs from most dementias, in which there is often damage to a large area of the cortex (the outer part of the brain). The major symptoms of Korsakoff's syndrome are: anterograde and retrograde amnesia, or severe memory loss; confabulation (invented events which to fill gaps in memory); apathy; in some case talkativeness, and repetitive behaviour in others. Other problems associated with heavy alcohol consumption include peripheral neuropathies (lack of sensation or pain in the limbs), 'alcohol dementia' and physical, immunological and psychological disorders. There appears to be a strong association between the degree to which an individual is dependent on alcohol and the severity of the problems experienced by the individual and this is independent of the amount of alcohol consumed.

ALCOHOL WITHDRAWAL SYNDROME

Alcohol dependence involves both physical and psychological dependence. The presence of physical dependence is shown when problem drinkers cease or reduce alcohol consumption. Alcohol withdrawal syndrome is a set of symptoms that individuals have when they suddenly stop drinking alcohol, following continuous and heavy consumption. Withdrawal symptoms rarely occur in individuals who are recreational

Table 7.4 Mild, moderate and severe withdrawal symptoms

Mild to moderate psychological symptoms	*Mild to moderate physical symptoms*	*Severe symptoms*
Feeling of shakiness	Headache	A state of confusion and
Feeling of anxiety	Sweating (palms and face)	hallucinations (visual or
Irritability or easily excited	Nausea	tactile) – delirium tremens
Emotionally volatile	Vomiting	Clouding of consciousness
Rapid emotional changes	Loss of appetite	Agitation
Depression	Insomnia	Disorientation of time and place
Fatigue	Paleness	Paranoid delusions
Difficulty with thinking clearly	Rapid heart rate (palpitations)	Fear, suspicion and anger
Bad dreams	Enlarged, dilated pupils	Suicidal behaviour
	Skin clammy	Elevated temperature
	Abnormal movements	Convulsions
	Tremor of hands	Blackouts
	Involuntary movements of the eyelids	

Source: Adapted from Finn, D.A. and Crabbe, J.C. (1997) Exploring alcohol withdrawal syndrome. *Alcohol Health & Research World*, 21, 2: 149–56

drinkers. Problem drinkers who have gone through withdrawal before are more likely to have withdrawal symptoms each time they stop drinking. Some individuals have the forms of syndrome including tremors, seizures and hallucinations, typically occurring within 6–48 hours after the last alcoholic drink. Withdrawals can be mild, moderate or severe (see Table 7.4). For most problem drinkers, alcohol withdrawal will not progress to the severe stage of delirium tremens (confusion and hallucination). When an individual has severe withdrawal symptoms, this can be a life-threatening condition and requires supervision under medical care.

SENSIBLE DRINKING

The effect of alcohol on an individual varies with age, diet, weight, health, gender, culture and religious belief. The recommendations of the *Sensible Drinking* report (Department of Health 1995) advise that men should not regularly drink more than 3–4 units of alcohol per day, and women should not regularly drink more than 2–3 units of alcohol per day. After heavy drinking, it is advised to have two alcohol-free days. For men over 40 and post-menopausal women, modest alcohol consumption (1 or 2 units per day) has a protective effect against coronary heart disease and stroke. This protective effect is estimated to prevent up to 22,000 deaths annually.

However the benefit is apparent at a consumption level of a drink every second day and there appears to be no additional benefit from drinking more than one to two drinks per day (Bondy *et al.* 1999).

Regularly drinking at levels greater than the recommended level is associated with progressive health risks. Sensible drinking also involves a personal assessment of the particular risks and responsibilities of drinking at the time: for example, it is sensible not to drink when driving, using machinery or taking certain medications. Guidelines and benefits of sensible drinking are shown in Table 7.5

Table 7.5 Guidelines for sensible drinking

	Men (over 40 years of age)	Women (post-menopausal)
Health benefits	1–2 units/day	1–2 units/day
No significant health risks	3–4 units/day (all ages)	2–3 units/day (all ages)
Harmful	5 or more units/day	3 or more units/day

WHAT IS A UNIT OF ALCOHOL?

One unit of alcohol = half a pint of ordinary strength beer, lager or cider (3–4% alcohol by volume ABV) = a standard pub measure (50ml) of fortified wine such as sherry or port (20% ABV) = a small glass of ordinary strength wine (12% ABV) = a small pub measure of spirits (40% ABV).

The exact number of units in a particular drink can be calculated by multiplying the volume of the drink (number of ml) by the % ABV (Alcohol by Volume) and dividing by 1,000. For example, the number of units in a strong beer of 500 ml with a 6% ABV = 500 × 6.0 divided by 1,000 = 3 units. Another way of calculating units is as follows. The percentage alcohol by volume (% ABV) of a drink equals the number of units in one litre of that drink. For example, strong beer at 6% ABV has 6 units in one litre. If you drink half a litre (500ml) – just under a pint – then you have had 3 units.

KEY POINTS

- Alcohol has become one of the most important risks to health globally.
- About 1.1 million people with alcohol dependence in Britain.
- Younger people were more likely to drink heavily above the daily recommendations.
- Males were three times more likely to misuse alcohol than females.
- Most of the alcohol-related deaths were caused by cirrhosis and chronic liver disease.
- Alcohol is absorbed in the mouth, oesophagus and stomach. This adds to the problem of poor malnutrition or vitamin deficiencies in heavy alcohol drinkers.
- Women do not metabolise alcohol as effectively as men and are more vulnerable to the consequences of alcohol drinking.
- A blackout is a memory impairment that occurs in anyone who drinks large amount of alcohol in one session.
- Chronic alcohol use may result in significant memory problems and cognitive impairment.
- Foetal alcohol syndrome is caused by prenatal alcohol exposure and can cause permanent damage to the baby's brain, resulting in neurological impairment of the executive functions.
- Alcohol withdrawal syndrome is a set of symptoms that individuals have when they suddenly stop drinking alcohol, following continuous and heavy consumption.
- Men should not regularly drink more than 3–4 units of alcohol per day, and women should not regularly drink more than 2–3 units of alcohol per day.

ACTIVITY 7.2

Please choose one correct answer to the following multiple-choice questions

Alcohol is a
a.   Stimulant
b.   Hallucinogen
c.   Depressant
d.   Opioid

In the UK, how many people die each year from their alcohol consumption?
a.   30,000
b.   22,000
c.   60,000
d.   10,000

The World Health Organization's (WHO 2004) estimate of diagnosable alcohol use disorders is
a.   33.3 million
b.   45.3 million
c.   66.3 million
d.   76.3 million

In England, the percentage of hazardous or harmful drinkers is
a.   33%
b.   43%
c.   23%
d.   53%

The number of people dependent on alcohol in England is
a.   2.1million
b.   0.5 million
c.   1.1 million
d.   1.5 million

The average rate of binge drinking in the UK is about
a.   Once every 10 days
b.   Once every 11 days
c.   Once every 12 days
d.   Once every 13 days

According to recent research, which of the following nations has the highest rate of binge drinking among men?
a.   UK
b.   Finland
c.   Italy
d.   France

Binge drinking refers to

a.   Men drinking more than 4 units and women drinking at least 3 units on at
      least one day in the last week
b.   Men drinking more than 5 units and women drinking at least 4 units on at
      least one day in the last week
c.   Men drinking more than 8 units and women drinking at least 6 units on at
      least one day in the last week
d.   Men drinking more than 10 units and women drinking at least 7 units on
      at least one day in the last week

**According to government statistics, which age group is most likely to drink heavily
– more than eight units a day for men or six units for women?**

a.   11–15-year-olds
b.   16–24-year-olds
c.   36–44-year-olds
d.   65 and over

Alcohol is nearly as addictive as which drug?

a.   Cocaine
b.   Heroin
c.   Cannabis
d.   Stimulants

Which of the following is a factor in alcohol's effect?

a.   Body weight, age and gender
b.   Gender, body weight and metabolism
c.   Gender, age and genetics
d.   Age, metabolism and genetics

How old do you have to be to legally buy alcohol at a pub in the UK?

a.   15
b.   16
c.   17
d.   18

When drinking the same amount of alcohol, women become

a.   Less intoxicated than men
b.   More intoxicated than men
c.   There is no difference
d.   More agitated than men

**How does the alcohol content of a pint of normal-strength beer compare with the
alcohol content of a double whisky?**

a.   More in the beer
b.   More in the whisky
c.   The same amount
d.   Cannot compare the content

What are the government's recommended daily alcohol limits for men in the UK?
a.   2 units
b.   3–4 units
c.   4–5 units
d.   5–6 units

What are the government's recommended daily alcohol limits for women in the UK?
a.   1 unit
b.   1–2 units
c.   2–3 units
d.   3–4 units

Drinking too much alcohol may increase the likelihood of which of these diseases?
a.   Liver cirrhosis
b.   Cancer
c.   Fertility problems
d.   All of the above

Alcohol misuse can cause cirrhosis of one of the main organs of the body. Which organ?
a.   Liver
b.   Heart
c.   Kidneys
d.   Stomach

Approximately how long does your liver take to process one unit of alcohol?
a.   30 minutes
b.   60 minutes
c.   90 minutes
d.   120 minutes

Is it true that drinking alcohol can be good for your heart?
a.   No – it doesn't benefit the heart at all
b.   No – in fact, drinking any alcohol increases your risk of heart disease
c.   Yes – alcohol consumption helps to protect all of us from heart disease
d.   Yes – moderate alcohol consumption does protect people from heart disease, but only for men over 40, and women who have gone through the menopause

Alcohol is broken down in the liver by the enzyme:
a.   Acetaldehyde hydrogenase
b.   Acetaldehyde dehydrogenase
c.   Acetyl choline
d.   Serotonin

Thiamine deficiency can cause:
a.   Alcohol psychosis
b.   Wernicke's encephalopathy

c.   Neuropthaties
d.   Depression

Alcohol withdrawal syndrome is present when a problem drinker:
a.   Ceases alcohol consumption
b.   Increases alcohol consumption
c.   Reduces alcohol consumption
d.   Ceases or reduces alcohol consumption

Withdrawal symptoms occur in individuals who are:
a.   Heavy drinkers
b.   Recreational drinkers
c.   Social drinkers
d.   Experimental drinkers

How many units of alcohol are in three pints of strong lager?
a.   3 units
b.   6 units
c.   9 units
d.   12 units

At what stage does drinking alcohol begin to impact upon your ability to drive safely? Is it after you have consumed:
a.   1 unit
b.   2 units
c.   3 units
d.   10 units

ACTIVITY 7.3

Safe drinking – How much do I drink?

Counting units of alcohol can help us to keep track of the amount we are drinking. The labels of many bottled drinks will tell you how many units of alcohol are in the bottle. One way of getting a picture of your drinking is to keep a drinking diary for a week or month. When you have an alcoholic drink, please fill the diary

Day	When	Where	Drinks
Sunday			
Monday			
Tuesday			
Wednesday			

Thursday

Friday

Saturday

Fill in the average number of drinks you have in a day (a 24-hour period) and calculate the number of units by using the calculations given in the text.

Alcoholic drinks	Volume	ABV	Total	Units
Bitter	1 pint	4.7%		
Stout	1 pint	4.5%		
Cider	1 pint	6.2		
Alcopop	275 ml	5%		
Low-strength beer or lager	1 pint	3.5–4%		
Wine (large)	250	12%		
Wine (small)	125 ml	12%		
Fortified wine (sherry/port)	50 ml	20%		
Spirits	35 ml	40%		

Volume (ml)   ×   Strength in %ABV   ×   ÷ 1000 =

The list below shows the number of units of alcohol in common drinks:

- A pint of ordinary-strength lager (Carling Black Label, Fosters) – 2 units
- A pint of strong lager (Stella Artois, Kronenbourg 1664) – 3 units
- A pint of ordinary bitter (John Smith's, Boddingtons) – 2 units
- A pint of best bitter (Fuller's ESB, Young's Special) – 3 units
- A pint of ordinary strength cider (Woodpecker) – 2 units
- A pint of strong cider (Dry Blackthorn, Strongbow) – 3 units
- A 175 ml glass of red or white wine at 13% strength – 2.3 units
- A pub measure of spirits – 1 unit
- An alcopop (Smirnoff Ice, Bacardi Breezer, WKD, Reef) – around 1.5 units

REFERENCES

Anderson, P. (2007) *Binge Drinking and Europe*. London: Institute of Alcohol Studies. London.

Anderson, P. and Baumberg, B. (2007) *Alcohol and Public Health in Europe*. London: Institute of Alcohol Studies. London.

Bondy, S.J., Rehm, J., Ashley, M.J., Walsh, G., Single, E. and Room, R. (1999) Low-risk drinking guidelines: the scientific evidence. *Canadian Journal of Public Health*, 90: 264–70.

Department of Health (1995) *Sensible Drinking*. London: Department of Health.

Department of Health (2004) Choosing Health Summaries Alcohol. *Summary of Intelligence on Alcohol*. London: Department of Health.

Department of Health (2005) *The Alcohol Needs Assessment Research Project* (ANARP). London: Department of Health.

Epstein, E.E., Rhine, K.C., Cook, S., Zdep-Mattocks, B., Jensen, N.K. and Mccrady, B.S. (2006) Changes in alcohol craving and consumption by phase of menstrual cycle in alcohol dependent women. *Journal of Substance Use*, 11, 5: 323–32.

Foster, T., Gillespie, K. and McClelland, R. (1997) Mental disorders and suicide in Northern Ireland. *British Journal of Psychiatry*, 170: 447–52.

Information Centre (2007) *Statistics on Alcohol: England 2007* [NS] http://www.ic.nhs.uk/statistics-and-data-collections/health-and-lifestyles/alcohol/statistics-on-alcohol:-england-2007 (accessed 15 June 2007).

Jefferis, B., Power, C. and Manor, O. (2005) Adolescent drinking level and adult binge drinking in a national birth cohort. *Addiction*, 100, 4: 543–9.

Matthews, S. and Richardson, A. (2005) *Findings from the 2003 Offending, Crime and Justice Survey: Alcohol-related Crime and Disorder*. Home Office Findings 261. London: Home Office.

National Statistics (2006) *Drinking: Adults' Behaviour and Knowledge*. Omnibus Surveys Report No. 31. London: HMSO.

Office for National Statistics (2001) *General Household Survey*. London: HMSO.

Office for National Statistics (2004) *General Household Survey 2003*. London: HMSO.

Office for National Statistics (2005) *Mortality Statistics. Cause. Review of the Registrar General on Deaths by Cause, Sex and Age, in England and Wales, 2005*. London: HMSO.

Prime Minister's Strategy Unit (2004). *Alcohol Harm Reduction Strategy for England (2004)*. London: Cabinet Office.

Richardson, A. and Budd, T. (2003) *Alcohol, Crime and Disorder: A Study of Young Adults*. Home Office Research Study 263. London: Home Office.

Road Casualties in Great Britain (2004) *Annual Report*. London: Department for Transport, 2006. Available at: www.dft.gov.uk/stellent/groups/dft_control/documents/contentserver template/dft_index.hcst?n=8290&l=4 (accessed 15 June 2007).

Sharkey, J., Brennan, D. and Curran, P. (1996). The pattern of alcohol consumption of a general hospital population in north Belfast. *Alcohol and Alcoholism*, 31, 3: 279–85.

Stanistreet, D. and Jeffrey, V. (2003). Injury and poisoning mortality among young men – are there common factors amenable to prevention? *Crisis*, 24, 3: 122–7.

Streissguth, A. and Kanter J. (1997). *The Challenge of Fetal Alcohol Syndrome: Overcoming Secondary Disabilities*. Washington: University of Washington Press.

WHO (2002) *Global Status Report on Alcohol 2002*. Geneva: World Health Organization.

WHO (2004) *Global Status Report on Alcohol 2004*. Geneva: World Health Organization.

OPIATES

TRENDS IN DRUG MISUSE

The British Crime Survey (Home Office Statistical Bulletin 2007) reported that the most commonly used drug in 2006/7 was cannabis, with 8.2% of adults. The next most commonly used drug was cocaine, with 2.6% of adults, followed by ecstasy (1.8%), amyl nitrite (1.4%), amphetamines (1.3%), hallucinogens (LSD and magic mushrooms)

(0.7%), tranquillisers (0.4%), ketamine (0.3%), glues (0.2%) and anabolic steroids (0.1%). Other more serious drugs are also very rarely used: opiate (heroin and methadone) use was reported by 0.2% of 16- to 59-year-olds. It is estimated that over 11.25 million people aged 16 to 59 in England and Wales have ever used illicit drugs. Cannabis remains the drug most likely to be used by 16- to 24-year-olds with 20.9% using cannabis in the last year. Cocaine is the next most commonly used drug with 6.1% reporting use, ecstasy use at 4.8%, amyl nitrite use at 4.3%, use of amphetamines at 3.5% and use of hallucinogens at 2.1%. Other drugs used are glues and tranquillisers at 0.6% and anabolic steroids at 0.2%. The trend in illicit drug use used by 16–59- and 16–24-year-olds is presented in Table 8.1.

OPIATES

The term 'opiate' refers to any psychoactive substance of either natural or synthetic origin that has an effect similar to morphine. Opium is the raw exudates of the opium poppy (Papaver somniferum) which is scraped from the scored seed head of the poppy, and contains a number of alkaloids including morphine and codeine. Morphine and codeine are extracted from opium and heroin is manufactured chemically from morphine. Raw opium is treated with lime and other compounds to leave partially refined morphine. With the addition of acetic anhydride, this produces a base form of diamorphine. This crude base form of the drug is what makes up the bulk of the UK market. Some of the commoner opiate drugs are: codeine, heroin (diacetylmorphine), pethidine, methadone, morphine and diconal. In England and Wales, the national estimate and prevalence rate for those using opiates for 2005/6 was between 280,000 and 300,000 amongst 15- to 64-year-olds.

The main source of street heroin in the UK is the Golden Crescent countries of south-west Asia, mainly Afghanistan, Iran and Pakistan. Heroin is usually sold as a powder; the colour ranges from white, off-white, yellowish, to reddish brown, the most

Table 8.1 Summary of trends in drug use in the last year amongst 16–59 and 16–24-year-olds, 1998 to 2006/7 (British Crime Survey)

Age group	Increase	Decrease	Stable
16–59 years	Any class A drug (overall), any cocaine (overall), cocaine powder	Any drug (overall), any hallucinogens (overall), amphetamines, cannabis, LSD, anabolic steroids, tranquillisers	Any opiates (overall), amyl nitrite, crack cocaine, ecstasy, glues, heroin, magic mushrooms, methadone
16–24 years	Any cocaine (overall), cocaine powder	Any drug (overall), any hallucinogens (overall), any opiates (overall), amphetamines, cannabis, LSD, magic mushrooms, tranquillisers	Any class A drug (overall), amyl nitrite, crack cocaine, ecstasy, glues, heroin, methadone, steroids

Source: Home Office Statistical Bulletin (2007)

prevalent type now on the market. Afghan-sourced brown heroin is the mainstay of the UK market. The myth that street heroin is commonly adulterated with dangerous substances has been refuted. Anecdotal evidence from drug workers, drug users, the police and politicians reports that adulteration of heroin is common but there is no foundation in forensic evidence. Recent research in the UK, the USA and Australia shows that the purity of drugs such as heroin is little different at street level than at importation (Coomber 1999). Most cutting does occur before importation, usually with other drugs such as paracetamol and caffeine.

Heroin is usually sold in small quantities, typically £10 bags. The street price of heroin was £47 per gram in 2007 (Drugscope 2007). Habitual users of heroin may generally consume half a gram to over 1 gram per day. The street names for heroin are smack, junk, gear, scag, H, scat, tiger, chi, elephant, harry, dragon etc. Methadone is also known as doll, red rock, juice or 'script'. A comparison of common opiates and their abuse potential is presented in Table 8.2.

LEGAL STATUS

Heroin, pethidine, morphine, dihydrocodeine and methadone are class A, controlled drugs. Codeine and dihydrocodeine are class B but class A if prepared for injection. Distalgesic, dextropoxyphene and buprenorphine (Temgesic) are class C.

THERAPEUTIC USES

The medical applications of opiates include effective relief of pain, treatment for diarrhoea and vomiting and as a cough suppressant. Morphine, for instance, is widely used for short-term acute pain resulting from myocardial infarction, sickle cell crisis, after surgery, fractures, burns and the later stages of terminal illnesses. Methadone is

Table 8.2 Common opiates – comparison chart

Drug	Trade/street name	Equivalent dose (mg)	Duration (hours)	Abuse potential
Opium	Omnopon	10–20	4–5	Moderate–High
Morphine	Generic	10	4–5	High
Codeine	Generic	120	4–5	Low
Diamorphine	Heroin	3	3–4	High
Buprenorphine	Temgesic	0.2–0.6	6–8	Low
Dihydrocodeine	DF118	30	4–5	Moderate
Dipipanone	Diconal	10	4–5	High
Dextromoramide	Palfium	5–10	4–5	High
Methadone	Physeptone	10	3–12	High
Dextropropoxyphene	Co-proxamol	60–120	4–5	Low
Pethidine	Generic	50–150	2–4	High
Pentazocine	Fortral	30–50	3–4	Low–Moderate

Source: http://www.idmu.co.uk/opiates2003.htm

often prescribed to heroin addicts for maintenance or withdrawal purposes. Some of the opiates such as pethidine, morphine, dihydrocodeine and methadone are highly addictive when compared to other substances; tolerance and physical and psychological dependences develop very rapidly. However, occasional use of heroin does not lead to symptoms of withdrawal.

NON-THERAPEUTIC USES

The most popular of opiates as an illicit drug of misuse is heroin. The drug is swallowed, or smoked, sniffed or injected either subcutaneously or intravenously. Diverted pharmaceutical opiates and opioids may be formulated for injection, oral use or occasionally as suppositories. Smoking is often called 'chasing the dragon', or more recently 'booting'. A small line of heroin is placed on a piece of silver foil, and heated from below. The heroin runs into a liquid, and gives off a curl of smoke, which is inhaled through a rolled tube of paper or foil. Tablets are sometimes crushed and injected. If heroin powder is injected it is generally acidified, using lemon juice, citric or ascorbic acid, heated with water, and then filtered prior to injecting.

Heroin's effects are dependent on the modes of administration. When heroin is taken orally, it is metabolised into morphine before crossing the blood-brain barrier; so the effects are the same as oral morphine. Snorting heroin results in an onset within three to five minutes. Smoking heroin results in an almost immediate, though mild effect which strengthens the longer it is used: 7 to 11 seconds. Intravenous injection results in rush and euphoria within 30 to 60 seconds; while intramuscular or subcutaneous injection takes longer, having an effect within three to five minutes.

CONTROLLED HEROIN USE

There is limited literature on the nature and pattern of occasional and controlled heroin users. Heroin use in many cases leads to heroin addiction. However, there are also many occasional or 'controlled' heroin (and other drug) users who are capable of using the drug with informal controls or constraints on their using behaviour, for example, using only at weekends, never on a working day, never alone, never with children around etc. In some cases such use can go on indefinitely with little physical harm accruing to the user. It is not uncommon for the drug use of such users to be unknown by those close to them.

The findings from a report from the Joseph Rowntree Foundation (Warbuton *et al.* 2005) showed that from a sample of 123 users, almost all respondents were in work or studying, more affluent than treatment samples and also had better accommodation. Their heroin-using careers varied. Some reported patterns of mid- or long-term non-dependent use. Others had moved from dependent and problematic use to non-dependent use. A third group maintained patterns of controlled dependence over the mid- to long term. Respondents took great care over where they used heroin and whom they used with. Most avoided using with people who were deeply immersed in the heroin subculture or involved in crime. A range of different strategies is used for avoiding dependence or for retaining control over dependence. Non-dependent users tended to follow rules that enabled them to restrict the frequency with which they used. Dependent users aimed to contain the amount of heroin that they used on a regular basis, to ensure that their use did not intrude into their everyday work and social routines. Contrary to popular beliefs about heroin use, the findings suggest that heroin use does not lead inevitably to dependence and that some people can bring their heroin use back under control.

SOUGHT-AFTER EFFECTS

In moderate doses, opiates produce a range of generally mild physical effects apart from the analgesic effect. They induce euphoria, which may wear off but use continues to avoid withdrawal symptoms. Heroin users report the ability of the drug to induce a relaxed detachment from pain and anxiety, a sense of calm, pleasure and profound well-being. The depressant effects reduce the activity of the nervous system including reflex functions such as coughing, respiration and heart rate. They also dilate the blood vessels, thus giving a feeling of warmth. Opiates such as heroin provide powerful relief from physical pain (for which they are used medically) and also from psychological pain. Methadone effects are similar to heroin and may be prescribed to prevent opiate withdrawal symptoms. Methadone tincture cannot be injected, thus reducing the risks associated with injecting behaviours.

ADVERSE EFFECTS

Users often experience nausea or vomiting on the first occasions that they use heroin, or when returning to use after a period of abstinence. Heroin dependence develops after repeated use over several weeks and sudden withdrawal leads to anxiety, nausea, muscle pains, sweating, diarrhoea and goose flesh. Tolerance develops quickly so that larger amounts of the same drug are needed to produce the same effect. During a period of abstinence (in treatment or prison), tolerance diminishes quickly so that individuals can easily overdose by taking their usual dose. Overdose occurs as a result of depression of the respiratory centre in the brain, which leads to respiratory and cardiac arrest and death unless immediate medical attention is received. Though stupor, coma and death can occur from overdoses, there is generally little effect on the motor skills and sensation. The user of opiates may appear detached or withdrawn with contraction of the pupils. Whilst pharmaceutical heroin is not especially toxic to human organs, adulterants in street heroin may well cause more damage, especially when they are injected. Injecting brings with it the risks of vein damage and collapse, local infections, abscesses, circulatory problems, ulcers, thrombosis, infections in heart valves and systemic infections. It also exposes users who share injecting equipment to blood-borne viruses including hepatitis B and C, and HIV. However, most complications arise from unsterile injections and adulterated street drugs. Heroin, taken by injection, is also a risk factor in contracting hepatitis B and C, HIV and septicaemia.

MECHANISM OF ACTION

When injected, swallowed or smoked, opiates enter the bloodstream and quickly affect the brain. In the brain the drug is converted into monoacetylmorphine and morphine. It is the morphine molecule that binds with opioid receptors in the brain. These receptors are specialised proteins on the surface of nerve cells that exist to detect the body's own opiate-like substances known as endorphins. This produces the subjective effects of the heroin high resulting in a sense of extreme well-being with the feeling centred in the gut. The body responds to heroin in the brain by reducing (and sometimes stopping) production of the endogenous opioids (endorphins) when heroin is present. The reduced endorphin production in heroin users creates a dependence on the heroin, and the cessation of heroin results in extremely uncomfortable symptoms including pain (even in the absence of physical trauma). This set of symptoms is called withdrawal syndrome and has an onset six to eight hours after the last dose of heroin.

DRUG-RELATED OVERDOSE

Death through overdose remains a significant cause of mortality amongst heroin users. Recorded rates of drug-related death due to overdose in the UK are among the highest in Europe (EMCCDA 2007). In the UK, acute drug-related deaths accounted for more than 7% of all deaths among those aged 15–39 years in 2004 (EMCCDA 2007). The np-SAD Annual Report for 2006 (Ghodse *et al.* 2006) shows that there were 1,644 drug-related deaths reported in 2005. Opiates or opioids (for example, heroin or morphine; methadone; other opiates or opioid analgesics), alone or in combination with other drugs, accounted for the majority (70%) of fatalities. Heroin or morphine alone or in combination with other drugs accounted for the highest proportion (48%) of fatalities. Deaths involving methadone were more likely to be the result of illicit use (60% or more) rather than prescribed drugs. The mentions of heroin and morphine on death certificates in 2004 were 1,042 for heroin or morphine and 314 for methadone. A significant proportion of deaths also occur among drug misusers who have just left prison. Deaths associated with methadone have significantly reduced over the past five years, probably reflecting implementation of supervised consumption of methadone prescriptions in the initial stages of drug treatment.

WITHDRAWAL SYNDROME

The withdrawal syndrome from heroin may become apparent 8 to 24 hours after the discontinuation of sustained use of the drug. This time frame can fluctuate with the degree of tolerance and the amount of the last consumed dose. Heroin must have been used daily for at least two to three weeks for physical withdrawals to occur. The withdrawal symptoms include anxiety, insomnia, diarrhoea, aches, tremor, sweating, muscular spasms and sneezing and yawning. The severity of withdrawal symptoms will depend on the extent of an individual's dependence. Common symptoms of withdrawal syndrome are presented in Table 8.3.

Table 8.3 Opiates withdrawal symptoms

- Sweating
- Malaise
- Feelings of heaviness
- Cramps
- Yawning
- Tears
- Cold sweats
- Chills
- Severe bone and muscle aches
- Nausea and vomiting

- Diarrhoea
- Goose-bumps
- Fever
- Anxiety
- Depression
- Insomnia
- Compulsive scratching
- Penile erection in males
- Extra sensitivity of genitals in females

METHADONE

Methadone is a synthetic opioid, used therapeutically as an analgesic and in the treatment of opiate addiction. Methadone maintenance is commonly used as a form of treatment for opiate addiction in the UK because it produces similar effects to heroin or morphine and could break the cycle of dependence on opiates. In heroin addiction, heroin releases an excess of dopamine in the body and causes users to need an opiate continuously to occupy the opioid receptor in the brain. Methadone occupies this receptor and provides a stabilising factor that enable opiate users on methadone treatment to change their life styles and behaviours. There is a tradition in the UK to prescribe injectable methadone to opiate addicts as treatment for their addition along with injectable heroin prescribing, and this approach is known as the 'British system'. Methadone is a class A drug and it is legal for a person to possess methadone only if it has been prescribed for that individual. If prescription for an individual involves drinking the methadone syrup within the clinic or pharmacy dispensing it, possession of the drug outside of those premises would constitute an offence – it would be unlawful possession.

Methadone is considered to be the best substitute drug for opiate-dependent drug users because it is easy to administer and long-acting. Methadone is usually prescribed as liquid syrup to be swallowed but it is also manufactured as tablets and ampoules for injection. It is almost as effective when administered orally as by injection. A majority of heroin users require 60 mg and 120 mg of methadone. There is evidence to suggest that maintenance of individuals on a daily dose between 60 mg and 120 mg and higher in exceptional cases is a critical factor in improving maintenance treatment outcomes (Gossop *et al.* 2001)

The effects of methadone last far longer than those of heroin or morphine. Methadone has a typical half-life of 24 hours or more, which allows an opiate addict to take methadone only once a day in methadone maintenance programmes without experiencing withdrawal symptoms. Methadone reduces the cravings associated with heroin use and blocks the high from heroin, but it does not provide the euphoric rush. As with other opiates, tolerance and dependence usually develop with repeated doses. Tolerance to the different physiological effects of methadone varies. Tolerance and dependence may develop, and withdrawal symptoms, although they develop more slowly and are less acutely severe than those of morphine and heroin, are more prolonged. Some heroin addicts feel that it is actually harder to quit methadone than heroin itself. Withdrawal symptoms are generally slightly less severe than those of morphine or heroin at equivalent doses but are significantly more prolonged. Methadone withdrawal symptoms can last for several weeks or more. The withdrawal symptoms of methadone are:

- nausea and vomiting
- increased lacrimation
- rhinnorrhea
- high temperature
- tremor
- chills
- sneezing
- tachycardia

Some problem drug users take extra methadone above the recommended dose or mix it with other depressants such as temazepam, alcohol or even heroin. This is very dangerous and may result in overdose or death. There were 314 mentions of methadone on death certificates in 2004 (Ghodse *et al.* 2006). There is evidence to suggest that oral methadone substitution treatment can help to reduce the use of heroin, avoids the risks of overdose, reduces death rates, reduces crime associated with heroin use, improves the health of drug users, improves social skills and functioning and has the potential to reduce the transmission of infectious diseases associated with heroin injection, such as hepatitis and HIV. However, the major benefits of methadone maintenance are to relieve opiate craving, suppress the abstinence syndrome, and block the euphoric effects associated with heroin (Joseph *et al.* 2000, Stimson and Metrebian 2001). The use of methadone is an important element in opiate treatment which includes comprehensive psychosocial and rehabilitation approaches.

In 2005, a pilot scheme, funded by both the Home Office and the Department of Health, was initiated in three clinics where addicts inject themselves with heroin (BBC News 2007). The injecting clinics, intended for hardened heroin addicts for whom conventional treatment has failed, have operated for about two years. Initial results show that about 40% of users had 'quit their involvement with the street scene completely', had more stability in their lives and reduced criminal activities. The benefits and risks of prescribing heroin to treat opiate dependence are presented in Table 8.4.

Table 8.4 Benefits and risks of prescribing heroin to treat opiate dependence

Benefits	Risks
• Engaging people who are not attracted by other treatments (such as methadone), and retaining them in treatment for longer • Helping people to stop or reduce their illicit heroin use • Ensuring that people dependent on heroin can use a drug of known quality and strength • Reducing the health problems such as overdose or using unsafe injecting practices • Reducing acquisitive crime to support drug habits • Providing a stepping stone to a gradual change from heroin use to methadone, and from injecting to oral use	• Prolonging the time that heroin users are drug-dependent and injecting by removing the motivation to stop using or injecting drugs • Adverse health consequences as a result of continued heroin injecting, including risk of overdose, infections, abscesses and blood-borne viruses • Heroin users presenting for treatment coming to expect heroin, thus making other therapeutic interventions less attractive • The potential for prescribed heroin being diverted into the illicit market

Source: Adapted from Stimson and Metrebian (2003)

ACTIVITY 8.1

There is only one correct answer to the following multiple-choice questions

Which three countries make up the Golden Crescent – an area known for its opium production?
a.   Afghanistan, Iran and Pakistan
b.   Burma, Laos and Thailand
c.   Sri Lanka, India and Pakistan
d.   England, Wales and Scotland

The brain's natural pain killers are known as
a.   Opioids
b.   Endorphins
c.   Aspirin
d.   Opiates

Which statement concerning endorphins is not true?
a.   Endorphins are only given in drug form
b.   Receptors for endorphins can be found in the synapse
c.   Endorphins are the body's natural pain killers
d.   Opiates are exogenous forms of endorphins

Heroin is manufactured chemically from
a.   Codeine
b.   Morphine
c.   Diconal
d.   Opium

In England and Wales, the national estimate and prevalence rate for those (15–64 years old) using opiates for 2005/6 was
a.   150,000 to 280,000
b.   280,000 to 300,000
c.   280,000 to 300,000
d.   350,000 to 400,000

Which statement concerning heroin is true?
a.   Heroin is commonly adulterated with dangerous substances
b.   Heroin differs little at street level and at importation
c.   Most cutting with adulterants occurs after importation
d.   Adulterants are made from heroin products

Heroin as a controlled drug is classified by law as
a.   Class D
b.   Class A
c.   Class C
d.   Class B

Which statement concerning the therapeutic uses of opiates is not true?
a. Relief of pain
b. Treatment for depression
c. Maintenance and withdrawal purposes
d. Treatment for diarrhoea

Heroin's effects are dependent on the modes of administration. Smoking heroin results in rush and euphoria
a. Within 3 to 5 minutes
b. Within 7 to 11 seconds
c. Within 20 to 30 seconds
d. Within 30 to 60 seconds

Which statement is not true regarding controlled heroin users?
a. They use the drug with informal controls
b. They use only at weekends
c. They use with heroin subculture
d. They use indefinitely with little physical harm

Which statement is not true? Injecting heroin brings with it the risks of
a. Vein damage and collapse
b. Contracting hepatitis B and C, HIV
c. Toxicity to human organs
d. Circulatory problems and systemic infections

Most of the health problems that stem from heroin use are due to
a. The chemical constituents of heroin
b. Injecting drug use
c. Oral administration
d. Toxicity of the drug

Research consistently shows that becoming addicted to heroin takes about
a. 2–3 days
b. 3–5 days
c. 6–9 days
d. 2–3 months

The withdrawal syndrome from heroin may become apparent within
a. 8 to 24 hours
b. 4 to 6 hours
c. 6 to 8 hours
d. 1 to 2 hours

Methadone is considered to be the best substitute drug for opiate-dependent drug users because
a. It is easy to administer and long-acting
b. It has fewer withdrawal effects
c. It is manufactured in tablet form
d. It is easy to administer and short-acting

When compared to heroin, tolerance and withdrawal symptoms of methadone develop
a.   Very quickly and more severe
b.   More slowly and less severe
c.   The same as heroin
d.   And last for a few hours or days

Which statement is not true? There is evidence to suggest that oral methadone substitution treatment can help to
a.   Reduce the use of heroin
b.   Avoid the risks of overdose
c.   Reduce the death rates
d.   Increase blood-borne infections

KEY POINTS

- The term 'opiate' refers to any psychoactive substance of either natural or synthetic origin that has an effect similar to morphine.
- There is a tradition in the UK to prescribe injectable methadone or injectable heroin to opiate addicts as treatment for their addition and this approach is known as the 'British system'.
- The body responds to heroin in the brain by reducing (and sometimes stopping) production of the endogenous opioids (endorphins) when heroin is present.
- Some of the commoner opiate drugs are codeine, heroin (diacetylmorphine), pethidine, methadone, morphine and diconal.
- The myth that street heroin is commonly adulterated with dangerous substances has been refuted.
- Recent research in the UK, the US and Australia shows that the purity of drugs such as heroin differs little between street level importation.
- The medical applications of opiates include effective relief of pain, treatment for diarrhoea and vomiting and as a cough suppressant.
- Heroin is swallowed or smoked, sniffed, or injected either subcutaneously or intravenously.
- Heroin's effects are dependent on the modes of administration.
- Contrary to popular beliefs, heroin use does not lead inevitably to dependence, that some people can bring their heroin use back under control.
- In moderate doses, opiates produce a range of generally mild physical effects apart from the analgesic effect. They induce euphoria, which may wear off but use continues to avoid withdrawal symptoms.
- Heroin dependence develops after repeated use over several weeks, and sudden withdrawal leads to anxiety, nausea, muscle pains, sweating, diarrhoea and goose flesh.
- Death through overdose remains a significant cause of mortality amongst heroin users.
- The withdrawal syndrome from heroin may become apparent 8 to 24 hours after the discontinuation of sustained use of the drug.

- Methadone maintenance is commonly used as a form of treatment for opiate addiction in the UK because it produces similar effects to heroin or morphine.
- Methadone is considered to be the best substitute drug for opiate-dependent drug users because it is easy to administer and long-acting.
- Some problem-drug users take extra methadone above the recommended dose or mix it with other depressants such as temazepam, alcohol or even heroin. This is very dangerous and may result in overdose or death.
- There are benefits and risks of prescribing heroin to treat opiate dependence.

REFERENCES

BBC News (2007) *A Fix on the State*. http://news.bbc.co.uk (accessed 19 November 2007).

Coomber, R. (1999) Cutting the crap: the reality of drug adulteration. *Druglink*, July/August, 14, 4: 19–21.

DrugScope (2007) *Street Drug Trends Survey 2007: Two Tier Cocain Market Puts Drug in Reach of More Users*. www.drugscope.org.uk/ourwork/pressoffice/pressreleases/drugscope-street-drug-survey.htm.

EMCDDA (2007) 2007 *Annual Report on the State of the Drugs Problem in Europe*. National Report (2005 data) to the EMCDDA by the Reitox National Focal Point United Kingdom. New Development, Trends and In-depth Information on Selected Issues. REITOX, Lisbon, EMCDDA. http://www.emcdda.europa.eu.

Ghodse, H., Corkery, J., Oyefeso, A., Schifano, F., Tonia, T. and Annan, J. (2006) *Drug Related Death in the UK: Annual Report 2006. Drug-related Deaths Reported by Coroners in England, Wales, Northern Ireland, Guernsey, Jersey and the Isle of Man and Police Forces in Scotland – Annual Report January–December 2005 and 17th Surveillance Report July–December 2005*, London: International Centre for Drug Policy, St George's Hospital Medical School.

Gossop, M., Marsden, J., Stewart, D. and Treacy, S. (2001) Outcomes after methadone maintenance and methadone reduction treatments: two-year follow-up results from the National Treatment Outcome Research Study. Drug and Alcohol Dependence, 62, 3: 255–64.

Home Office (2007). *National and Regional Estimates of the Prevalence of Opiate Use and/or Crack Cocaine Use 2005/06: A Summary of Key Findings* Home Office Online Report 21/07. http://www.homeoffice.gov.uk/rds/pdfs07/rdsolr2107.pdf (accessed 20 June 2007).

Home Office Statistical Bulletin (2007) *Drug Misuse Declared: Findings from the 2006/07 British Crime Survey*. www.homeoffice.gov.uk/rds/index.htm (accessed 20 June 2007).

Joseph, H. Stancliff, S. and Langrod, J. (2000). Methadone maintenance treatment (MMT): a review of historical and clinical issues. *Mount Sinai Journal of Medicine*, 67, 5–6: 347–64.

Stimson, G.V. and Metrebian, N. (2003) *Prescribing Heroin: What Is the Evidence?* London: Joseph Rowntree Foundation.

Warburton, H., Turnbull, P.J. and Hough, M. (2005) *Occasional and Controlled Heroin Use Not a Problem?* London: Joseph Rowntree Foundation. Available at www.jrf.org.uk.

Wikipedia contributors (2007), Heroin *Wikipedia, The Free Encyclopedia*. http://en.wikipedia.org/w/index.php?title=Heroin&oldid=174302275 (accessed 29 November 2007),

CHAPTER 9

CANNABIS

OBJECTIVES

- Discuss the therapeutic and non-therapeutic uses of cannabis.

- Describe briefly the mechanism of action of cannabis.

- Describe cannabis effects on the different modes of administration.

- Discuss the sought-after effects of cannabis.

- Discuss the psychological and physical effects of cannabis.

- Discuss cannabis as a gateway drug.

- List the symptoms of the amotivational syndrome.

Cannabis is the most commonly used psychoactive substance in the world. It is derived from a bushy plant, Cannabis sativa, which is easily cultivated in the United Kingdom. It is used as a relaxant or mild intoxicant. The street names for the substance can vary around the country: bhang, black, blast, blow, blunts, Bob Hope, bush, dope, draw, ganja, grass, hash, hashish, hemp, herb, marijuana, pot, puff, Northern Lights, resin, sensi, sinsemilla, shit, skunk, smoke, soap, spliff, wacky backy, weed, zero. Some names are based on where it comes from, for example, Afghan, homegrown, Moroccan etc.

The EMCDDA (2006) reports that cannabis is the most commonly used substance in all European countries. Prevalence of cannabis use in the year prior to interview was highest in Spain (11.3%), France (9.8%), England and Wales (9.7%). In England and

Wales, cannabis remains the most widely used drug. The 2005/6 British Crime Survey (Roe and Mann 2006) indicates that 8.7% of 16- to 59-year-olds reported using cannabis in the last year. By the age of 16, a majority of young people may have tried cannabis at least once and between 20 and 25% may be regular users. Cannabis is the largest illicit worldwide drug market by far, with roughly 160 million annual consumers. Cannabis production is taking place in at least 172 countries and territories (UNDOC 2007). The production of cannabis resin (also known as hashish) is concentrated in North Africa (Morocco) and in the south-west Asia and Middle East region, particularly in Afghanistan and Pakistan.

Cannabis contains more than four hundred chemicals and one of the main active ingredients, Delta-9 tetrahydrocannabinol (THC), is concentrated in the resin at the top of the plant. 'Skunk' (which has a particularly strong smell), 'sinsemilla' (a bud grown in the absence of male plants and which has no seeds) and 'netherweed' contain on average two to three times the amount of the active compound, THC as other strains of cannabis do. Hash or hashish is resin which is scraped from the plant and then compressed into blocks. Herbal cannabis, also known as marijuana or grass, is a weaker preparation of dried plant material. The strongest preparation, cannabis oil, prepared from the resin, is less common in the UK.

Usually these substances are mixed with tobacco and smoked. Sometimes they are smoked in a pipe, brewed in a drink or mixed with food. Smoking allows the user to regulate the dose because the effect is very rapid when used in this way. Cannabis is usually retailed in ounces (28 grams) or fractions of ounces, quarter ounce (7 grams), half ounce (14 grams). Generally about half a gram of resin is used to make a couple of joints. The retail price varies depending on whether it is sold in herbal (grass) or resin form.

MECHANISM OF ACTION

Cannabis has two powerful active ingredients – THC and CBD (cannabidiol) and both substances are classed as cannabinoids. The substances produce psychoactive effects by binding with special receptors which are extraordinarily abundant all over the brain and body. The brain makes its own natural cannabinoid – anandamide – which is thought to be involved in pain sensations and immune system and memory regulation. THC is absorbed into the bloodstream through the walls of the lungs (if cannabis is smoked), or through the walls of the stomach and intestines (if eaten). The THC level in the blood gets redistributed in areas of high fat content in the body such as the brain and the testes for men. The physiological properties of THC acts like a hypnosedative, has an anti-convulsant activity and acts as an analgesic. The time of onset of eating cannabis is usually between one and two hours but the effects last considerably longer, around four hours. Taking oral cannabis may produce undesired psychedelic experiences. Cannabis gets into the bloodstream more quickly when inhaled than when eaten.

LEGAL STATUS

Cannabis was banned in 1928 after it was linked to 'harder' drugs like heroin and opium. Cannabis is not frowned on by society as much now, and its medical benefits are starting to look attractive. Being caught in the UK with a small amount of cannabis is more likely to get you a caution than a jail sentence. Cannabis is controlled under the Misuse of Drugs Act (class C), making it illegal to cultivate, produce, supply or possess the drug, unless a Home Office licence has been issued for research use or other special purposes. It is an offence to allow any premises to be used for cultivating, producing, supplying, storage or smoking of cannabis. Cannabis is to be reclassified to a class B drug if approved by parliament. The classification would take effect in 2009.

THERAPEUTIC USE

Compared with all other drugs controlled under the Misuse of Drugs Act, cannabis has the greatest non-medical usage. However, cannabis is indicated for the treatment of anorexia associated with weight loss in patients with AIDS, and to treat mild to moderate nausea and vomiting associated with cancer chemotherapy. Cannabis is effective in treating the loss of appetite and physical wasting associated with AIDS, glaucoma (a serious eye disease), muscle spasms occurring in multiple sclerosis and other disorders that produce involuntary muscle contractions, chronic pain and migraine headaches. A synthetic extract of cannabis has been shown to relieve symptoms of anorexia in patients with Alzheimer's disease, glaucoma, pain relief, arterial blockage and multiple sclerosis.

SOUGHT-AFTER EFFECTS

The desired effects experienced by users are talkativeness, cheerfulness, relaxation and greater appreciation of sound and colour. Cannabis users often describe the experience of smoking as initially relaxing and mellow, creating a feeling of haziness and light-headedness. Users may become more aware of their senses and this is known as being 'high' or 'stoned'. Cannabis is also famous for stimulating the appetite: hunger pangs are common and are known as 'getting the munchies'.

SHORT-TERM USE

The active chemical in cannabis will normally stop having an effect after about four hours. However, traces of it remain in the urine and hair for much longer. Cannabis lowers the blood pressure which is why some users experience an intense feeling of relaxation. However, it increases the heart rate, which may contribute to the feelings of paranoia or panic. The following are common effects: talkativeness, bouts of hilarity, relaxation and greater sensitivity to sound and colour. There is no hangover of the type associated with alcohol use. Whilst under the influence of cannabis, concentration and mental and manual dexterity are impaired, making tasks such as driving or any procedure requiring accuracy or precision both difficult and dangerous. The effects derived depend to a large extent on expectations, motivation and mood of the user. The effects of cannabis usually start just a few minutes after smoking and last from about one hour to several hours depending on how much is consumed. There is also a risk that using cannabis may trigger mental health problems. In the short term, none of these effects is dangerous in its own right, and, if in a relaxed environment, will quickly pass as long as the consumption of cannabis is low.

LONG-TERM USE

Cannabis is so often taken alongside tobacco, and so the effects of tobacco on the heart and lungs must also be considered. Like tobacco smoking, frequently and chronically inhaled cannabis smoke probably causes bronchitis and other respiratory problems and may also contribute to the development of lung cancer. The concentration of one cancer-producing agent, benzopyrene, in cannabis smoke is even higher than in tobacco smoke. Other respiratory conditions such as emphysema, and heart disease, while not inevitable, are definite possibilities for anyone who regularly smokes tobacco. It can also make asthma worse and is a risk factor for anyone with cardiovascular problems. Researchers have found that THC impairs immune system function in laboratory animals, but the doses in those studies were extremely high. Frequent use of cannabis can cut a man's sperm count and suppress ovulation in women. Using cannabis during pregnancy may affect the baby. Research suggests there may be a link between cannabis use during pregnancy and subtle cognitive problems in children. Cannabis smoke contains many of the same chemicals found in cigarette smoke, which are dangerous to the foetus.

Cannabis does not cause muscle spasms. On the contrary, it can ease muscle spasms. That is why people suffering from multiple sclerosis, for example, find that cannabis has a beneficial effect on their condition. Cannabis use also causes short-term memory problems. This is due to THC's actions in the hippocampus, part of the nervous system involved in memory. When THC interferes with its normal functioning, trouble recalling recent events can be the result.

Perceptual distortion may also occur, especially with heavy use. If the drug is used while an individual is anxious or depressed, these feelings may be accentuated leading to a feeling of panic. People chronically intoxicated on cannabis appear apathetic and sluggish, and neglect their appearance. There may be particular risks for people with respiratory or heart disorders. Heavy use, particularly if strong varieties such as some forms of skunk are used regularly, can lead to psychosis. Heavy users of cannabis with personality disturbance or psychiatric problems may experience a temporary exacerbation of symptoms. In 2007, a study published in *The Lancet* showed that a growing number of medical health practitioners are convinced that cannabis use increases susceptibility to mental illness, accounting for 14% of UK psychosis cases (Moore *et al*. 2007). However, the risk to an individual smoking cannabis is increased only by 2% (Morral *et al*. 2002)

Opinion varies about the effects of long-term cannabis use. This may be partly because slowly developing and infrequent effects need large longitudinal samples to arrive at conclusive results, and these studies are rare. While there is little evidence that

Table 9.1 Psychological and physical effects of cannabis

Psychological effects	Physical effects
• Euphoria	• Increased heart rate
• Changes in perception	• Dry mouth
• Anxiety	• Red eyes
• Panic	• Impaired motor co-ordination
• Paranoia	• Hunger
• Hallucinations	• Increased desire for sweets
• Depression	• Bronchitis
• Lethargy	• Emphysema
• Loss of communication skills	• Bronchial asthma
• Impaired problem-solving abilities	• Lung cancer
• Impaired judgement	• Reduced sperm production
• Impaired memory-storing new information	• Disruption menstrual cycle
• Low motivation	• Suppression immune system

cannabis can produce a physical dependence, regular use can produce a psychological need for the drug and some individuals may come to rely on it as a 'social lubricant'. On the basis of current research cannabis cannot be said to provide as clear a withdrawal pattern as other drugs of misuse, such as opiates (Smith 2002). A summary of the psychological and physical effects of cannabis is presented in Table 9.1.

CANNABIS AS A GATEWAY DRUG

Generally people who smoke cannabis are more likely to use other drugs, and people who smoke tobacco and drink are also more likely to try cannabis. However, there is no evidence that the use of one drug actually causes people to use another (Escalation theory). Studies have shown that tobacco smoking is a better predictor of concurrent illicit hard drug use than smoking cannabis (Ellgren 2007). The cause and effect of cannabis have been debated, and the purported relationship between cannabis and more illicit drugs, as proposed by the 'gateway theory', is methodologically flawed (Kandel 2003). The RAND study (Morral *et al.* 2002) demonstrates that associations between cannabis and hard drug use could be expected even if cannabis use has no gateway effect. Instead, the associations can result from known differences in the ages at which youths have opportunities to use cannabis and hard drugs, and known variations in individuals' willingness to try any drugs.

AMOTIVATIONAL SYNDROME

The concept of amotivational syndrome in relation to the long-term effects of cannabis remains a controversial entity in the literature. According to the lexicon of alcohol and drug terms published by the World Health Organization, amotivational syndrome is a constellation of features said to be associated with substance use, including apathy, loss of effectiveness, diminished capacity to carry out complex or long-term plans, low tolerance for frustration, impaired concentration and difficulty in following routines. The existence of this condition is controversial. It has been reported principally in connection with cannabis use, and may simply reflect chronic cannabis intoxication. The symptoms may also reflect the user's personality, attitudes or developmental stage. However, most reports of the amotivational syndrome originated in the 1960s in North America and some are based on case reports, case studies and animal experimental studies.

KEY POINTS

- Cannabis is the most commonly used psychoactive substance in the world.
- In England and Wales, cannabis remains the most widely used drug.
- Herbal cannabis, also known as marijuana or grass, is a weaker preparation of dried plant material.
- Cannabis has two powerful active ingredients – THC and CBD (cannabidiol) and both substances are classed as cannabinoids.
- Taking oral cannabis may produce undesired psychedelic experiences. Cannabis gets into the bloodstream more quickly when inhaled than when eaten.
- It is an offence to allow any premises to be used for cultivating, producing, supplying, storage or smoking of cannabis.
- Cannabis lowers the blood pressure, which is why some users experience an intense feeling of relaxation.
- People chronically intoxicated on cannabis appear apathetic and sluggish, and neglect their appearance.
- The alleged relationship between cannabis and more illicit drugs, as proposed by the 'gateway theory', is methodologically flawed.
- The concept of amotivational syndrome in relation to the long-term effects of cannabis, remains a controversial entity in the literature. It may simply reflect chronic cannabis intoxication.

ACTIVITY 9.1

There is only one correct answer to the following multiple-choice questions

When was cannabis outlawed in Britain?
a.   1928
b.   1968
c.   1938
d.   1948

What is THC?
a.   A cannabis cigarette
b.   The psycho-active ingredient in cannabis

c.   A cannabis pressure group in favour of legalisation
d.   Treatment for cannabis

The effects of cannabis last for a maximum of how long?
a.   14 hours
b.   48 hours
c.   4 hours
d.   24 hours

A common form of cannabis is
a.   Marijuana
b.   Hashish
c.   Hash oil
d.   All of the above

What is the name of the active chemical in cannabis?
a.   Delta-9 ethanol dehydrogenase
b.   Delta-Fos-9
c.   Delta-9 tetrahydrocannabinol
d.   Delta Gamma

Which of the following statements is the most accurate?
a.   Cannabis has little effect on ability to drive a car
b.   Cannabis is less damaging on ability to drive a car than alcohol
c.   It is safe to get in a car if the driver has been smoking marijuana
d.   Cannabis impairs co-ordination and judgement resulting in an inability to drive

How does the risk of lung cancer for a marijuana smoker compare to a tobacco smoker's risk?
a.   Cannabis causes little risk of lung cancer
b.   Cannabis contains more of the cancer-causing chemical benzopyrene than tobacco
c.   Cannabis contains less of the cancer-causing chemical benzopyrene than tobacco
d.   Cannabis contains the same amount of cancer-causing chemical benzopyrene as tobacco

Can cannabis use affect your mental health?
a.   No
b.   Yes
c.   It is a risk factor especially if predisposed to schizophrenia
d.   Only if you take another psychoactive substance

How does cannabis affect the brain?
a.   THC affects memory and learning
b.   Changes in the sensory information processing
c.   The information-processing centre of the brain is suppressed
d.   All of the above

Cannabis is

a.   Physically addictive
b.   Psychologically addictive
c.   More addictive than tobacco
d.   More addictive than alcohol

Cannabis is

a.   Gateway drug
b.   Not a gateway drug
c.   Leads to heroin use
d.   Leads to dependence

Cannabis is

a.   Central nervous system stimulant
b.   Central nervous system depressant
c.   Not an appetite stimulant
d.   Not a bronchodialator

When cannabis is smoked

a.   The onset of the effect takes between 1 and 2 hours
b.   The onset of the effect takes between 2 and 3 hours
c.   The onset of the effect is almost immediate
d.   The onset of the effect may last several hours

Large doses of potent cannabis

a.   When swallowed can cause 'toxic psychosis'
b.   When smoked can cause 'toxic psychosis'
c.   Raise blood pressure
d.   Decrease risk of heart attack

Research suggests that

a.   There is a link between cannabis use and pregnancy
b.   Cannabis smoke contains fewer chemicals than tobacco
c.   Cannabis does not affect the foetus
d.   There is no link between cannabis use and pregnancy

The scientific name for cannabis is

a.   Cannabis sativa
b.   Cannabis
c.   Cotton candy
d.   Cannabis B

The majority of young people who enter drug treatment have problems associated with

a.   Cocaine
b.   Heroin
c.   Ecstasy
d.   Cannabis

The chemical in cannabis that causes the user to feel 'high' is
a.   Dopamine
b.   Cannabis sativa
c.   Tetrahydrocannabinol (THC)
d.   Serotonin

Tetrahydrocannabinol, the active ingredient in marijuana, acts on the brain by
a.   Coating the nervous system
b.   Binding to specific receptors
c.   Causing brain tissue to grow
d.   Decreasing fat tissue in the brain

Memory problems associated with marijuana use are due to THC's actions in which part of the brain?
a.   Cerebellum
b.   Hippocampus
c.   Cerebrum
d.   Basal ganglia

Cannabis affects the brain function of first-time users differently than it does experienced users because
a.   It causes a decrease in blood flow to the brain
b.   It causes an increase in blood flow to the brain
c.   Its effects vary with age and gender
d.   It affects the nervous system of men and women differently

Which statement is true?
a.   Men are more likely than women to become daily users of cannabis
b.   Women are more likely than men to become daily users of cannabis
c.   There is no difference between the prevalence rates of women and men
d.   Cannabis is healthier than tobacco

ACTIVITY 9.2

*   What are the therapeutic uses of cannabis?
*   What experiences do users of cannabis seek?
*   What are the short-term effects of cannabis?
*   What are the long-term effects of cannabis?
*   What is meant by 'gateway drug'?
*   What is 'amotivational syndrome'?

REFERENCES

Ellgren, M. (2007) *Neurobiological Effects of Early Life Cannabis Exposure in Relation to the Gateway Hypothesis*. Karolinska Institute. http://diss.kib.ki.se/2007/978-91-7357-064-0/ (accessed 25 June 2007).

EMCDDA Statistical Bulletin (2007) *European Monitoring Centre for Drugs and Drug Addiction (EMCDDA)*. Available at http://stats06.emcdda.europa.eu/en/homeen.html (accessed 25 June 2007).

Kandel, D.B. (2003) Does marijuana use cause the use of other drugs? *Journal of the American Medical Association*, 289, 4: 427–33.

Moore, T., Zammit, S., Lingford-Hughes, A., Barnes, T., Jones, P., Burke, M. and Lewis, G. (2007) Cannabis use and risk of psychotic or affective mental health outcomes: a systematic review. *The Lancet*, 370, 9584: 319–28.

Morral, A.R., McCaffrey, D.F. and Paddock, S.M. (2002) Reassessing the marijuana gateway effect. *Addiction*, 97, 1: 1493–1504.

Roe, S. and Mann, L. (2006) *Drug Misuse Declared; Findings from the 2005/06 British Crime Survey – England and Wales*. London: Home Office. Available at www.homeoffice.gov.uk/rds/pdfs06/hosb1506.pdf(accessed 25 June 2007).

Smith, N.T. (2002) Review of the published literature into cannabis withdrawal symptoms in human users. *Addiction* 97, 6: 621–32.

UNDOC (2007) *World Drug Report 2007*. http://www.unodc.org/india/world_drug_report_2007.html (accessed 25 June 2007).

CHAPTER 10

STIMULANTS: AMPHETAMINES, COCAINE AND KHAT

OBJECTIVES

■ Discuss the therapeutic and non-therapeutic uses of amphetamine.

■ Describe briefly the mechanism of action of stimulants.

■ Describe amphetamine effects on the different modes of administration.

■ Discuss the sought-after effects of stimulants.

■ Discuss the psychological and physical effects of amphetamines and cocaine.

■ List the withdrawal symptoms of amphetamine.

■ List the withdrawal symptoms of cocaine.

■ Discuss the phases in cocaine withdrawal.

■ Discuss the physiological and psychological effects of khat.

Stimulants are synthetic powders available in a variety of tablets and capsules, sometimes in combination with other drugs. Stimulants are psychoactive substances that cause an increase in activity in various parts of the central nervous system or directly increases muscle activity and are often referred to as 'uppers'. There are both legal and illegal stimulants. Caffeine is a mild stimulant which is considered relatively safe. Another legal stimulant is nicotine (found in tobacco products).

Stimulants such as methylphenidate are prescribed to increase alertness and physical activity. The most widely used illegal stimulants are amphetamines, cocaine and crack. Ritalin (methylphenidate) and diethylproprion (Tenuate, Apisate) have a similar effect to amphetamine, but are less potent.

Historically, stimulants were used to treat asthma and other respiratory problems, obesity and neurological disorders. In the 1950s and 1960s they were widely prescribed for symptoms of depression, and as appetite suppressants. These drugs may be taken orally or sniffed in powder form, smoked or dissolved in water and injected. This chapter focuses on amphetamine, cocaine and khat.

LEGAL STATUS

All amphetamines and similar stimulants are 'prescription'-only drugs under the Medicines Act. Most are also controlled under the Misuse of Drugs Act with the exception of some mild stimulants. Amphetamine, dex- and methyl-amphetamine, phenmetrazine and methylphenidate are in class B, but if prepared for injection the increased penalties of class A apply. Diethylpropion and other amphetamine-like stimulants are in class C. Cocaine, its derivative salts and the leaves of the coca plant come under class A. As in the case of some opiates, a doctor must be licensed by the Home Office before prescribing cocaine. Such prescribing is, however, very uncommon.

AMPHETAMINES

Amphetamine, dextroamphetamine and methamphetamine are collectively referred to as amphetamines. The name 'Amphetamine' is derived from its chemical name: alpha-methylphenethylamine. The chemical properties of synthetic amphetamine, dextroamphetamine and methamphetamine and actions are very similar. However, natural amphetamine and methamphetamine compounds have been found in Acacia species in Texas in the United States (Clement et al. 1997, 1998). Amphetamine was first synthesised in 1887 by Lazar Edeleanu at the University of Berlin and was first marketed in the 1930s as benzedrine in an over-the-counter inhaler to treat nasal congestion. During the Second World War, amphetamine was widely used to combat fatigue and increase alertness in soldiers. During the past decades, amphetamine has become popular as a recreational drug and performance enhancer amongst young people. The most common type is amphetamine sulphate, which is relatively easy to produce. Recently amphetamine has experienced a revival in its uses. Amphetamines are often manufactured in home-made laboratories in a matter of hours, mixing the main ingredient, pseudo-ephedrine (a cold remedy) with a cocktail of about fifteen chemicals. This process is highly toxic and dangerous.

The 2006/7 British Crime Survey report (Roe and Mann 2006) indicates that 1.3% of 16- to 59-year-olds reported using amphetamine in England and Wales. Compared to cocaine, amphetamine is cheaper and has a long-lasting effect. Most 'street stimulants' are illicitly manufactured amphetamine sulphate powder. Illicit amphetamine heavily diluted with adulterants (often to 15% purity) is easily available. In 2007, amphetamine was being sold at £9.80 per gram (Druglink 2007). An occasional user may take a few weeks to consume half a gram while a heavy user might consume up to 6 grams per day of relatively impure substance. Crystal amphetamine (methamphetamine hydrochloride), the street form of the drug methamphetamine, comes in clear, chunky crystals and is heated and smoked. Smokable methamphetamine, usually called 'ice', is off-white, grey or pinkish powder which is usually smoked in a glass pipe. Amphetamines – known as speed, whizz, sulph, uppers, ice, crystal, glass, amph, billy or sulphate – are swallowed, sniffed, smoked or injected (by crushing the tablets).

Mechanism of action

Amphetamine has been shown to release high levels of dopamine in the brain, a neurotransmitter that is associated with pleasurable or rewarding experiences. The transmitter dopamine is the one most affected by stimulants and many other psychoactive drugs. The increase of dopamine is the primary mechanism for its behavioural-stimulant effects with intense pleasure and increase energy.

The intensity of amphetamine is based on the amount of the drug taken and routes of administration. In very low doses, amphetamine increases attention spans and decreases impulsiveness whereas in higher doses it decreases appetite and brings on weight loss. In oral form, the user experiences increased wakefulness and physical activity, and decreased appetite. If it is smoked and injected, the user immediately experiences an intense 'rush' (also called a 'flash') that causes intense pleasure but lasts only a few minutes. With repeated use, stimulants can decrease dopamine, dampening users' ability to feel pleasure and the development of tolerance.

Sought-after effects

Amphetamines create arousal and activate the user in a manner similar to adrenalin which the body produces naturally. Heart and respiratory rate are speeded up, pupils widen and appetite lessens. The user feels more energetic, confident and cheerful. The experience of these effects creates the possibility of psychological dependence. As the individual's energy is depleted, the predominant feelings may be anxiety, irritability and restlessness. Snorting produces effects within three to five minutes, and oral ingestion takes 15 to 30 minutes to produce effects. These methods produce a euphoric effect, but not the intense rush of the rapid-onset methods. The duration of the effect can vary and depends on the quantity ingested, but can last up to 12 hours. By contrast, the body processes cocaine much more quickly, with 50% of the substance removed in the first hour after consumption.

Therapeutic uses

Amphetamines are sometimes prescribed therapeutically for a number of conditions. They are commonly used to treat attention-deficit hyperactivity disorder (ADHD) in adults and children. They are also used to treat symptoms of traumatic brain injury, symptoms of narcolepsy and chronic fatigue syndrome. Amphetamines can also be used as a supplement to antidepressant therapy in depressive conditions.

Adverse effects

Short-term physiological effects vary greatly, depending on dosage and the method in which the drug is taken. Long-term use of amphetamine may cause violent behaviour, anxiety, confusion, and insomnia. Heavy users may also display a number of psychotic features, including paranoia, auditory hallucinations, mood disturbances and delusions known as amphetamine psychosis. The paranoid delusion may result in homicidal or suicidal thoughts. In most people, these effects disappear when they stop using the drug. Heavy prolonged use also exposes the individual to the risk of cardiovascular problems. This applies particularly to people with hypertension and anyone who does strenuous exercise while taking the drug (for example, athletes).

Amphetamine can also cause a variety of problems, including rapid heart rate, irregular heartbeat, stroke, high blood pressure, shortness of breath, nausea, vomiting, diarrhoea and physical collapse. There may also be an increase in body temperature and convulsions, which can be lethal if not treated as an emergency. Some users believe that methamphetamine can increase their sex drive. However, research indicates that long-term methamphetamine use may be associated with decreased sexual functioning, at least in men (National Institute on Drug Abuse 1998). A list of physical and psychological effects is presented in Table 10.1.

The effects of a single dose last about three to four hours, leaving the user feeling tired and depleted. It can take a couple of days for the body to recover fully. Chronic users of amphetamines typically snort or resort to drug injection to experience the full-intensity effects of the drug with the added risks of infection, vein damage and higher risk of overdose. The use of amphetamine is highly addictive, and, with chronic abuse, tolerance develops very quickly. Repeated amphetamine use can produce 'reverse tolerance', or sensitisation to some psychological effects. Many amphetamine users will repeat the amphetamine cycle by taking more of the drug during the withdrawal. This leads to a very dangerous cycle and may involve the use of other drugs to get over the withdrawal process. Withdrawal, although not physiologically threatening, is an unpleasant experience. How severe and prolonged these withdrawal symptoms are depends on the degree of abuse. Key withdrawal symptoms of amphetamine are presented in Table 10.2.

ACTIVITY 10.1

Please choose one correct answer for the following multiple choice questions

Which of these drugs is a stimulant?
a.   Speed
b.   Crack/Cocaine
c.   Caffeine
d.   All of these

Snorting cocaine effects are produced
a.   Within 3 to 5 minutes
b.   Within 15 to 20 minutes

Table 10.1 Physical and psychological effects of amphetamine

Physical effects	Psychological effects
Short-term	**Short-term**
• Decreased appetite	• Alertness
• Increased stamina	• Euphoria
• Increased sexual drive	• Increased concentration
• In some cases, decreased sexual drive	• Rapid talking
• Teeth-grinding	• Increased confidence
• Hyperactivity	• Increased social awareness
• Agitation	• Hallucinations
• Nausea	• Loss of REM sleep
• Itchy	• Insomnia
• Greasy skin	
• Tachycardia	
• Irregular heart rate	
• Hypertension	
• Headaches	
• Fatigue	
• Nystagmus	
Long-term	**Long-term**
• Tolerance	• Irritability
• Deterioration of the lining of the nostrils	• Anxiety
• Difficulty in breathing	• Depression
• Tremor	• Aggressiveness
• Restlessness	• Obsessive behaviours
• Fatigue	• Delusions
• Changes in sleep patterns	• Paranoia
• Poor skin condition	• Dependence
• Twitching	• Withdrawal symptoms
• Gastric flactuations and/or pain	
• Cardiovascular problems	
• Stroke	
• Damage to lung, kidney and liver	
• Erectile dysfunction	

Table 10.2 Withdrawal symptoms of amphetamine

• Cravings	• Hyperventilation
• Nausea	• Convulsions
• Irritability	• Irregular heart beat
• Depression	• Insomnia
• Loss of energy	• Depression
• Sweats	• Long periods of sleep
• Fatigue	• Paranoia
• Decreased libido	• Delusions
• Decreased self-confidence	

c.   Within 20 to 25 minutes
d.   Within 35 to 45 minutes

In very low doses, amphetamine
a.   Decreases attention spans and wakefulness
b.   Increases attention spans and decreases impulsiveness
c.   Decreases appetite and brings on weight loss
d.   Increases appetite and wakefulness

Amphetamine causes
a.   A decrease in heart and respiratory rate
b.   An increase in heart and respiratory rate
c.   Low confidence and energy
d.   An increase in heart rate and low anxiety

Amphetamines are sometimes prescribed therapeutically. Which condition is not treated with amphetamine?
a.   Attention-deficit hyperactivity disorder
b.   Traumatic brain injury
c.   Narcolepsy
d.   Cardiovascular disorder

Withdrawal from amphetamine
a.   Is not physiologically threatening
b.   Is physiologically threatening
c.   Is psychologically threatening
d.   Is both physiologically and psychologically threatening

ACTIVITY 10.2

Please state whether the following statements are true or false. Reflect on the statements and give reason(s) for choosing a particular option (if appropriate)

	True	False
Stimulants have been used to treat asthma and other respiratory problems, obesity and neurological disorders		
The most common type of amphetamine is amphetamine sulphate		
Amphetamine users quickly develop a tolerance		
Amphetamine is a depressant psychoactive substance		
Amphetamines keep people awake for a long period of time		
There are no dangerous withdrawal symptoms with amphetamines		
Heavy users of amphetamines can experience unpleasant side effects like disturbed sleep and loss of appetite		

Crack is a smokable form of cocaine

Smoking a powerful drug like cocaine may cause respiratory problems

With crack cocaine, the user may feel tired and depressed in the period immediately after stopping using the drug

Cocaine is physically addictive

Crack cocaine is considered a class A drug (Misuse of Drugs Act)

Caffeine is a mild stimulant

Cocaethylene is produced when alcohol and cocaine are consumed together

---

ACTIVITY 10.3

- What are the short-term effects of amphetamine?
- What are the long-term effects of amphetamine?
- What are the psychological and physiological effects of amphetamine?
- What is meant by 'amphetamine psychosis'?
- What are the features of withdrawal from amphetamine?

COCAINE

Cocaine is a drug with powerfully stimulant properties. It is a white powder derived from the leaves of the Andean coca shrub. The street names for the drug can vary around the country. For powder cocaine, the street names are coke, Charlie, C, white, Percy, snow and toot. In Europe and North America, the most common form of cocaine is a white crystalline powder. Cocaine is a stimulant but is not normally prescribed therapeutically for its stimulant properties, although it sees clinical use as a local anaesthetic, particularly in ophthalmology. A small amount of the drug is usually 'sniffed' or 'snorted' up the nose through a tube and absorbed through the nasal membranes, although sometimes the substance is injected. There are three forms of cocaine: cocaine hydrochloride, freebase and crack cocaine.

Freebasing consists of smoking cocaine base (or crack). Crack cocaine (rocks, ready wash, ice, base, freebase, stones) is whitish in colour and looks like irregular lumps of sugar. Crack is made by heating cocaine hydrochloride with baking soda or ammonia in water. Smoking cocaine base is a more potent way of administration than snorting and produces a 'rush' similar to the experience of injecting cocaine. Many cocaine and crack users also take other drugs, including heroin. A highly dangerous practice is the injecting of a mixture of heroin and soluble cocaine (known as snow-balling or speedballing). Alcohol is often mixed with cocaine to produce coca-ethylene, which is highly toxic.

In recent years, there has been considerable concern regarding rises in cocaine use in recreational settings (for example, discos and clubs) and among young people in general in some European countries. Cocaine is the second most commonly used illicit drug in Europe, after cannabis (ECMDDA 2007). Among young people in Europe (15–34 years), an estimated 7.5 million have used cocaine at least once in their lives, 3.5 million in the last year and 1.5 million in the past month. Targeted studies in dance music settings have observed lifetime prevalence of cocaine use of up to 60%. Cocaine powder is generally used by socially integrated recreational users, while crack cocaine remains very rare, being mainly consumed by more marginalised groups (for example, homeless people or sex workers). In many cases, cocaine users are polydrug users, often consuming cocaine with alcohol and tobacco, with other illicit drugs such as other stimulants and cannabis, or with heroin (EMDDCA 2007). In England and Wales, the 2006/7 British Crime Survey estimated that 6.1% of 16- to-24-year-olds had used cocaine of any form in the previous year (Roe and Mann 2006).

Therapeutic uses

In July 1884, Sigmund Freud, the father of psychoanalysis, published 'Über Coca', a paper in which he enthusiastically reported on the therapeutic uses of coca and its alkaloid, cocaine. Freud expected that cocaine would be used as a substitution therapy for morphine addiction and as a euphoriant in cases of melancholia. Cocaine had been used as a local anaesthetic in ophthalmology and dentistry. Cocaine was also used in the treatment of asthma, cramps, mountain-sickness, sea-sickness and vomiting in pregnancy. Today most of the therapeutic uses of cocaine are now obsolete with the development of safer drugs.

Mechanism of action

Cocaine modifies the action of dopamine in the brain. It acts on the brain's 'reward pathways' or pleasure centre to prevent the reabsorption of the neurotransmitter dopamine after its release from nerve cells. This causes a build-up of dopamine in the synapse which results in strong feelings of 'high' and euphoria. When cocaine level use is reduced completely the dopamine levels return to normal. During the withdrawal symptoms of cocaine, such as craving, the user experiences a very strong need for the drug to get the level of dopamine back up. Cocaine also blocks the re-uptake of norepinephrine in the nervous system, resulting in increased stimulation of the sympathetic nervous system. This results in tachycardia, hypertension, sweating, dilation of the pupils and tremors associated with cocaine use. In high doses, cocaine can cause depression, disturbed sleep, hallucinations, delusions and paranoia.

The intensity and the duration of the effects of cocaine are influenced by the route of administration. A traditional way of taking cocaine is chewing coca leaves mixed with an alkaline substance (such as lime or bicarbonate). The leaves, with the alkaline substance, are chewed into a bolus that is retained in the mouth between gum and cheek and its juices are sucked. The alkaloids are rapidly absorbed into the bloodstream through the stomach. The effect of chewing coca leaves is felt within 15 to 20 minutes with the increase of alertness, awareness, feeling of well-being; there is an increase in activity or the desire to do something. The effect of chewing is strong at the start but it disappears progressively and it is necessary to increase the intake slowly to maintain the effect. Alternatively, coca leaves can be infused in liquid and consumed like tea. Mate de coca or coca-leaf infusion is often recommended in coca-producing countries, such as Peru and Bolivia, to ameliorate some symptoms of altitude sickness.

With oral administration, cocaine takes approximately 30 minutes to enter the bloodstream. Given the uptake of cocaine in the bloodstream and the slow rate of absorption, the effects are reached approximately 60 minutes after cocaine is administered and these effects are prolonged for approximately 60 minutes after their peak is attained. Snorting, 'sniffing' or 'blowing' (insufflations) is the most common method of ingestion of cocaine. Snorting cocaine produces maximum physiological effects within 40 minutes and an activation period is between 5 to 10 minutes, which is similar to oral use of cocaine. Compared to ingestion, the faster absorption of snorting cocaine results in rapid onset of maximum drug effects. With smoking freebase the cocaine is absorbed immediately into the blood, reaching the brain in about five seconds. The intensity of the 'rush' is more powerful than snorting the same amount of cocaine nasally, but the effects are short-lived. The peak of the freebase rush is rapid and the high typically lasts 5–10 minutes afterwards. These effects are similar to those that can be achieved by injecting cocaine hydrochloride, but without the risks associated with injecting drug use.

Cocaethylene is produced when alcohol and cocaine are consumed together. Cocaethylene is active in the brain, and has a similar effect to cocaine, but the subjective perception of the cocaine 'high' and its heart effects are not increased – instead they decline in intensity.

Sought-after effects

The sought-after effects of cocaine are:

- a rapid feeling of intense high
- increase in alertness and energy
- a feeling of well-being
- delay of hunger and fatigue
- increase of confidence
- stimulation of sex drive.

Adverse effects

Several quickly repeated doses can lead to extreme agitation, panic attacks and feelings of restlessness, irritability, and anxiety. Chronic use of cocaine results in ongoing rhinitis (runny nose) and damages the nasal septum. Many users report a burning sensation in the nostrils after cocaine's anaesthetic effects wear off. Cocaine has an effect on the constriction of blood vessels and prevents adequate blood supply to that area. Cocaine users may also experience paranoia, auditory hallucination or a full-blown cocaine psychosis. With cocaine psychosis, the symptoms may take the person several months to recover fully. The long-term use of cocaine can cause debilitation due to lack of sleep and food, leading to lowered resistance to illness generally.

Hyperthermia (elevated body temperature) and convulsions occur with cocaine overdoses, and if not treated immediately, can result in death. Excessive doses, whether snorted, injected or smoked, can lead to overdose, which can lead to sudden death from respiratory or heart failure. Cocaine-related deaths are often a result of cardiac arrest or seizures followed by respiratory arrest. The physical symptoms of cocaine overdose may include chest pain, nausea, blurred vision, fever, muscle spasms, convulsions and coma. Some of the physical and psychological effects of low to moderate dose, excessive dose and chronic use of cocaine are presented in Table 10.3.

Withdrawal syndrome

Cocaine users can develop a tolerance to the euphoric effects of cocaine very rapidly. This makes it necessary to take more and more cocaine to get the same desired effect. In contrast, regular cocaine users may develop a 'reverse tolerance', whereby they experience the adverse effects of cocaine more intensely. Cocaine causes both physical

Table 10.3 Physical and psychological effects of cocaine

Dose	Physical effects	Psychological effects
Low to moderate dose	• Loss of appetite • Dry mouth • Tachycardia • Raised heart rate • Hypertension • Sweating • Dilated pupils • Reduced appetite • Reduced need for sleep • Impaired motor skills • Reduced lung function • Erratic or violent behaviour • Increased desire for sex	• Euphoria • Sense of well-being • Impaired reaction time • Increased self-confidence • Suspiciousness • Increased sensory awareness • Sense of superiority
Excessive doses	• Convulsions • Heart failure • Stroke • Cerebral haemorrhage • Respiratory arrest • Exhaustion	• Anxiety • Irritability • Insomnia • Depression • Paranoia • Aggressiveness • Delusions • Disorientation • Indifference • Reduced psychomotor function
Chronic Use	• Destruction of nasal septum (snorting) • Nasal eczema (snorting) • Chest pains • Muscle spasm • Respiratory problems (smoking) • Contraction of infection (injected cocaine) • Abscesses (injected cocaine) • Weight loss • Malnutrition • Sexual impotence	• Tolerance • Psychological dependence • Cocaine psychosis

and psychological dependence, the severity of which depends on the route of administration. The psychological dependence is more of a problem than physical withdrawal symptoms. It is more severe when the drug has been injected or smoked. Withdrawal leads to strong craving and drug-seeking behaviour, followed by a withdrawal syndrome. However in a study of cocaine abstinence in an outpatient population, Coffey *et al.* (2002) found that craving is relatively mild during cocaine withdrawal compared to other drugs of abuse, and that cocaine withdrawal symptoms decrease steadily over time. In addition, the authors reported that unlike earlier subjects of inpatient studies of cocaine withdrawal and research on alcohol withdrawal, these patients did not report significant disruptions in sleep.

Stages in cocaine withdrawal

Cocaine withdrawal generally occurs in three phases: the 'crash', the 'withdrawal' and the 'extinction'. Not all cocaine users may go through the three distinct phases as this may be influenced by the level of consumption, the set and the setting.

The crash

The crash occurs in the first few days when a person who has used cocaine for an extended period suddenly stops using cocaine. Even first-time users of cocaine can experience the crash, depending on dosage and length of use. The withdrawal symptoms experienced can last between nine hours and four days. The withdrawal symptoms can include:

- agitation
- depression
- anxiety
- anorexia
- intense craving for cocaine
- uncontrollable appetite
- insomnia or prolonged but disturbed sleep
- extreme fatigue and exhaustion.

Withdrawal

The withdrawal phase may last up to ten weeks from the end of the crash. During this early stage of this phase, there is a gradual return to normal sleep and mood, often accompanied by a low level of cocaine craving and low level of anxiety. This may last from one to ten weeks. In the middle phase of the withdrawal, severe cravings for cocaine are experienced. This may be reinforced by cues such as cocaine paraphernalia or other environmental cues which may lead to intense craving. This may induce physiological responses such as runny nose, taste sensations and fidgetiness. Other withdrawal symptoms during this phase include:

- low energy
- anhedonia (inability to feel pleasure)

- anxiety
- angry outbursts.

Extinction

The final phase of cocaine withdrawal is called the extinction phase. This may for some cocaine users last for at least six months and for others indefinitely. Some cocaine users may experience craving when faced with strong cues. This is in response to people, places or objects that are conditioned cues and provoke memories of taking the drug. These cravings may surface months or years after cocaine use has stopped. The person returns to a normal mood but still feels an occasional craving for cocaine. Relapse is high because of continued cravings.

ACTIVITY 10.4

There is only one correct answer to the following multiple-choice questions

What plant does cocaine come from?
a.   Coca leaves
b.   Cola leaves
c.   Poppy leaves
d.   Caffeine leaves

Which one of the following countries produces coca?
a.   Mexico
b.   Bolivia
c.   Argentina
d.   Brazil

The trend in cocaine use in Europe as reported by EMCDA has
a.   Decreased
b.   Remained steady
c.   Been the same as heroin
d.   Increased

The traditional method of coca consumption to alleviate altitude sickness is
a.   Ingesting
b.   Injecting
c.   Smoking
d.   Mate de coca

Cocaine
a.   Comes from coca leaves
b.   Is made synthetically
c.   Comes from coca leaves or is made synthetically
d.   None of the above

Forms of cocaine include
a.   Crack and cocaine hydrochloride
b.   Cannabis and crack
c.   Heroin and cocaine
d.   Sulphate and freebase

The therapeutic use of cocaine is as
a.   Anaesthetic
b.   Stimulant
c.   Appetite suppressant
d.   Depressant

The popularity of crack cocaine is known as the
a.   Cocaine epidemic
b.   Crack epidemic
c.   Speedball endemic
d.   Drug epidemic

What is the route of administration of cocaine?
a.   Injecting
b.   Snorting
c.   Smoking
d.   All of the above

Snorting cocaine produces effects
a.   Within 3 to 5 minutes
b.   Within 5 to 8 minutes
c.   Within 8 to 10 minutes
d.   Within 10 to 20 minutes

Crack is
a.   A form of cocaine
b.   Chemically altered cocaine
c.   Deadlier than other forms of cocaine
d.   All of the above

Which is a long-term effect of cocaine?
a.   Seizures
b.   Increased heart rate
c.   Blood vessel constriction
d.   Insomnia

A 'Speedball' is a combination of which two drugs?
a.   LSD and heroin
b.   Alcohol and cocaine
c.   Cocaine and heroin
d.   Amphetamines and alcohol

Which is a long-term effect of crack?
a. Cardiac arrest
b. Hallucinations
c. Seizures
d. Paranoia

Cocaine and crack users report being 'hooked' after
a. One use
b. Five uses
c. Never
d. Using continually for one week

Freebasing is
a. The sale price of the drug
b. A method of cutting the drug
c. A method of taking cocaine or crack
d. Mixing cocaine and crack

What are some of the effects of cocaine?
a. Euphoria
b. Arousal
c. Anxiety
d. All of the above

The active psychoactive substance in the coca plant is
a. Cocoa
b. Crack
c. Cocaine
d. All the above

Cocaine's mechanism of action works by
a. Blocking the chemical in the brain
b. Blocking the re-uptake of dopamine
c. Breaking down the blood barrier
d. None of the above

The immediate effect of crack has an influence on the
a. Respiratory system
b. Circulatory system
c. Excretory system
d. Central nervous system

One of the effects of crack cocaine is the feeling of euphoria. How long does this effect last?
a. 15 minutes
b. 30 minutes
c. 60 minutes
d. 180 minutes

ACTIVITY 10.5

- Briefly describe the mechanism of action of cocaine.
- What are the adverse effects of cocaine?
- What are the features of the withdrawal syndrome of cocaine?
- Describe the stages in cocaine withdrawal.

KHAT

Khat (also spelled quat, qat and kat) acts as a social lubricant in mostly Muslim countries, with links to (especially) the Yemen, Ethiopia or Somalia. It is an evergreen shrub (Catha edulis) that grows in parts of East Africa and the Middle East. It is transported to the UK by air and is generally preferred fresh as the leaves from the plant are most powerful when fresh. The users usually chew about two ounces of leaves or stems for a number of hours, swallowing the juice. Dryness of the mouth is caused by the juice so large amounts of liquid are also drunk. Effects start about a quarter of an hour into chewing and finish up to two hours after stopping. The main active substances in khat are cathine and cathinone: these are closely related to amphetamine but are of less potency. The prevalence data on the use of Khat range from 34% to 67% of the Somali community who identify themselves as current users of khat (ACMD 2005). Khat is used also by the small Yemeni communities and communities from the horn of Africa. Khat users appear to have very low levels of other drug or alcohol use. There is no evidence that khat use is a gateway to the use of other stimulant drugs, although there is, however, high associated tobacco use (ACMD 2005).

Legal status

The khat plant is legal, but its active ingredients cathinone and cathine are class C.

Sought-after effects

Khat generally produces talkativeness, mild euphoria and hallucinations. In many countries it has social and cultural significance and it is mostly used as a social stimulant on festive occasions.

Adverse effects

Effects start after approximately 30 minutes with stimulation and talkativeness. This is followed by a relaxed and introspective state that can last up to five hours, often with insomnia. This is then followed by periods of lethargy, irritability and general hangover. Dependence can develop and heavy use can be problematic. Nausea, vomiting, mouth ulcers, abdominal pain, headache, palpitations, increased aggression and hallucinations can occur. Continued use can lead to cycles of sleeplessness and irritability and can in

Table 10.4 Khat: risks to physical and psychological health

Risks to physical health	Risks to psychological health
• Increase in blood pressure • Risk factor for oral cancer • Risk factor for myocardial infarction • Affects reproductive heath • Delivery of low-birth-weight babies • Lower sperm motility • Increase libido • Decrease libido (Chronic use) • Residual pesticides	• Low mood • Dependence • ? Psychosis

the longer term lead to psychiatric problems such as paranoia and possibly psychosis. Digestive problems such as constipation and stomach ulcers have frequently been reported to affect regular users. Khat is also often used with tobacco and hypno-sedatives such as benzodiazepines: this brings additional associated risks. The physical and psychological risk associated with khat are presented in Table 10.4.

ACTIVITY 10.6

Are the statements below true or false?

	True	False
Khat is a depressant		
The main active substances in khat are cathine and cathinone		
Effects start about a quarter of an hour into chewing and finish up to two hours after stopping		
The khat plant is illegal in the UK		
Khat generally produces talkativeness, mild euphoria and hallucinations		
The onset of the effect of khat is immediate		

- List the physical risks associated with khat
- List the psychological risks associated with khat

KEY POINTS

- Amphetamine, dextroamphetamine and methamphetamine are collectively referred to as amphetamines.
- The increase of dopamine is the primary mechanism for its behavioural-stimulant effects with intense pleasure and increased energy.

- Chronic users of amphetamines typically snort or resort to drug injection to experience the full intensity effects of the drug.
- Injecting cocaine has the added risks of infection and vein damage, and higher risk of overdose.
- Many amphetamine users will repeat the amphetamine cycle by taking more of the drug during the withdrawal.
- Cocaine is the second most commonly used illicit drug in Europe, after cannabis.
- Smoking cocaine base is a more potent way of administration than snorting and produces a 'rush' similar to the experience of injecting cocaine.
- Many cocaine and crack users also take other drugs, including heroin. Alcohol is often mixed with cocaine to produce cocaethylene, which is highly toxic.
- Cocaine users are polydrug users, often consuming cocaine with alcohol and tobacco, with other illicit drugs such as other stimulants and cannabis, or with heroin.
- During the withdrawal symptoms of cocaine, such as craving, the user experiences a very strong need for the drug to get the level of dopamine back up.
- The intensity and the duration of the effects of cocaine are influenced by the route of administration.
- Cocaine users may also experience paranoia, auditory hallucination or a full-blown cocaine psychosis.
- Withdrawal leads to strong craving and drug-seeking behaviour followed by a withdrawal syndrome.
- Cocaine withdrawal generally occurs in three phases: the 'crash', the 'withdrawal' and the 'extinction'.
- Khat generally produces talkativeness, mild euphoria and hallucinations.
- Khat users appear to have very low levels of other drug or alcohol use.
- Nausea, vomiting, mouth ulcers abdominal pain, headache, palpitations, increased aggression and hallucinations can occur.

REFERENCES

Advisory Council on the Misuse of Drugs (ACMD) (2005) *Khat (Qat): Assessment of Risk to the Individual and Communities in the UK.* London: Home Office.

Clement, B.A., Goff, E.A.B., Christina, M., Forbes, T. and David, A. (1997) Toxic amines and alkaloids from Acacia berlandieri. *Phytochemistry,* 46, 2: 249–54.

Clement, B.A., Goff, E.A.B., Christina, M., Forbes, T. and David A. (1998) Toxic amines and alkaloids from Acacia rigidula. *Phytochemistry,* 49, 5: 1377–80.

Coffey, S.F., Dansky, B.S., Carrigan, M.H. and Brady, K.T. (2000) Acute and protracted cocaine abstinence in an outpatient population: a prospective study of mood, sleep and withdrawal symptoms. *Drug and Alcohol Dependence,* 59, 3: 277–86.

Coffey, S.F., Saladin, M.E., Drobes, D.J., Brady, K.T., Dansky, B.S. and Kilpatrick, D.G. (2002) Trauma and substance cue reactivity in individuals with comorbid posttraumatic stress disorder and cocaine or alcohol dependence. *Drug and Alcohol Dependence,* 65: 115–27.

Druglink (2007) *Average UK National Street Drug Price.* London: Druglink. http://www.drugscope.org.uk.

EMCDDA Statistical Bulletin (2007) European Monitoring Centre for Drugs and Drug Addiction (EMCDDA). *Cocaine and Crack Cocaine: A Growing Public Health Issue.* Available at http://stats06.emcdda.europa.eu/en/homeen.html (accessed 21 June 2007).

National Institute on Drug Abuse (1998) *Mind Over Matter: Stimulants*. Bethesda, MD: NIDA, NIH. DHHS, NIH Publication No. 03-3857. Printed 1997, reprinted 1998, 2000, 2003. http://teens.drugabuse.gov/mom/mom_stim6.asp. Retrieved May 2008.

National Institute on Drug Abuse (2002) *NIDA Research Report – Methamphetamine Abuse and Addiction*. NIH Publication No. 02-4210. http://www.drugabuse.gov/ResearchReports/methamph/methamph.html (accessed 21 June 2007).

Roe, S. and Man, L. (2006) *Drug Misuse Declared: Findings from the 2005/06 British Crime Survey – England and Wales*. London: Home Office. Available at: www.homeoffice.gov.uk/rds/pdfs06/hosb15 (accessed 26 June 2007).

CHAPTER 11

HALLUCINOGENS

OBJECTIVES

- State the meaning of hallucinogens.

- Understand the legal aspects of hallucinogens.

- Describe the physiological effects of LSD, ecstasy, GHB, ketamine, psilocybin and PCP.

- Describe the psychological effects of LSD, ecstasy, GHB, ketamine, psilocybin and PCP.

- List the withdrawal symptoms of ecstasy.

- Describe the risks factors in using ecstasy.

- List the withdrawal symptoms of GHB.

ACTIVITY 11.1

Please choose one answer for the following multiple-choice questions. There is only one correct answer

Hallucinogens refer to
a.   A group of drugs causing hyperactivity
b.   A group of drugs causing hallucinogenic experiences

c.   A group of synthetic drugs
d.   A group of natural drugs

The following drugs are hallucinogens
a.   LSD, alcohol, cannabis, PCP
b.   LSD, alcohol, PCP, GHB
c.   LSD, PCP, GHB, ecstasy
d.   LSD, PCP, heroin, cocaine

Most hallucinogenic drugs
a.   Cause hallucinations
b.   Do not cause hallucinations
c.   Cause changes in mood or thoughts
d.   Do not change mood or thoughts

The effects of LSD start
a.   About 10 minutes after taking it
b.   About 20 minutes after taking it
c.   About 30 minutes after taking it
d.   Immediately

Acid, microdots, dots, tabs or trips are slang names for
a.   PCP
b.   GHB
c.   Ecstasy
d.   LSD

LSD is associated with
a.   Physical dependence
b.   Withdrawal symptoms
c.   Dependence
d.   Tolerance

Ecstasy refers to which of the following drugs?
a.   Alcohol
b.   Cocaine
c.   MDMA
d.   Steroids

Ecstasy tablets contain
a.   MDMA
b.   Amphetamine
c.   Caffeine
d.   Heroin

The effects of ecstasy start
a.   About 10 minutes after taking it
b.   About 20 minutes after taking it

c. About 30 minutes after taking it
d. Immediately

Which of the following are considered 'club drugs'?
a. Ecstasy
b. Rohypnol
c. Ketamine
d. All of the above

The effects of ecstasy may cause
a. Physical dependence
b. Psychological dependence
c. No dependence
d. Both physical and psychological dependence

GHB (Gammahydroxybutyrate) is a
a. Class A drug
b. Class B drug
c. Class C drug
d. Class D drug

The effects of GHB start
a. Anything from 10 to 30 minutes after taking it
b. Anything from 10 to 60 minutes after taking it
c. Anything from 30 to 60 minutes after taking it
d. Immediately

In terms of physical and social harm, GHB
a. Is more dangerous than alcohol
b. Is less dangerous than alcohol
c. Is equally dangerous as alcohol
d. Causes no harm

Regular use of GHB can cause
a. Physical dependence
b. Psychological dependence
c. No dependence
d. Both physical and psychological dependence

Special K is the street name for
a. GHB
b. PCP
c. Ketamine
d. Cannabis

The effects of injecting ketamine start
a. Anything from 10 to 15 minutes after taking it
b. Anything from 30 to 60 minutes after taking it

c.   Anything from 30 to 40 minutes after taking it
d.   Immediately

Psilocybin is known as
a.   Angel dust
b.   PCP
c.   Magic mushrooms
d.   Special K

The effects of injecting psilocybin start
a.   Anything from 10 to 20 minutes after taking it
b.   Anything from 30 to 50 minutes after taking it
c.   Anything from 50 to 60 minutes after taking it
d.   Immediately

Phencyclidine (PCP) is known as
a.   Angel dust
b.   PCP
c.   Magic mushrooms
d.   Special K

Regular use of PCP can cause
a.   Physical dependence
b.   Psychological dependence
c.   No dependence
d.   Both physical and psychological dependence

This chapter deals with a group of substances known as hallucinogens or hallucinogenic drugs. The term hallucinogens refers to a diverse group of drugs, natural or synthetic, that induce an alteration in perception, thought, emotion and consciousness. Some hallucinogens occur naturally, in trees, vines, seeds, fungi and leaves, and others are manufactured in laboratories. Lysergic acid diethylamide, known as LSD, is derived from an alkaloid (ergot) which is a synthetic. Other hallucinogens include psilocybin (liberty cap mushrooms), Amanita muscaria (fly agaric mushrooms), morning glory seeds and mescaline (peyote cactus), PCP (phencyclidine), ketamine, ecstasy (MDMA and related drugs, in high doses) and cannabis (in high quantities).

Unlike other psychoactive substances, hallucinogens induce subjective experiences that are qualitatively different from those experienced in normal consciousness. Hallucinogens are a diverse group of substances that have different chemical structures, mechanisms of action and adverse effects. Most hallucinogenic drugs do not consistently cause hallucinations but are more likely to cause a modification of normal perception with changes in mood or in thought than actual hallucinations. Some less common drugs, such as dimethyltryptamine and atropine, may cause hallucinations in the proper sense.

The widespread experimentation with LSD and other hallucinogens in the sub-culture of the 1960s resurfaced in the late 1980s. Experimentation with the drug in recent times has been associated with the advent of the rave scene or club drugs. In England and Wales, the 2006/7 British Crime Survey (Roe and Man 2006) indicates that 1.8% of 16- to 59-year-olds reported using ecstasy, and the use of hallucinogens (LSD and magic mushrooms) in the last year was reported by 0.7%. Use of ketamine in the past year was reported by 0.3%. When looking at specific types of drugs, it is estimated that just over 550,000 people used ecstasy in the last year. Over the past decade, the trends in the use of hallucinogens among 16- to 59-year-olds show an overall decrease. Among young people (16–24 years old), it is estimated that 4.8% had used ecstasy; use of amphetamines at 3.5%, use of hallucinogens at 2.1% and use of ketamine at 0.8% in the past year was reported by 16- to 24-year-olds. Since 1998 there has been a decrease in the use of magic mushrooms amongst 16- to 24-year-olds.

MECHANISM OF ACTION

The exact mechanism of action of hallucinogens remains unclear but there is some evidence that hallucinogens bind with one type of serotonin receptor (5-HT_2) in the brain. Serotonin is involved in the control of mood, hunger, body temperature, sexual behaviour, muscle control and sensory perception. The binding of a hallucinogenic compound with serotonin receptors induces the blockage of serotonin from those receptor sites. This results in the increase of serotonin in the nervous system, producing a distortion of the senses of sight, sound, and touch, disorientation in time and space, and alterations of mood. LSD appears to enhance the effect of several neurotransmitters such as serotonin, dopamine, and norepinephrine which may contribute to the hallucinogenic effect of the drug. Ecstasy (MDMA) mechanism of action also involves the serotonin and dopamine systems and other neurochemical transmitters.

LSD (LYSERGIC ACID DIETHYLAMIDE)

Lysergic acid diethylamide, known as LSD, is derived from an alkaloid (ergot), a fungus that grows on rye and other grains. In pure state, LSD is an odourless, colourless, and tasteless powder. LSD usually comes in the form of liquid, tablets or capsules, squares of gelatine or blotting paper. The blotting paper is divided into small decorated squares, with each square representing one dose. LSD can be swallowed, sniffed, injected or smoked. LSD is taken by mouth in extremely small doses (50–150 micrograms) which are usually on small paper squares. The effects tend to start about half an hour after taking it and last up to 12 hours or sometimes even longer, depending on the dosage. LSD is also known as acid, microdots, dots, tabs or trips.

Legal status

LSD is a class A controlled drug.

Therapeutic use

In ancient cultures the plants and the extracts were used during religious rituals and witchcraft, and were employed as intoxicants in medicine. Hallucinogens have been investigated as potential therapeutic agents in treating several disorders including depression, obsessive-compulsive behaviour, alcohol dependence and opiate addiction. In recent times, LSD has been used occasionally in psychotherapy.

Sought-after effects

The effects of the drug are dependent on the user's prior experience, mood, expectations and setting. It is much stronger in effect than psychedelic mushrooms or mescaline. A moderate dose will produce profound alteration in mood, sensation and consciousness, intensified sensory experiences and perceptual distortions. Confusion of time, space, body image and boundaries can occur with what have been called the blending of sight and sound. The user may 'see' sounds and 'hear' colours. Mushrooms are similar to LSD, but the trip is often milder and shorter.

Adverse effects

The drug may cause panic, confusion, impulsive behaviour and unpleasant illusions (bad trip) and flashbacks, and may precipitate psychotic reactions. In a 'bad trip', the user may experience strong feelings of anxiety, paranoia, panic or fear. The hallucinations can be unpleasant, such as feeling as if insects are crawling on the skin. A lack of control and ability to stop the experience can cause panic. LSD users often underestimate the length of a trip and feel exhausted physically and psychologically after a 12–36 hour experience. LSD can produce physiological effects including elevated heart rate, increased blood pressure, dilated pupils, higher body temperature, sweating, loss of appetite, sleeplessness, dry mouth and tremors. Sensations may seem to 'cross over' for the user, giving the feeling of hearing colours and seeing sounds. If taken in a large enough doses, the drug produces delusions and visual hallucinations. Feelings of panic, paranoia and fear can lead to risky behaviour that can cause injury, such as running across a busy street or jumping out of a window. Although cases of accidental death due to impaired judgement have occurred, this is extremely rare. The negative and unpleasant effects are much more likely to arise if the user is in a negative mood or situation, or mixes hallucinogens with other drugs or alcohol. There is a strong risk to precipitate relapse in those already susceptible to schizophrenia. Table 11.1 presents the physical and psychological effects of LSD.

Tolerance, dependence and withdrawal

Frequent, repeated doses of LSD are unusual and therefore tolerance is not commonly seen. Tolerance to the euphoric and psychedelic effects of hallucinogens develops after 3–4 daily doses. Any tolerance developed quickly goes away once regular use is stopped. There is no physical dependence or withdrawal symptoms associated with recreational

Table 11.1 Physical and psychological effects of LSD

Physical effects	Psychological effects
Short-term effects	
• Dilated pupils	• Heightened senses (sight, sound and touch)
• Lowered body temperature	• Distorted perception of depth, time, and the size and
• Nausea	shape of objects
• Vomiting	• Hallucinations (stationary objects appear to be moving)
• Profuse sweating	• Anxiety
• Rapid heart rate	• Depression
• Hypertension	• Dizziness
• Convulsions	• Disorientation
• Loss of appetite	• Paranoia
• Sleeplessness	• Panic
• Impaired coordination	
• Risk of accidents	
Long-term effects	
• ? Organic brain damage	• Tolerance
	• Flashbacks
	• Disorientation
	• Anxiety
	• Distress
	• Prolonged depression
	• Increased delusions
	• Psychosis

use of LSD. LSD is not considered an addictive drug since it does not produce compulsive drug-seeking behaviour.

ACTIVITY 11.2

- What is LSD (lysergic acid diethylamide)?
- What are the sought-after effects of LSD?
- What are the physiological effects of LSD?
- What are the psychological effects of LSD?

ECSTASY (MDMA)

3,4-methylenedioxymethamphetamine is better known as ecstasy (E, Adam, XTC, doves, 'Dennis the Menace', 'rhubarb and custard', 'New Yorkers', 'love doves', 'disco burgers', E, pills, brownies, Mitsubishis, Rolexes, dolphins, or 'Phase 4'). It is a synthetic, psychoactive drug with hallucinogenic and amphetamine-like properties. It is often categorised as a hallucinogen, as in some respects it resembles LSD. MDMA is manufactured from the components of methylamphetamine and safrole (a nutmeg derivative). It usually comes in tablet form, in powder or in capsules with different shapes and colours. Swallowing is the most common way that ecstasy is taken. Ecstasy tablets are also crushed and snorted or taken in a liquid form through injection.

The main use of ecstasy has been as a 'dance' or 'raves culture' drug. In the early 1990s it was given much publicity in the media, supposedly emphasising the dangers of the drug. A strong youth culture developed involving ecstasy, 'house music' and all-night 'raves'. The effects of ecstasy take about half an hour to kick in and tend to last between three and six hours, followed by a gradual comedown. The strength and contents of ecstasy tablets cannot be known accurately as all ecstasy available on the street is produced in unregulated black market laboratories. Ecstasy is sometimes cut with amphetamines, caffeine and other substances. Less than 1% remains in the body after 48 hours and this amount will not be detectable in blood or urine samples. However, ecstasy users may test positive for amphetamines in the standard drug test.

A 2007 street drug trends survey (Drugscope 2007) reported that the bottom has fallen out of the ecstasy pill market with the average street price of a pill now as low as £2.40, with pills most commonly sold in batches of three to five for £10. Pills sold as 'ecstasy' often contain no MDMA and are instead made from an amphetamine ('speed') base. In response more drug users are willing to pay a premium for crystal or powder MDMA at an average price of £38 per gram.

Legal status

Ecstasy is a class A drug.

Therapeutic use

Ecstasy was first manufactured in Germany in 1914 as an appetite suppressant, although it was never actually marketed for this purpose. It has been used in a limited way as an adjunct to various types of psychotherapy in order to facilitate the therapeutic process. In addition, the drug has also been used to some extent with terminally ill patients in order to help them come to terms with their situation and to communicate or ventilate their feelings more easily.

Sought-after effects

The effects start after about 20–60 minutes after use and can last several hours. Users describe ecstasy as making them empathetic, producing a temporary state of openness with an enhanced perception of colours and sound. The user experiences euphoric feelings, and feelings of empathy, relaxation and meaningfulness. Tactile sensations are enhanced for some users, making physical contact with others more pleasurable. The user experiences feelings of euphoria which plateau for two to three hours before wearing off. Ecstasy can also cause mild hallucinogenic effects.

Effects

There are usually three phases associated with ecstasy use. There is the 'coming up' effect when the user experiences a sudden amphetamine-like rush. This rush is accompanied by mild nausea. It is immediately followed by the plateau of intoxication where the user may feel good, happy and relaxed. The final phase is the 'coming down' where the user may feel physically exhausted, depressed, irritable. The effects of ecstasy usually begin within 20 minutes of taking the drug, and may last up to six hours. The physiological effects can develop that include dilated pupils, a tingling feeling, tightening of the jaw muscles, raised body temperature, increased heart rate, muscle tension, involuntary teeth clenching, nausea, blurred vision, rapid eye movement, faintness and chills or sweating. The psychological effects can include anxiety, panic attacks, depression, sleep problems, drug craving, confused episodes and paranoid or psychotic states. The physiological and psychological effects of ecstasy are presented in Table 11.2.

Table 11.2 Immediate and adverse effects of ecstasy

Physiological	Psychological
Immediate effects	
• Increased physical energy	• Relaxation
• Increased heart rate	• Euphoria
• Increased body temperature	• Empathy
• Increased blood pressure	• Increase in emotion energy
• Nausea	• Increased ability to interact with others
• Sweating	• Increased confidence
• Ataxia	• Heightened sensitivity
• Involuntary jaw clenching	• Increased responsiveness to touch
• Teeth-grinding	• Changes in perception
• Loss of appetite	• Feelings of insight
• Dilated pupils	• Anxiety
	• Short-term memory lapses
Adverse effects	
• Decreased ability to perform tasks	• Increased restlessness
• Tachycardia	• Confusion
• Hyperthermia	• Depression
• Hyponatremia	• Sleep problems
• Nystagmus	• Attentional dysfunction
• Convulsions	• Panic attacks
• Vomiting	• Floating sensations
• Motor rituals	• Impairment of cognitive functions
• Headaches	• Poor memory recall
	• Increased anxiety
	• Depressed mood
	• Depersonalisation
	• Irrational or bizarre behaviour
	• Hallucinations
	• Catatonic stupor

Adverse effects

The adverse effects of ecstasy include tiredness, confusion, anxiety and depression. With higher doses the user can feel anxious and confused, and co-ordination can be impaired, making driving or similar activity very dangerous. If ecstasy is taken regularly over the period of a few days the user can experience panic attacks, temporary paranoia or insomnia. The use of this particular drug may be more hazardous with individuals having heart conditions, hypertension, blood clotting disorders, a history of seizures or any type of psychiatric disorder. Ecstasy should not be used in combination with amphetamines, mono amine oxidase inhibitors, alcohol or diuretics. Recent research findings also link MDMA use to long-term damage to those parts of the brain critical to thought and memory. It is believed that the drug causes damage to the neurons that use the chemical serotonin to communicate with other neurons.

Overdose and death

Overdose from ecstasy can occur. It is usually characterised by very high body temperature and blood pressure, hallucinations and an elevated heartbeat. This is especially dangerous for those who have an existing heart condition or breathing problems, and for people with depression or other psychological disorder. Sudden death through overheating, dehydration, heavy alcohol consumption or drinking too much water has led to collapse, convulsions or renal failure. However, drinking too much water in an attempt to stay 'safe' is more dangerous. Some, often inexperienced, users have died after drinking as much water (dilutional hyponatremia) as they physically could. The excess water causes the brain to swell inside the skull, which puts pressure on the brain stem and leads to coma and death. Because of these ill-effects, users are advised to wear light, loose clothing, and to drink plenty of non-alcoholic fluids as well as to stop dancing when feeling exhausted in order to help reduce the possible complications of the drug. There is always a danger of the drug being contaminated by other substances such as amphetamine mixtures, LSD and ketamine. About ten ecstasy-related deaths have been reported in the UK each year for the past several years. Although the number of deaths is relatively low compared to drugs such as heroin or alcohol, there is still cause for concern.

Tolerance and dependence

Some people may develop tolerance to the effects of ecstasy: using larger amounts will increase the severity of undesirable effects, rather than increase the pleasurable effects. There is evidence that people can become psychologically dependent on ecstasy and it can be very difficult for them to stop or decrease their use. At present, there is no conclusive evidence that people can become physically dependent on ecstasy.

ACTIVITY 11.3

- What is ecstasy (MDMA)?
- What are the sought-after effects of ecstasy?
- What are the physiological effects of ecstasy?
- What are the psychological effects of ecstasy?
- What are the risks associated with ecstasy?

GHB

GHB (gammahydroxybutyrate), also known as liquid ecstasy, GBL, BDO, Blue Nitro, Midnight Blue, Renew Trient, Reviarent, SomatoPro, Serenity, Enliven, is a central nervous depressant. It is a colourless liquid, with a slightly salty taste. GHB is also produced as a result of fermentation and so is found in small quantities in some beers and wines, particularly fruit wines, with limited effect. The drug is usually sold in small 30 ml plastic containers (approximately £15) and consumed in capfuls. It is sometimes sold as 'liquid ecstasy', but is not related to ecstasy. In the last few years, GHB has become popular on the club scene, with users enjoying an alcohol-like high with potent positive sexual effects. The drug can take anything from ten minutes to an hour to take effect and the effects can last from one and a half to three hours or even longer. GHB causes intoxication resembling alcohol or ketamine intoxication and can lead to respiratory depression and death, especially when combined with alcohol. The drug has been referred to in the media as a date rape drug, in much the same way as alcohol and Rohypnol. As it is colourless and odourless, GHB has been described as 'very easy to add to drinks' and been used in many cases of drug-related sexual assault. GHB is also used by body-builders and athletes. GHB is difficult to trace because it quickly leaves the body and may be difficult to detect.

A Science and Technology Committee report found the use of GHB to be less dangerous than tobacco and alcohol in social harms, physical harm and addiction (Stationery Office 2006).

Legal status

As of 30 June 2003, GHB, or gammahydroxybutyrate, is categorised as a class C drug in the UK, with dealers facing up to five years in jail and possession punishable by up to two years

Therapeutic use

GHB has been used historically as a general anaesthetic, as a hypnotic in the treatment of insomnia, to treat depression and to improve athletic performance. In Italy, GHB is used in the treatment of acute alcohol withdrawal and medium- to long-term detoxification.

Sought-after effects

GHB affects the release of dopamine in the brain, causing effects ranging from relaxation to sleep at low doses. A small capful can make you feel uninhibited, exhilarated, relaxed and feeling good with the effects lasting as long as a day, although it is difficult to give a clear 'safe' dose, as the concentration of the liquid will vary. Regular alcohol users break down GHB faster than people who do not drink alcohol.

Adverse effects

Adverse effects with the dosage increase can lead to disorientation, nausea, confusion, a numbing of the muscles or muscle spasms and vomiting. At high doses, convulsions, coma and respiratory collapse can occur. The drug also lowers blood pressure and in some cases people find breathing difficult. Combining GHB and any other sedative, especially alcohol, is extremely dangerous. When in a GHB sleep, convulsions can occur, often requiring emergency care. Driving or operating machinery while under the influence of GHB increases the risk of physical injury or accident to the user and to others. The long-term effects of GHB remain unknown. Table 11.3 presents the effects of GHB related to dosage.

Overdose and death

Overdosing can lead to a loss of consciousness and coma. It is not recommended that asthmatics or those with any form of respiratory or low blood pressure disorders take

Table 11.3 Doses and effects of GHB

Doses	Effects
Recreational	• Euphoria • Increased enjoyment of movement and music • Increased libido • Increased sociability • Intoxication
Higher	• Nausea • Vomiting • Desire to sleep • Giddiness • Slurred speech • Dizziness • Respiratory depression • Drowsiness • Agitation • Visual disturbances • Depressed breathing • Amnesia • Convulsions • Unconsciousness • Death

this drug. Most deaths have occurred when GHB was taken with alcohol or other drugs. When taken in combination with other psychoactive substances, the effects of GHB are more intense and the risk of toxic effects and overdose increases. Users may vomit while sleeping and choke.

Dependence and withdrawal

Regular use of GHB can cause physical dependence. Withdrawal effects may include insomnia, restlessness, anxiety, tremors, sweating, loss of appetite, tachycardia, chest pain, high blood pressure, muscle and bone aches, sensitivity to external stimuli and inability to sleep. The withdrawal symptoms will subside after 2–21 days depending on the doses and frequency of use. Withdrawal from GHB may cause symptoms similar to acute withdrawal from alcohol or barbiturates (delirium tremens) and can cause convulsions, paranoia and hallucinations.

ACTIVITY 11.4

- What is GHB?
- What are the sought-after effects of GHB?
- What are the adverse effects of GHB?
- What are the risks associated with GHB?
- What are the withdrawal effects of GHB?

KETAMINE

Ketamine (Special K, green, super K, vitamin K), in powder form, appears similar to that of pharmaceutical cocaine and can act as a depressant and a hallucinogen. It is sold in either powdered or liquid form. Ketamine can be inhaled, injected or mixed in drinks. The effects are evident in about 10–15 minutes and last about one hour. It is also possible to smoke ketamine mixed with cannabis and tobacco. The drug is often mixed with other psychoactive substances such as cocaine and ecstasy to enhance their potency. With intravenous use, the onset of the effects of ketamine is immediate and reaches peak effects within minutes. Ketamine is odourless and tasteless, so it can be added to beverages without being detected, and it induces amnesia.

Ketamine is now a significant player in the UK drugs market and has widened its appeal to a larger group of partygoers. Owing to growing concern about the rising popularity as a recreational drug in Europe, Asia and North America and the misuse of the drug by medical personnel in a number of countries, the World Health Organization (WHO) Expert Committee on Drug Dependence in its thirty-third report (2003) recommended research into its recreational use or misuse. The British Crime Survey (Roe and Man 2006) reported that use of ketamine in the past year was reported by 0.3% of 16- to 59-year-olds in England and Wales. Use of ketamine in the past year was reported by 0.8% of 16- to 24-year-olds.

Legal status

Ketamine is a class C drug, which means that it is illegal to possess it and to supply it.

Therapeutic use

Ketamine is currently used in human anaesthesia and veterinary medicine.

Sought-after effects

Ketamine users report sensations ranging from a pleasant feeling of floating to being separated from their bodies. A giddy euphoria occurs with lower doses, often followed by bursts of anxiety or mood lability. Some ketamine users' experiences involve a terrifying feeling of almost complete sensory detachment that is likened to a near-death experience. These experiences, similar to a 'bad trip' on LSD, are called the 'K-hole'.

Adverse effects

Higher doses produce a withdrawn state (disassociation); when doses are higher still, disassociation (known as a 'K-hole') can become severe with ataxia, dysarthria, muscular hypertonicity, and myoclonic jerks. With very high doses, coma and severe hypertension may occur; deaths are unusual. Acute effects generally fade after 30 minutes. Ketamine may impair memory and aggravate existing psychosis, anxiety or depression. Prolonged use may cause disorientation and gradual detachment from the world. Ketamine produces only mild respiratory depression, and cardiovascular status is usually unaffected. In addition, ketamine has both analgesic and amnesic properties and is associated with less confusion, irrationality and violent behaviour than PCP.

A few deaths have occurred through overdose, heart or respiratory failure. With large or repeat doses hallucinations occur, for example, loss of sense of time, feeling disconnected from the body, near-death experiences. Large doses can lead to loss of consciousness. In a study of ten ketamine users, there was some evidence to suggest that long-term use may result in damage to the liver or urinary bladder, or even acute renal failure (Chu *et al.* 2007). However, the researchers suspect that the damage 'may be due to other toxins that the "street ketamine" has been contaminated with'. A summary of the physiological and psychological effects of ketamine is shown in Table 11.4.

ACTIVITY 11.5

- What is ketamine?
- What are the sought-after effects of ketamine?
- What are the adverse effects of ketamine?

Table 11.4 Physiological and psychological effects of ketamine

Dose	Physiological effects	Psychological effects
Low	• Vertigo • Ataxia • Slurred speech • Slow reaction time	• Euphoria
Higher	• Analgesia • Movement difficult • Muscular hypertonicity • Hypertension • Mild respiratory depression • Coma	• Amnesia • Dissociation (K-hole) • Disorganised thinking • Speech unintelligible • Altered body image • Feeling of unreality • Visual hallucinations

PSILOCYBIN

Psilocybin ('magic mushrooms') is the hallucinogenic chemical that occurs in some mushrooms. In its pure form, psilocybin is also a white powder, but it is usually sold as dried mushrooms or in substances made from mushrooms. There is a variety of wild growing fungi native to the UK and the most common one is the liberty cap. International varieties are becoming more widely available through specialist shops and the internet. Psilocybin is from the same chemical family as LSD so its effects are similar. The mushrooms can be eaten fresh, cooked or brewed into a 'tea'. It usually takes about 30–50 mushrooms to produce a hallucinogenic experience similar to that experienced with LSD. Physical effects of psilocybin are usually experienced within 20 minutes of ingestion and can last for six hours. Other hallucinogens include Amanita muscaria (fly agaric mushrooms) and mescaline which is derived from the peyote cactus.

Legal status

Psilocybin or psilocybin-containing mushrooms are now a class A drug under the Drugs Act 2005 and 'fungus (of any kind) which contains psilocin or an ester of psilocin'. This does not include fly agaric, which is still legal.

Sought-after effect

The sought-after effects are similar to LSD, but the hallucinogenic trip is often milder and shorter.

Adverse effects

Small quantities cause relaxation and slight changes in mood but larger quantities can cause stomach pain, nausea and vomiting, shivering, a numbing of the mouth, muscle weakness, dizziness, drowsiness and panic reactions. The adverse effects can include stomach pains, sickness and diarrhoea. Higher doses cause perceptual changes, distortion of body image and hallucinations. Some people eat poisonous mushrooms thinking they are mushrooms containing psilocybin. This can be very dangerous as some poisonous mushrooms can cause death or permanent liver damage within hours of ingestion. Fly agaric mushrooms often cause nausea and stomach pain. Tolerance builds up with mushrooms in so far as the user needs to space out 'trips' to get the desired effects.

ACTIVITY 11.6

- What is psilocybin?
- What are the sought-after effects of psilocybin?
- What are the adverse effects of psilocybin?

PCP

PCP (phencyclidine), a pure white crystalline powder, is most often called 'angel dust'. It was first developed as an anaesthetic in the 1950s but discontinued for therapeutic use because of its hallucinatory effects. PCP has a distinctive bitter chemical taste and comes in a variety of tablets, capsules and coloured powders. It can be swallowed, smoked, sniffed or injected. PCP is sometimes sprinkled on cannabis, mint or parsley and smoked. PCP has been sold as mescaline THC, or other psychoactive drugs.

Legal status

PCP is a class A substance in the United Kingdom.

Sought-after effect

The user experiences alterations in thought, mood, sensory perception and changes in body awareness. However, the drug has been known to alter mood states in an unpredictable fashion. For some users, PCP in small amounts acts as a stimulant, speeding up bodily functions, and for others it acts as a depressant. A drug-taking episode may produce feelings of detachment from reality, including distortions of space, time and body image; another episode may produce hallucinations, panic, and fear.

Adverse effects

The effects of PCP use are unpredictable, can be felt within minutes of ingestion, and can last for many hours. Some users report feeling the effects of the drug for a number of days. A low to moderate amount of PCP often causes the user to feel detached, distant and estranged from the environment. Other effects include numbness, slurred speech, loss of co-ordination, rapid and involuntary eye movements, exaggerated gait, shallow and rapid breathing, increased blood pressure, elevated heart rate, and increased temperature. Nausea, blurred vision, dizziness and decreased awareness can also occur. High doses of PCP can cause convulsions, coma, hyperthermia and death. Long-term users report memory loss, difficulties with speech and thinking, depression and weight loss. Interactions with other central nervous system depressants, such as alcohol and benzodiazepines, can lead to coma and death (though death more often results from accidental injury or suicide during PCP intoxication). A temporary schizophrenic-type psychosis may last for days or weeks. Auditory hallucinations, image distortion, severe mood disorders and amnesia may also occur.

Dependence and tolerance

PCP causes the development of tolerance and strong psychological dependence. The repeated abuse can lead to craving and compulsive PCP-seeking behaviour. Recent research suggests that repeated or prolonged use of PCP can cause withdrawal syndrome when drug use is stopped. Symptoms such as memory loss and depression may persist for as long as a year after a chronic user stops taking PCP.

Table 11.5 Physiological and psychological effects of PCP

Dose	Physiological effects	Psychological effects
Low to moderate	• Shallow rapid breathing • Increased blood pressure • Elevated heart rate • Increased temperature • Sweating • Nausea • Blurred vision • Dizziness • Numbness of extremities • Loss of muscular co-ordination	• Decreased awareness • Detached, distant and estranged from surroundings
High	• Decreased blood pressure • Decreased pulse rate • Decreased respiration • Nystagmus • Drooling • Loss of balance • Dizziness • Convulsions • Hyperthermia • Coma • Death	• Disordered thinking • Disordered speech • Delusions • Delirium • Suicide • Violent behaviour • Hallucinations • Paranoia • Catatonia

ACTIVITY 11.7

- What is PCP?
- What are the sought-after effects of PCP?
- What are the adverse effects of PCP?

KEY POINTS

- Hallucinogens are a diverse group of substances that have different chemical structures, mechanisms of action and adverse effects.
- LSD is an odourless, colourless and tasteless powder. It can be swallowed, sniffed, injected or smoked.
- The effects of LSD may cause panic, confusion, impulsive behaviour and unpleasant illusions (bad trip) and flashbacks, and may precipitate psychotic reactions.
- The ecstasy user experiences euphoric feelings, and feelings of empathy, relaxation and meaningfulness.
- The adverse effects of ecstasy include tiredness, confusion, anxiety and depression.
- Some people may develop tolerance to the effects of ecstasy: using larger amounts will increase the severity of undesirable effects, rather than increase the pleasurable effects.
- GHB causes intoxication resembling alcohol or ketamine intoxication and can lead to respiratory depression and death, especially when combined with alcohol.
- At high GHB doses, convulsions, coma and respiratory collapse can occur.
- Most deaths have occurred when GHB was taken with alcohol or other drugs.
- Withdrawal from GHB may cause symptoms similar to acute withdrawal from alcohol or barbiturates (delirium tremens) and can cause convulsions, paranoia and hallucinations.
- Some ketamine users' experiences involve a terrifying feeling of almost complete sensory detachment that is likened to a near-death experience.
- With very high ketamine doses, coma and severe hypertension may occur; deaths are unusual.
- Psilocybin usually takes about 30–50 mushrooms to produce a hallucinogenic experience similar to that experienced with LSD.
- Higher psilocybin doses cause perceptual changes, distortion of body image and hallucinations.
- Some people eat poisonous mushrooms thinking they are mushrooms containing psilocybin.
- High doses of PCP can cause convulsions, coma, hyperthermia and death.
- Long-term PCP users report memory loss, difficulties with speech and thinking, depression and weight loss.
- Recent research suggests that repeated or prolonged use of PCP can cause withdrawal syndrome when drug use is stopped.

REFERENCES

Chu. P.S.K., Kwok, S.C., Lam, K.M., Chu, T.Y., Chan, S.W.H., Ma, W.K., Chui, K.L., Yiu, M.K., Chan, Y.C., Tse, M.L. and Lau, F.L. (2007) Street ketamine – associated bladder dysfunction: a report of ten cases. *Hong Kong Medical Journal*, 13: 311–13.

Drugscope (2007) *Street Drug Trends Survey 2007*. London: Drugscope. www.drugscope.org.uk.

Roe, S. and Man, L. (2006) *Drug Misuse Declared: Findings from the 2005/06 British Crime Survey – England and Wales*. London: Home Office. Available www.homeoffice.gov.uk/rds/pdfs06/hosb15 (accessed 26 June 2007).

Stationery Office (2006) *Science and Technology Committee Report Drug Classification Making a Hash of it?* Fifth Report of Session 2005–6. London: The Stationery Office.

CHAPTER 12

ANABOLIC STEROIDS, AMYL AND BUTYL NITRITE, HYPNO-SEDATIVES, VOLATILE SUBSTANCES, OVER-THE-COUNTER DRUGS, SMART AND ECO DRUGS

OBJECTIVES

- Describe the therapeutic and adverse effects of anabolic steroids.

- Describe the therapeutic and adverse effects of amyl nitrite.

- Describe the therapeutic and adverse effects of hypno-sedatives.

- Describe the short-term and long-term effects of volatile substances.

- Identify the use and misuse of over-the-counter drugs.

- Aware of the risk of using smart and eco drugs.

ANABOLIC STEROIDS

Steroids are hormones that occur naturally in the body and control the development and functioning of the reproductive system. The term 'anabolic' means to chemically build up, or muscle-building. Steroids are typically used without prescription by athletes and body-builders in order to build up muscle mass, to reduce the fatigue involved in training regimes and to improve physical appearance. A survey of 20 UK towns and cities found that the use of anabolic steroids is becoming mainstream as young men turn to the drugs to boost self-confidence and improve body image (Daly 2006). The findings from the survey indicate that drug workers are seeing young professionals, building site workers and students, aged between 16 and 25, using steroids for purely aesthetic reasons – a shortcut to the muscled, toned physique of their sporting heroes. Anabolic steroids are taken orally or injected, typically in cycles of weeks or months (referred to as 'cycling'), rather than continuously. Synthetic anabolic steroids, in particular the modified male sex hormone, testosterone, form the main market supplies. Anabolic steroids can be taken orally, by injection, or as skin patches.

Legal status

Anabolic steroids are a class C drug under the Misuse of Drugs Act 1971. They are, however, prescription-only drugs and intent to supply can be an offence under the Medicines Act. Anabolic steroid law in the United Kingdom allows body-builders to possess anabolic steroids for their own personal use.

Therapeutic use

Only two anabolic steroids are available on prescription in the UK. These are nandrolone (Durabolin) and stanozol (Stromba). Anabolic steroids have an effect on muscle building and are medically used in the treatment of thrombosis, anaemia and muscle wasting. These drugs are available legally only by prescription, to treat conditions that occur when the body produces abnormally low amounts of testosterone, such as delayed puberty and some types of impotence. They are also prescribed to treat body wasting in patients with AIDS and other diseases that result in loss of lean muscle mass. Abuse of anabolic steroids, however, can lead to serious health problems, some irreversible.

Sought-after effects

The sought-after effects of steroids are to build up muscle size and body strength to enhance performance. In addition, for some users, it is about physical appearance or body image. Anabolic steroids increase the retention of nitrogen by the body, allowing this to be used to build muscle. Steroids also aid in the production of red blood cells, which has led to the belief that they might be helpful in increasing endurance. There is, however, no empirical evidence to support this.

Adverse effects

As anabolic steroids are modelled chemically on male hormones they can have a masculinising effect. Women may have an increase in body hair, a deepened voice, enlargement of the clitoris and decrease in breast size. Men may suffer from a decrease in sperm production and testes size and development of breast tissue. Some of these effects may be permanent and therefore irreversible. The major adverse effects from misusing anabolic steroids include liver tumours and cancer, jaundice, oedema, high blood pressure, increases in LDL (bad cholesterol) and decreases in HDL (good cholesterol). Other side effects include kidney tumours, severe acne and trembling. In addition, there are some gender-specific side effects (see Table 12.1).

Table 12.1 Adverse effects of anabolic steroids

Common adverse effects	Male	Female
• Acne	• Testicular atrophy	• Growth of facial hair
• Premature baldness	• Breast development	• Deepened voice
• Headaches	• Baldness	• Changes in menstrual cycle
• Increased aggression	• Impotence	• Enlarged clitoris
• Aching joints	• Infertility	• Breast reduction
• Oedema of feet and ankles	• Enlarged prostate	• Potential damage to foetus
• High blood pressure	• Reduced sperm count	
• Reduced in HDL (good cholesterol)		
• Cardiovascular disease		
• Coronary heart disease		
• Sudden cardiac death		
• Liver disease		
• Liver cancer		
• HIV (sharing needles)		
• Aggression		
• Manic-like symptoms		
• Paranoid jealousy		
• Delusions		

The increase in aggression is welcome by athletes but sometimes the associated steroid mania has been blamed for violent crimes. Steroids misuse can also be associated with mental health problems such as manic-like symptoms and depression. They affect mood and can cause aggression and paranoia. There is a high level of injecting, but users do not engage with substance misuse services for clean equipment, bringing associated dangers of injecting with the added risk of contracting or transmitting HIV/AIDS or hepatitis. Physical dependence does not seem to be a problem but users have reported depression, delusions, lethargy and impaired judgements after stopping their use.

ACTIVITY 12.1

Please choose one correct answer to the following multiple-choice questions

Steroids are synthetic versions of
a.   Bacteria
b.   Testosterone
c.   Estrogen
d.   Hormone

Steroids are hormones that occur naturally in the body
a.   To control the digestive system
b.   To control the respiratory system
c.   To control the reproductive system
d.   To control the circulatory system

Steroids are typically used
a.   To stimulate muscle growth
b.   To increase intelligence
c.   To decrease performance
d.   To increase low confidence

Which organ is the first to be affected with heavy use of steroids?
a.   Kidneys
b.   Liver
c.   Heart
d.   Brain

Steroid abuse can cause
a.   Brain tumours
b.   Heart tumours
c.   Liver tumours
d.   Kidney tumours

Which of the following cannot steroids do?
a.   Increase muscle mass
b.   Improve visual acuity
c.   Increase stamina
d.   Increase strength

Female steroid misusers become more masculine. Among other things, their voice
a.   Deepens
b.   Gets lower
c.   Gets higher
d.   Gets hoarse

Male steroid misusers may suffer from
a.   A decrease in sperm production
b.   An increase in testes size
c.   An increase in sperm production
d.   None of the above

ACTIVITY 12.2

State whether the statements are true or false

	True	False
Anabolic steroids are classified as a class C drug under the Misuse of Drugs Act 1971		
Only two anabolic steroids are available on prescription in the UK		

Anabolic steroids can be taken orally, injected or via skin patches

The sought-after effects of steroids are to enhance physical appearance or body image

Steroids can cause hair loss, acne, breast development and low sperm production

Steroids misuse affect mood and can cause aggression and paranoia

Physical dependence is common in steroid users

ACTIVITY 12.3

- What are the physical effects of anabolic steroids?
- What are the psychological effects of anabolic steroids?

AMYL AND BUTYL NITRITE

Amyl and butyl nitrites are stimulants and are known collectively as alkyl nitrites. They are chemically related to nitrous oxide or laughing gas. They are clear, yellow, volatile and inflammable liquids with a sweet smell when fresh. When stale, the drug degenerates to a smell often described as 'smelly socks'. The vapour is inhaled through the nose or mouth from a small bottle or tube. To users, the alkyl nitrites are known as 'poppers'. In the UK, drugs such as butyl nitrite are on sale in sex shops, pubs, bars and clubs. As a street drug, butyl nitrite comes in small bottles with screw or plug tops. It is sold mainly, but not exclusively, to the gay community.

Legal status

Butyl nitrite is not classified as a drug and has no restrictions on its availability under current medicine or drug legislation. However, other laws such as the Offences Against the Persons Act 1861 may be used to restrict distribution of these substances.

Therapeutic use

Medically, amyl nitrite has been used in the treatment of angina and as an antidote to cyanide poisoning. Butyl nitrite has no therapeutic medical uses.

Sought-after effects

Once inhaled, the effects are virtually instantaneous and last for two to five minutes. The blood vessels dilate, heart rate increases and the blood rushes to the brain. Those using the drug to enhance sexual pleasure report a slow sense of time, prolonged sensation of orgasm and the prevention of premature ejaculation. Alkyl nitrites are also used for the relaxation of the anal sphincter, easing anal intercourse.

Adverse effects

There are a number of effects of using nitrites, including dizziness, relaxation of muscles, increased heart rate, low blood pressure, feeling flushed, blurred vision, headaches, vomiting, burning feeling (mouth and nose) and death due to existing heart problems or low blood pressure. Anyone with cardiovascular problems, glaucoma and anaemia should avoid using nitrites. There appear to be no serious long-term effects of the drug as it is excreted rapidly from the body in healthy individuals, but there are reports that it may suppress the immune system. Taking after drinking alcohol, cannabis or cocaine may worsen adverse effects. The immediate and long-term effects of nitrites are presented in Table 12.2.

Tolerance to the drug develops within two to three weeks of regular use, but after a few days of abstinence this tolerance is lost. There are no reports of withdrawal symptoms or psychological dependence. Overdose symptoms include nausea, vomiting, hypotension, hypoventilation, shortness of breath, and fainting. The effects set in very quickly, typically within a few seconds and disappearing soon after (within a minute).

Table 12.2 Immediate and long-term effects of amyl nitrite

Immediate effects	Long-term effects
• Dizziness	• Reduced resistance to infections
• Relaxation of muscles	• Suppressed immune system
• Increased heart rate	
• Low blood pressure	
• Feeling flushed	
• Blurred vision	
• Headaches	
• Vomiting	
• Burning feeling (mouth and nose)	
• Death (due to existing heart problems or low blood pressure)	

ACTIVITY 12.4

Please choose one correct answer for the following multiple choice questions

Amyl and butyl nitrites, known collectively as alkyl nitrites, are
a.   Depressants
b.   Hallucinogenic
c.   Stimulants
d.   Hypno-sedatives

The therapeutic use of amyl nitrite is for
a.   The treatment of angina
b.   The treatment of cancer
c.   Has no therapeutic medical uses
d.   The treatment of liver disease

The effects of amyl nitrite, once inhaled, are
a.   Slow and take about 35 minutes
b.   Immediate and last for 2–5 minutes
c.   Fast and take about 15 minutes
d.   Immediate and last for 20–25 minutes

Tolerance to the drug develops
a.   Within two to three weeks of regular use
b.   After a few days of abstinence
c.   Within four to five weeks of regular use
d.   Within two days of occasional use

HYPNO-SEDATIVES

The hypno-sedatives include both hypnotics and minor tranquillisers. The barbiturates are tuinal, membutal, sodium amytal, phenobarbitone etc.; the minor tranquillisers (benzodiazepines) are: valium (diazepam), librium, ativan, mogadon, temazepam etc. Others include heminevrin, chloral hydrate etc. The street names are downers, barbs and tranx. Hyno-sedatives are drug of misuse not only among the illicit drug population but in the population in general. Benzodiazepines are usually taken by mouth but are sometimes ground up and injected. Temazepam has again become the drug of choice to inject along with heroin, especially in Scotland.

Legal status

Benzodiazepines and barbiturates are prescription-only medicines and are class C and class B controlled drugs respectively. It is illegal to supply and supply these psychoactive substances.

Therapeutic use

Barbiturates have been used medically in anaesthesia and in the treatment of epilepsy and, rarely nowadays, insomnia. Minor tranquillisers are often prescribed for the relief of anxiety and stress.

Adverse effects

Barbiturates are depressant drugs and their effects are similar to alcohol intoxication: slurred speech, stumbling, confusion, reduction of inhibition, lowering of anxiety and tension, and impairment of concentration, judgement and performance. The common reactions from minor tranquillisers include fatigue, drowsiness and ataxia. In addition, other effects may include constipation, incontinence, urinary retention, dysarthria, blurred vision, hypotension, nausea, dry mouth, skin rash and tremor. In case of overdose, respiratory failure and death may result if these drugs are mixed with alcohol or with each other. Injecting these drugs is particularly hazardous, with increased risk of overdose, gangrene and abscesses. Barbiturates and minor tranquillisers are highly addictive and withdrawal symptoms include anxiety, headaches, cramps in the abdomen, pains in the limbs and even epileptic fits. Withdrawal of barbiturates can be dangerous and should always be medically supervised.

ACTIVITY 12.5

State whether the statements are true or false

	True	False
The hypno-sedatives include both hypnotics and major tranquillisers		
Benzodiazepines cannot be injected		
Benzodiazepines and barbiturates are not controlled drugs		
Barbiturates have been used medically in anaesthesia and in the treatment of epilepsy		
Minor tranquillisers are prescribed for psychotic disorders		
Barbiturates and minor tranquillisers are not addictive		
Withdrawal of barbiturates can be dangerous		

- What are the effects of hypno-sedative drugs?

VOLATILE SUBSTANCES

Some organic-based substances produce effects similar to alcohol or anaesthetics when their vapours are inhaled. Lighter fuel refills, glues, aerosols and typewriter correction fluids or thinners, dry cleaning fluids, de-greasing compounds etc. are products which are subjected to misuse. Deliberate inhalation of a volatile substance achieves a change in mental state. Sniffers of volatile substances heighten the desired effect by increasing the concentration of the vapour and excluding air, for example by sniffing from a bag or by placing a plastic bag over the head while inhalation takes place.

Solvent misuse seems to occur in very localised areas, for example in a particular housing estate, school or group. Many young people who sniff these substances have accidents while they are intoxicated and suffer serious health consequences. Approximately one in ten secondary schoolchildren try sniffing. Some of these go on to become heavy and frequent solvent misusers. The pattern of use includes children from all areas and social classes and both genders. There is some evidence that girls are less likely to become chronic users, and prevalence is higher in inner-city areas. The peak age of experimentation is approximately 13–14 years. A report (St George's, University of London 2007) reveals that in 2005 there were 45 deaths in the UK associated with volatile substance abuse. This is the lowest annual total recorded since 1980. In 2005, butane from all sources accounted for 36 of the 45 deaths and of these butane cigarette lighter refills formed the largest group. Deaths were generally sudden and in 2005 were three times more common in males than females. Of the 45 deaths in 2005, nine were suicides involving the inhalation of a volatile substance.

Legal status

The Intoxicating Substances Supply Act (England and Wales), passed in 1985, makes it an offence to supply a young person under 18 years with a substance which the supplier knows or has reason to believe will be used 'to achieve intoxication'. The law is mainly directed to shopkeepers but could also be applied to anyone who sells or gives a young person a sniffable product. In Scotland, the common law provides for a similar offence of 'recklessly' selling solvents to children knowing they are going to inhale them. An amendment to the Consumer Protection Act (The Cigarette Lighter Refill (Safety) Regulations 1999) made it an offence to 'supply any cigarette lighter refill canister containing butane or a substance with butane as a constituent part to any person under the age of eighteen years'.

Sought-after effects

After inhalation of volatile substances, effects are experienced within a matter of minutes. Users typically experience sensation akin to taking alcohol – being giggly and disorientated, possibly being unco-ordinated and feeling dizzy. Nausea is not uncommon.

Adverse effects

The inhaled solvent vapours are absorbed quickly through the lungs and rapidly reach the brain. Part of the effect is the reduction in oxygen intake. Respiratory rate and heart rate are depressed and repeated or deep inhalation can result in an 'overdose', causing disorientation, loss of control and unconsciousness. The experience is similar to being drunk, and experienced sniffers try to achieve a dream-like state. The effects appear quickly and disappear, usually within 45 minutes of sniffing being stopped. There may be a hangover effect with headache and poor concentration for about a day.

There is considerable risk of accidental injury or death if the individual becomes intoxicated in a hazardous environment. During vomiting, there is the risk of choking if the sniffer has been intoxicated to the point of unconsciousness. If a plastic bag has been placed over the head in order to assist inhalation of the substance, suffocation becomes a real risk. Some volatile substances such as aerosol gases and cleaning fluids can sensitise the heart, causing heart failure, especially if exertion takes place at the same time. Some gases squirted directly into the mouth can cause death from suffocation. Sniffing from small bags held to the mouth or nose has caused fewer deaths than the practice of inhaling butane and similar gases with plastic bags placed over the head.

Long-term heavy solvent abuse can result in moderate and lasting impairment of brain function, particularly affecting the control of movement. Chronic misuse of aerosols and cleaning fluids can cause renal and hepatic damage. The practice of sniffing leaded petrol can cause lead poisoning. Chronic misuse can affect general performance, along with evidence of weight loss, depression and tremor. These symptoms usually clear when sniffing ceases. Tolerance can develop but physical dependence does not constitute a significant problem. Psychological dependence occurs in susceptible youngsters with concomitant family or personality problems. These individuals are also more prone to become 'lone sniffers' instead of the usual pattern of sniffing in groups. The short-term and long-term effects are presented in Table 12.3.

Table 12.3 Effects of volatile substances

Short-term effects	Long-term effects
• Depressed respiration rate	• Damage to brain, kidneys and liver
• Depressed heart rate	• Exhaustion
• Loss of co-ordination	• Amnesia
• Disorientation	• Loss of concentration
• Loss of consciousness	• Weight loss
• Drowsy	• Depression
• Hangover	
• Accidental death	
• Heart failure	

ACTIVITY 12.6

Tick true or false for the following statements

	True	False
Volatile substances produce effects similar to alcohol or anaesthetics		
Volatile-substance misuse is the deliberate inhalation of a volatile substance to achieve a change in mental state		
Sniffers of volatile substances heighten the desired effect by decreasing the concentration of the vapour and including air		
The pattern of use includes children from all lower social classes		
The peak age of experimentation is approximately 17–18 years		
There were more deaths from volatile substances compared to other illicit psychoactive substances		
The use of volatile substances is more common in women than in men		

Anyone can buy solvents in the local shop

After inhalation of volatile substances, effects are experienced within a matter of minutes

The experience of taking volatile substances is like being drunk on alcohol

Tolerance does not develop with volatile substances

Psychological dependence may develop with volatile substances

- What are the short-term effects of volatile substances?
- What are the long-term effects of volatile substance?

OVER-THE-COUNTER DRUGS

Several medicinal preparations are available without prescription and are sold in chemists' shops and are purchased for their non-medical therapeutic effects. These are depressants such as codeine linctus, Colles Browne's mixture, Gee's Linctus and Kaolin and Morphine. The stimulants include Fenox, Mercocaine Lozenges, Sinutads, Sudafed and Do-Do. Travel sickness remedies such as Kwells containing hallucinogenic compounds are also available over the counter.

Legal status

No prescriptions are required to purchase these substances.

Therapeutic use

Many of the medical preparations are used for relief of pain, coughs, the common cold, treatment of diarrhoea and respiratory conditions.

Effects

Some of these substances are taken in large doses and often combined with other drugs to obtain the desired effects. Antihistamines may be used for their sedative effect and or mixed with methadone or heroin. The amphetamine derivatives in decongestants may be used as a stimulant, and cough linctuses and diarrhoea drugs may be used for their opiate content.

SMART AND ECO-DRUGS

Smart drugs, smart products and eco-drugs are new substances that are composed of multiple ingredients. Smart drugs are substances taken with the purpose of enhancing cognitive functions and may have stimulating, sedating or hallucinogenic effects. These drugs are often promoted as mind enhancers, mind boosters, brain boosters, intelligence boosters etc. However, some of the smart drugs are reported to enhance sexual behaviour, physical endurance, muscle power and emotional intelligence. They are promoted as safe, healthy and harmless substitutes for illicit drugs. Cognitive enhancers have been used to treat people with neurological or mental disorders, but there are a growing number of healthy individuals who use these substances in hopes of getting smarter. These substances are classified as:

- smart drugs – improving cognitive functions
- smart drinks and nutrients
- smart products – herbal mixtures and food additives which mimic the effects of illicit drugs such as ecstasy
- eco-drugs – herbs, plants and mixtures of both: some hallucinogenic or euphoric effects are linked with their use
- energising drinks: high caffeine content with guarana and taurine.

Their effects can vary considerably. Some smart products are highly stimulating, and others induce a mild form of excitement and/or euphoria. Eco-drugs, such as hallucinogenic mushrooms, kava kava and yohimbe are vegetable substances that can produce a psychotropic or physical effect. It is not always clear which laws and regulations apply to these substances. In addition, there is limited evidence about the effects of these substances and the risks involved in using them.

ACTIVITY 12.7

State whether the statements are true or false

	True	False
Codeine linctus, Colles Browne's mixture, Gee's Linctus and Kaolin and Morphine are stimulants		
Some travel sickness tablets contain hallucinogenic compounds		
Antihistamines may be used as sedatives and or mixed with methadone or heroin		
Amphetamine derivatives in decongestants may be used as a depressant		
Smart drugs are reported to enhance sexual behaviour, physical endurance, muscle power and emotional intelligence		
Eco-drugs such as kava kava and yohimbe are vegetable substances that can produce a psychotropic or physical effect		

KEY POINTS

- Anabolic steroids can be taken orally, injected, or used as skin patches.
- Anabolic steroids are a class C drug under the Misuse of Drugs Act 1971.
- The sought-after effects of steroids are to build up muscle size and body strength to enhance performance.
- Abuse of anabolic steroids can lead to serious health problems, some irreversible.
- Amyl and butyl nitrites are stimulants and are known collectively as alkyl nitrites.
- The effects of using nitrites may lead to sudden death if the individual has existing low blood pressure or heart conditions.
- Hyno-sedatives are drugs of misuse not only among the illicit drug-using population but in the population in general.
- Benzodiazepines and barbiturates are prescription-only medicines and are class C and B controlled drugs respectively.
- Barbiturates are depressant drugs and their effects are similar to alcohol intoxication.
- Some organic-based substances produce effects similar to alcohol or anaesthetics when their vapours are inhaled.
- After inhalation of volatile substances, effects are experienced within a matter of minutes.
- Of the 45 deaths in 2005 involving the inhalation of a volatile substance, nine were suicides.
- Over-the-counter drug substances are taken in large doses and often combined with other drugs to obtain the desired effects.
- The amphetamine derivatives in decongestants may be used as a stimulant; cough linctuses and diarrhoea drugs treatment may be used for their opiate content.
- Smart drugs are substances taken with the purpose of enhancing cognitive functions and may have stimulating, sedating or hallucinogenic effects.

REFERENCES

Daly, M. (2006) Street drug prices 2006. *Druglink*. September/October, 21, 5: 26.

St George's, University of London (2007) *Trends in Death Associated with Abuse of Volatile Substances 1971–2005*. London: Division of Community Health Sciences, Report No. 20.

CHAPTER 13

NICOTINE ADDICTION

OBJECTIVES

▦ Have an awareness of the government strategy in relation to tobacco smoking.

▦ Understand the mechanism of action of tobacco smoking.

▦ Describe briefly the harmful constituents of tobacco smoke.

▦ List the medical effects of nicotine addiction.

▦ List the psychological effects of nicotine addiction.

▦ Describe the withdrawal symptoms associated with nicotine addiction.

Tobacco smoking is highly addictive, and cigarettes contain the most toxic and carcinogenic substances. Smoking is the single greatest cause of preventable illness and premature death in the UK. It is responsible for one-third of cancer, one-seventh of cardiovascular disease and most chronic lung disease in adults. There are multiple impacts on non-smokers and children exposed to tobacco smoke. Tobacco is the single largest cause of social inequalities in health and aggravates poverty among poor smokers (Royal College of Physicians 2002). Smoke from cigarettes, cigars and pipes contains thousands of chemicals, including nicotine. Nicotine is found also in chewing tobacco.

In the European Union, it is estimated that tobacco consumption kills 650,000 people a year while a further 80,000 are killed by passive smoking (Europa-Eu 2007). Almost one in three smokers has tried to give up at least once in the last 12 months. The highest percentage of quit attempts (46%) has been reported in the UK. Smoking kills over 120,000 people in the UK a year – more than 13 people an hour (Callum 1998). In England, in 2001, 27% of adults aged 16 and over smoked cigarettes, 28% of men and 25% of women (Statistical Bulletin 2003). In 2001, the prevalence of cigarette smoking continued to be higher for people in manual than in non-manual socio-economic groups (32% compared with 21%). In 2001, 66% of smokers in England wanted to give up smoking.

The UK has high rates of death due to smoking compared to most other countries in the EU. Women under 65 in the UK have the worst death rate from lung cancer of all EU countries except Denmark. They also have the second worst death rate from heart disease after women in Ireland. Men under 65 in the UK have a lower than average death rate from lung cancer, but the third worst death rate from heart disease, after men in Finland and Ireland (WHO 1998). The prevalence of regular smoking in the UK is higher among girls than in most other European countries but UK smoking rates among boys are among the lowest in Europe (ACMD 2006). Smoking has been declining in many European countries but the rate of decline is now slowing. Women are now smoking as much as men in many European countries and girls often smoke more than boys (Allender *et al.* 2008). The burden of the sequelae of tobacco smoking is estimated to cost the National Health Service up to £1.7 billion every year in terms of general practitioner visits, prescriptions, treatment and operations (Buck *et al.* 1997)

STRATEGY ON TOBACCO SMOKING

The health and risk factors associated with active cigarette smoking include cancer, cardiovascular disease, respiratory diseases and problems with sexual health and maternal health. It is clear that the harmful effects of smoking are not confined to smokers: data on the health effects of cigarette smoking documents adverse effects of 'second-hand' or passive smoking. It is against this background that the government aims to improve the health of the population as a whole by increasing the length of people's lives and the number of years people spend free from illness and to narrow the health gap (Stationery Office 1999a).

In the report *Smoking Kills – A White Paper on Tobacco* (Stationery Office 1999b), the government's strategy is to see a reduction in smoking to improve health in Britain. The strategy in tackling tobacco smoking aimed to reinforce the key goals for public health improvement and had three clear objectives:

- to reduce smoking among children and young people
- to help adults – especially the most disadvantaged – to give up smoking
- to offer particular help to pregnant women who smoke.

In addition, the White Paper also sets out our proposals to help the seventh out of every ten smokers who say they want to quit, with a comprehensive NHS service to help smokers to give up with added treatment including nicotine replacement therapy. The *Department of Health Public Service Agreement* (Department of Health 2004) provides new target in tackling the underlying determinants of ill-health and health inequalities by reducing adult smoking rates to 21% or less by 2010, with a reduction in prevalence among routine, casual and manual workers to 26% or less.

LEGAL STATUS

It is illegal to sell tobacco products to anyone under the age of 18.

MECHANISM OF ACTION

Nicotine, one of the harmful constituents of tobacco smoke, is readily absorbed in the body including the lung and the systemic arterial blood. The systemic arterial blood distributes the nicotine quickly throughout the body and it takes about 10–19 seconds for nicotine to reach the brain. Nicotine has a half-life of about 10–20 minutes depending on the dosage of nicotine. Nicotine from chewing tobacco and snuff is absorbed through the oral and/or nasal mucosa, and nicotine concentrations rise more slowly with these products than with cigarettes. Research has shown how nicotine acts on the brain to produce a number of effects. Of primary importance to its addictive nature are findings that nicotine activates reward pathways – the brain circuitry that regulates feelings of pleasure. In recent years, the effects of nicotine on dopamine release from receptors have been studied extensively. Research has shown that nicotine, like cocaine, heroin, and marijuana, increases the level of the neurotransmitter dopamine, which affects the brain pathways that control reward and pleasure. These studies have shown clearly that nicotine preferentially stimulates dopamine release of the receptors in the reward circuits in the mid-brain. This reaction is similar to that seen with other drugs of misuse, and is thought to underlie the pleasurable sensations experienced by many smokers.

NICOTINE ADDICTION

There is evidence to suggest that tobacco smoking is addictive. The Report of the US Surgeon General on nicotine addiction (USDHHS 1988) states that 'the pharmacologic and behavioural processes that determine tobacco addiction are similar to those that determine addiction to drugs such as heroin and cocaine'. The World Health Organization *International Classification of Diseases* (ICD)-10 (WHO 1992) and the *Diagnostic and Statistical Manual of Mental Disorders* (DSM-IV) (American Psychiatric Association 1995) provide a suitable framework for determining the addictive or dependent nature of nicotine and smoking. Nicotine dependence is considered to be a psychoactive substance use disorder. With the application of the criteria listed in the DSM-IV or ICD-10 definitions, the features of nicotine addictions include:

- a strong desire to take the drug
- a higher priority given to drug use
- continued use despite harmful consequences
- tolerance
- withdrawal.

On present evidence, it is reasonable to conclude that nicotine delivered through tobacco smoke should be regarded as an addictive drug, and tobacco use as the means of nicotine self-administration (Royal College of Physicians 2000). Nicotine's pharmacokinetic properties also enhance its abuse potential.

Sought-after effects

Tobacco, like many of psychoactive substances, is subjectively pleasurable and the effects often produce rewarding effects in the relief of stress, and in enhancing mood and performance. The rapid absorption of nicotine from cigarette smoking, and the high arterial levels which reach the brain as a result, allow for rapid behavioural reinforcement from smoking.

HARMFUL CONSTITUENTS OF TOBACCO SMOKE

The burning of tobacco or cigarette produces different gases and chemicals and the main components include tar, nicotine and carbon dioxide.

Tar

Tar comprises four thousand different organic chemicals, including carcinogens, and on exhalation the brown sticky substance remains in the lungs causing irritation and damage. Tar tends to increase as the cigarette is burnt down, which can mean that the end of a cigarette may contain as much as twice the amount of tar as the first puffs. Smokers could be forgiven for believing that low-tar cigarettes deliver less tar to the smoker's lung. However, the actual tar exposure, and hence health risk, from smoking low-tar brands may be almost the same as for conventional cigarettes (Jarvis and Bates 1999). In fact, smokers modify their behaviour to ensure they inhale enough smoke to achieve satisfactory nicotine 'hit'. But by increasing their intake of nicotine, smokers also take in more tar. The various components of tar are cancer-initiating and cancer-accelerating. Tar in cigarette smoke paralyses the cilia in the lungs and contributes to lung diseases such as emphysema, bronchitis and lung cancer.

Nicotine

Nicotine, a main toxic component of cigarette smoking, is highly addictive. The average cigarette yields at least 8 mg to 20 mg of nicotine (depending on the brand), while a cigar may contain up to 40 mg of nicotine. However, only approximately 1 mg is actually absorbed. Although nicotine is poisonous it is not delivered rapidly enough to prove fatal to the individual as the substance is absorbed very slowly when it is inhaled. Nicotine is broken down in the liver to produce cotinine and is also metabolised in the lungs to cotinine and nicotine oxide. Cotinine has a 24-hour half-life, so you can test whether or not someone has been smoking in the past day or two by screening his or her urine for cotinine. This addictive substance acts on the nervous system and increases the heart rate and blood pressure. Nicotine can increase the stickiness of the blood platelets and in patients with established coronary heart disease it can precipitate an episode of arrhythmia (irregular heartbeat).

Carbon monoxide

Carbon monoxide is a colourless, odourless gas which is one of the harmful gases included in tobacco smoke. It rapidly enters the blood stream, and its toxicity stems from its binding to haemoglobin to form carboxyhaemoglobin. Thus, habitual smokers have a reduced amount of haemoglobin available and an increased number of red blood cells. In smokers, where the oxygen-carrying capacity of the blood is reduced, disease of the peripheral circulation can have adverse health effects.

MEDICAL EFFECTS

The addictive nature of nicotine contributes to toxic or adverse effects resulting in high morbidity and mortality rates. Smoking is the most important modifiable risk factor for coronary heart disease in young and old. The fact that smokers of whatever age, sex or ethnic group have a higher risk of heart attacks than non-smokers has been known for a quarter of a century. All these effects have also been demonstrated in those exposed to smoking. The acute effects of nicotine include headache, dizziness, insomnia, abnormal dreams, nervousness, gastrointestinal (GI) distress: dry mouth, nausea, vomiting, dyspepsia, diarrhoea and musculoskeletal symptoms. The main health concerns over chronic effects of nicotine include the following.

Cardiovascular disease

Smoking causes one out of every seven deaths from heart disease – 40,300 deaths a year in the UK from all circulatory diseases. Coronary heart disease is one of the major cause of deaths from tobacco smoking. Coronary heart disease, including acute myocardial infarction and chronic ischemic heart disease, occurs frequently in women who smoke. Both nicotine and carbon monoxide in cigarette smoke can precipitate angina attacks. Smoking is an important risk factor for stroke when it occurs in association with other risk factors such as high blood pressure. Smoking tends to increase blood cholesterol levels, hypertension and arteriosclerosis.

Respiratory diseases

Eighty three per cent of deaths from chronic obstructive lung disease, including bronchitis, are related to smoking. There is a close relationship between cigarette smoking and chronic cough and mucus hyper-secretion. The majority of patients suffering from chronic bronchitis, pulmonary emphysema and bronchial asthma are cigarette smokers.

Cancer

Smoking causes 84% of deaths from lung cancer. Smokers taking 20 or more cigarettes a day have 20 times the risk of lung cancer in comparison to non-smokers. It is estimated that at least 80% of lung cancer is associated with smoking, with some 27,000 deaths a year. Smoking also increases the risks of cancers of the mouth, pharynx, larynx, bladder, pancreas, kidney, stomach, and is associated with cancer of the cervix. Smoking is the number one cause of mouth and oesophageal cancers, and together with alcohol, causes about nine in ten cases of these cancers.

Sexual health

Tobacco smoking might impair fertility in both women and men. Smokers take longer to conceive than non-smokers. Smokers are more likely to have an early menopause than smokers. Women smokers who take oral contraceptives have approximately ten times the risk of a heart attack, stroke or other cardiovascular disease compared to non-smokers.

Effects of maternal smoking during pregnancy

Maternal smoking during pregnancy is associated with increase foetal and perinatal mortality, and low birth weight. Smoking during pregnancy hinders the blood flow to the placenta, which reduces the amount of nutrients that reach the baby. There is also evidence that women exposed to second-hand smoke during pregnancy have lighter babies. Smoking during pregnancy has also been linked to other pregnancy complications including miscarriage, stillbirth, ectopic pregnancy and cot death. Maternal smoking during pregnancy exerts a direct growth-retarding effect on the foetus and delays physical and mental development of infants. Women who continue to smoke tobacco in pregnancy have increased risk of miscarriages. The effects of smoking in pregnancy may adversely affect the child's long-term growth, behavioural characteristics and educational achievement.

PSYCHOLOGICAL EFFECTS OF TOBACCO SMOKING

The main psychological effects of tobacco smoking are summarised below. Smokers' self-reports indicate that tobacco smoking

- acts as a kind of mood regulator and increases pleasure
- acts as a relief in highly stressful situations and periods of strong emotion and reduces aggression and irritability
- increases performance and concentration on minor tasks
- increases anxiety disorders
- increases depression.

SMOKING AND DIABETES TYPE 2

A recent study (Willi *et al.* 2007) found that smoking is linked to a significantly increased risk of developing type 2 diabetes. Researchers from the University of Lausanne looked at 25 studies involving 1.2 million patients. They found that smokers had a 44% increased risk of type 2 diabetes compared with non-smokers – the risk rising with the number of cigarettes smoked. The increased risk of diabetes type 2 for those who smoked at least 20 cigarettes a day rose to 61%. For lighter smokers the risk was 29% higher than for a non-smoker. The increased risk of developing diabetes in former smokers was 23%. However, it should be noted that research did not prove that smoking contributed to the development of diabetes. Previous research has linked smoking to insulin resistance – a condition which often leads to diabetes.

HEALTH BENEFITS OF SMOKING

Some studies have discovered a reduction in the occurrence of some diseases, but all such studies stressed that the benefits of smoking did not outweigh the risks. These include risk of ulcerative colitis reduced and interferance with the development of Kaposi's sarcoma, breast cancer among women and allergic asthma. Evidence suggests that non-smokers are up to twice as likely as smokers to develop Parkinson's disease or Alzheimer's disease.

NICOTINE WITHDRAWAL SYMPTOMS

The withdrawal symptoms of nicotine dependence happen with the sudden stopping or reduction of smoking or other tobacco use. The extent of withdrawal symptoms of nicotine is dependent on the duration of smoking and number of cigarettes smoked. These symptoms may begin within a few hours after the last cigarette, quickly driving people back to tobacco use. Symptoms peak within the first few days of smoking cessation and may subside within a few weeks. For some people, however, symptoms may persist for months. While withdrawal is related to the pharmacological effects of nicotine, many behavioural factors can also affect the severity of withdrawal symptoms. For some people the times, places or situations associated with the pleasurable effects of smoking can make withdrawal or craving worse. The physiological and psychological effects of nicotine withdrawal are presented in Table 13.1.

A milder form of nicotine withdrawal, involving some or all of these symptoms, can occur when a smoker switches from regular to low-nicotine cigarettes or significantly cuts down on the number of cigarettes smoked. The symptoms of nicotine withdrawal can mimic, disguise or aggravate the symptoms of other psychological problems. Depressed smokers appear to experience more withdrawal symptoms on quitting, are less likely to be successful at quitting and are more likely to relapse.

Table 13.1 Effects of nicotine withdrawal

Physiological effects	Psychological effects
• Dryness of the mouth	• Craving
• Nausea	• Restlessness
• Sore throat	• Feeling of loneliness
• Drowsiness	• Inability to concentrate
• Cough problems	• Anger
• Headache	• Irritability
• Tiredness	• Anxiety
• Postnasal drip	• Depression
• Bleeding in the gums	
• Stomach pain	
• Constipation	
• Hunger pangs	
• Increased appetite	
• Increased weight gain	
• Insomnia	
• Tightness or stiffness in the chest	

ACTIVITY 13.1

There is only one correct answer to the following multiple-choice questions

Today, worldwide, how many smokers are there?
a.   Over 1 billion
b.   10 million
c.   100 million
d.   200 million

Which country produces the most tobacco?
a.   USA
b.   India
c.   China
d.   France

How many regular smokers are there in the UK?
a.   100,000
b.   1 million
c.   10 million
d.   13 million

In what year was the first No Smoking Day?
a.   1990
b.   1984
c.   2004
d.   2007

Which of the following substances can be found in a cigarette?
a. Tar
b. Carbon monoxide
c. Nicotine
d. All of the above

Around how many chemicals are found in cigarette smoke?
a. 1,500
b. 4,000
c. 500
d. 2,000

Which of these diseases is NOT linked to tobacco use?
a. Hypertension
b. Stomach ulcers
c. Crohn's disease
d. Cancer

Smokers are more likely to suffer from cancer. Compared to non-smokers, how much more often are they affected?
a. 2 times
b. 1.5 times
c. 3 times
d. 4 times

After quitting, a smoker will have the same risk of coronary heart disease as that of a non-smoker after
a. 1 year
b. 2 years
c. 5 years
d. 15 years

Smoking is the primary cause of
a. Emphysema
b. Degenerative disease
c. Parkinson's disease
d. Alllergic asthma

By how much does smoking reduce women's fertility?
a. 30%
b. 50%
c. 10%
d. 20%

Which cancer is twelve times more common among smokers?
a. Oral cancer
b. Lung cancer

c.   Prostate cancer
d.   Liver cancer

Heavy smokers are especially vulnerable to which of the following mood disorders?
a.   Depression
b.   Anxiety
c.   Panic disorder
d.   All of the above

Which of these gynaecological disorders is especially common among women who smoke?
a.   Infertility
b.   Early menopause
c.   Pelvic inflammation
d.   All of the above

ACTIVITY 13.2

State whether the following statements are true or false. Give reasons for your answers

	True	False
Tobacco smoking is not addictive		
Smoking can hamper the sexual function of both men and women		
Smoking causes stomach ulcers		
Smoking helps to reduce a person's stress level		
Chewing tobacco does not have health risks because it is smoke-free		
Switching to light or low-tar cigarettes will save me		
Smoking a cigar is better for you than smoking a cigarette		
Some people gain weight when they quit smoking		
Chewing tobacco does not have the same adverse effects as smoking tobacco		
Even when a smoker inhales, two-thirds of the smoke from the cigarette goes into the environment		
Children who breathe second-hand smoke are more likely to develop asthma		
When one person smokes in a room, everyone smokes because they are inhaling second-hand smoke		
Second-hand smoke is more dangerous for children than adults because children breathe faster and their lungs are not as developed		

ACTIVITY 13.3

- Why is tobacco considered an addictive psychoactive substance?
- What are the medical effects of tobacco smoking?
- What are the psychological effects of tobacco smoking?
- What are the effects of withdrawal symptoms of nicotine addiction?

KEY POINTS

- Tobacco smoking is highly addictive, and cigarettes contain the most toxic and carcinogenic substances.
- There are multiple impacts on non-smokers and children exposed to tobacco smoke.
- The UK has high rates of death due to smoking compared to most other countries in the EU.
- The government's strategy is to see a reduction in smoking among children and young people and to offer particular help to pregnant women who smoke.
- There is evidence to suggest that tobacco smoking is addictive.
- Smokers could be forgiven for believing that low-tar cigarettes deliver less tar to the smoker's lung.
- Nicotine, a main toxic component of cigarette smoking, is highly addictive.
- The health and risk factors associated with active cigarette smoking include cancer, cardiovascular disease, respiratory diseases, and problems with sexual health and maternal health.
- There is an increased risk of diabetes type 2 for those who smoke at least 20 cigarettes a day.
- Nicotine withdrawal symptoms happen with the sudden stopping or reduction of smoking or other tobacco use.
- The extent of withdrawal symptoms of nicotine is dependent on the duration of smoking and number of cigarettes smoked.

REFERENCES

ACMD (2006) *Pathways to Problems: Hazardous Use of Tobacco, Alcohol and Other Drugs by Young People in the UK and Its Implications for Policy*. London: Home Office. http://drugs.homeoffice.gov.uk/publication-search/acmd/pathways-to-problems/Pathwaystoproblems.pdf.

Allender, S., Scarborough, P., Peto, V., Rayner, M., Leal, J., Luengo-Fernandez, R. and Gray, A. (2008) *European Cardiovascular Disease Statistics 2008*. Oxford: British Heart Foundation Health Promotion Research Group, Department of Public Health, University of Oxford.

American Psychiatric Association (1995) *Diagnostic and Statistical Manual of Mental Disorders*, 4th edn. Washington: APA.

Buck, D., Godfrey, C., Parrott, S. and Raw, M. (1997) University of York Centre for Health Economics. *Cost Effectiveness of Smoking Cessation Interventions*. London: Health Education Authority.

Callum, C. (1998) *The UK Smoking Epidemic: Deaths in 1995*. London: Health Education Authority.

Department of Health (2004) *DH Public Service Agreement 2004 Improvement, Expansion and Reform – The Next 3 Years: Priorities and Planning Framework 2003–2006*. London: Department of Health.

Europa-Eu (2007) http://europa.eu (accessed 12 December 2007).

Jarvis, M. and Bates, C. (1999) *Why Low Tar Cigarettes Don't Work and How the Tobacco Industry Has Fooled the Smoking Public*, 1999 edition. http://oldash.org.uk/html/regulation/html/big-one.html (accessed 12 December 2007).

Royal College of Physicians (2000) *A Report of the Tobacco Advisory Group*. London: The Royal College of Physicians.

Royal College of Physicians (2002) *Protecting Smokers, Saving Lives*. London: The Royal College of Physicians.

Statistical Bulletin (2003) *Statistics on Smoking: England, 2003/21*. London: Department of Health.

Stationery Office (1999a) *Saving Lives: Our Healthier Nation*. CM4386. London: The Stationery Office.

Stationery Office (1999b). *Smoking Kills – A White Paper on Tobacco*. CM4177. London: The Stationery Office.

US Department of Health and Human Services (1988) *Nicotine Addiction: A Report of the Surgeon General*. Washington, DC: USDHHS.

WHO (1992) *International Statistical Classification of Diseases and Related Health Problems*, 10th revision. Geneva: World Health Organization.

WHO (1998) *Health for All. Database: European Region*. Geneva: World Health Organization.

Willi, C., Bodenmann, P., Ghali, W.A., Faris, P.D. and Cornuz, J. (2007) Active smoking and the risk of type 2 diabetes. A systematic review and meta-analysis. *Journal of the American Medical Association*, 298, 22: 2654–64.

PART 3

SPECIAL ISSUES AND POPULATIONS

CHAPTER 14

BLOOD-BORNE INFECTIONS

OBJECTIVES

■ Relate to practice the impact of stigma and discrimination towards people with blood-borne viruses.

■ Define terminology used in relation to HIV and hepatitis C and hepatitis B.

■ Describe current trends in HIV, hepatitis C and hepatitis B infection in England.

■ Relate transmission routes of HIV, hepatitis C and hepatitis B to risk behaviours.

■ Relate the risks of injecting drug use to the transmission of blood-borne viruses.

■ Describe the process of HIV pre-discussion and post-test counselling.

■ Explore effective prevention measures to minimise blood-borne virus infection.

■ Understand current treatment and vaccinations available for viral infections.

BLOOD-BORNE VIRUSES

Blood-borne viruses (BBVs) are mainly found in blood or bodily fluids. Blood-borne infection is any infection which is transmitted from the bloodstream of one individual to the bloodstream of another. Blood-borne infection is transmitted by infected blood or bloodstained body fluids coming into contact with an open lesion on the skin and by injury with a sharp object contaminated with infected blood. However, the risk of transmission of BBV depends on a number of factors, including the frequency and scale of contact with blood and body fluids, the behaviour of different persons, the type of material contact is made with and the infectious nature of person or material. BBVs, especially the human immunodeficiency virus (HIV) and hepatitis viruses B and C (HBV, HCV), pose major risks to the health of people who inject illicit drugs. This is largely because of transfer of blood through sharing of contaminated injecting equipment or of environmental contamination in injecting settings. The main BBVs are human immunodeficiency (HIV), hepatitis B and hepatitis C.

NATIONAL STRATEGY FOR SEXUAL HEALTH AND HIV

In England, in response to the HIV epidemic, a National Strategy on sexual health and HIV, 'Better prevention, better services, better sexual health' (Department of Health 2001a) was published. It aims to address the rising prevalence of sexually transmitted infections and of HIV. The broad sexual health strategy covers a wider sexual health agenda, including HIV, sexually transmitted infections (STIs) and unintended pregnancies in areas of prevention, testing, treatment and care, stigma and discrimination.
    In relation to HIV and STIs, the Strategy aims to:

- reduce the transmission of HIV and STIs
- reduce the prevalence of undiagnosed HIV and STIs
- improve health and social care for people living with HIV
- reduce the stigma associated with HIV and STIs.

The Strategy proposes providing clear information so that people can take informed decisions about preventing STIs, including HIV; ensuring there is a sound evidence base for effective local HIV/STI prevention; setting a target to reduce the number of newly acquired HIV infections; developing managed networks for HIV and sexual health services; and evaluating the benefits of more integrated sexual health services, including pilots of one-stop clinics, primary care youth services and primary care teams with a special interest in sexual health.

WHAT IS HIV?

HIV stands for Human Immunodeficiency Virus. HIV is the virus that causes AIDS (Acquired Immune Deficiency Syndrome). HIV is a retrovirus that attacks CD4 host cell receptors. CD4 receptors are found on macrophages, microglial cells and most importantly certain lymphocytes (T4 – helper cells). The HIV replicates within the cell

Table 14.1 Opportunistic infections and tumours in the late stage of AIDS

Bacterial	Viral	Fungal	Protozoal	Tumours
• Mycobacterial tuberculosis • *Mycobacterium avium* complex • *Salmonella* • *Shigella*	• *Papovaviruses* • *Cytomeglovirus* • Herpes (*Simplex* and *Zoster*)	• *Candida* • *Cryptococcus* • *Aspergillus*	• *Pneumocystis carrini* • Toxoplasmosis • *Cryptosporidium isospora*	• Kaposi's sarcoma • Non-Hodgkin's lymphoma • Cervical cancer

and then destroys it. When the immune system loses too many CD4 cells and becomes impaired, the infected person becomes susceptible to opportunistic infections and unusual tumours. AIDS is a collection of rare infections and cancers that people with HIV can develop. A person is diagnosed with AIDS when the individual has fewer than 200 CD4 cells and/or one of 21 AIDS-defining Opportunistic infections. Some of the opportunistic infections and tumours in the late stage of AIDS are presented in Table 14.1.

HIV TRANSMISSION

Blood, blood products, semen, vaginal secretions, donor organs and tissues and breast milk have been implicated in the transmission of infection. There is good evidence from studies of household contacts of infected people that HIV is not spread by close social contact. Most HIV transmission occurs:

- through unprotected vaginal or anal intercourse
- through sharing contaminated needles and syringes
- through transfusion of contaminated blood and blood products
- from mother to baby in utero, at birth or via breast feeding.

NATURE AND EXTENT OF HIV INFECTION

AIDS is among the leading causes of death globally and remains the primary cause of death in Africa. However, new data show that global HIV prevalence (the percentage of people living with HIV) has levelled off and that the number of new infections has fallen, in part as a result of the impact of HIV programmes (UNAIDS and WHO 2007). However in 2007, 33.2 million people were estimated to be living with HIV, 2.5 million people became newly infected and 2.1 million people died of AIDS.

The number of people dying from AIDS-related illnesses has declined in the last two years, partly as a result of the life-prolonging effects of antiretroviral therapy. In the UK, in 2006 there were an estimated 73,000 persons of all ages living with HIV; approximately 21,600 were unaware of their infection (Health Protection Agency 2007). Two-fifths of newly diagnosed persons in 2006 probably acquired their infection in the UK, of whom approximately two-thirds were men who have sex with men. There is concern regarding the steady increase in heterosexual HIV transmission especially in the Black ethnic minority and transmission of HIV among injecting drug users. The prevalence of HIV among injecting drug users (IDUs) attending specialist drug agencies in England and Wales and who had injected during the previous four weeks remained higher at 1.3% in 2006 compared with 0.7% in 2000.

A survey (National AIDS Trust 2005) found that one in three people living with HIV in the UK did not know that they were infected, and there is still stigma attached to being tested for HIV. People are also less aware of the risks of HIV transmission than they were ten years ago. In addition, the survey found that one in five people were not aware of the risk of HIV infection through sex without a condom, the most common route of transmission in the UK.

TESTING FOR HIV

In order to ascertain whether an individual is infected with HIV, an 'HIV-antibody test', or 'HIV test' is undertaken. The standard HIV test looks for antibodies in a person's blood. So if a person has antibodies to HIV in their blood, it means they have been infected with HIV, except if it is an HIV-negative baby born to a positive mother. Babies retain their mother's antibodies for up to 18 months and may test positive on an HIV antibody test, even if they are actually HIV-negative. Most individuals will develop detectable HIV antibodies within 6 to 12 weeks of infection but may take up to six months in very rare cases. If a test is taken earlier than three months after infection, this may result in an unclear test result, as an infected person may not yet have developed antibodies to HIV.

HIV testing can take place in a number of settings including genito-urinary (GU) clinics, primary care services, open-access same-day test clinics, drug units, antenatal clinics, TB (tuberculosis) clinics and acute hospitals. However, despite recommended guidance, much HIV testing still takes place in GU clinics and in antenatal care, and there is a failure to test in TB clinics (National Aids Trust 2007). People are tested for a number of reasons. Some come forward for testing if they feel they may have been at risk of contracting HIV, and women are offered testing at antenatal clinics. People may present with symptoms that relate to immunodeficiency, and HIV testing may be indicated in order to plan appropriate care, treatment and management. In addition, people who are HIV-positive can receive counselling and health information in order to take action to prevent further transmission, for example by practising safe sex and informing past sexual partners. The early detection of HIV infection allows women who may have been infected to seek advice and make decisions about conception, the management of pregnancy and breast feeding. All women in England are now offered and recommended an HIV test as part of their antenatal care, not just those in high prevalence areas.

PRE-TEST DISCUSSION AND POST-TEST COUNSELLING

Guidelines on pre-test discussion and post-test counselling are available (Expert Advisory Group on AIDS 2002), and informed consent must be obtained before a person is tested. The United Kingdom Health Departments recommend that named testing for evidence of HIV infection should be undertaken only with informed consent, individuals having received information about how HIV is transmitted, the significance of both positive and negative results, and following a discussion of the particular needs and interests relevant to the individual. Key components of the pre-test discussion are presented in Table 14.2.

Post-test counselling should be available for both those diagnosed as HIV-negative and those diagnosed positive. The main features of post-test counselling are outlined in Table 14.3. The contents and the timing of the discussion will depend on the patients' reactions to their positive result.

Table 14.2 Pre-test discussion

Pre-test contents	Discussion
Nature of HIV	Modes of transmission
	Difference between HIV and AIDS
	Methods to reduce transmission
	Provision of materials of risk reduction strategies
Risk activities / need for test	Unsafe sexual practices
	History of drug use
	Injecting behaviour
	History of exposure to blood or blood products
	Tattooing
	Occupational risk
	Overseas travel with exposure to high risk activity
Advantages of testing	Allow individual to form strategies to protect sexual partners
	Allow interventions to reduce vertical transmission (pregnant women)
	Allow for appropriate medical care
	Allow effective prophylactic care
	Allow decisions for future plan
	Reduction of needless anxiety about HIV infection
Disadvantages of testing	Psychological complications
	Possible adverse impact on relationships (family, partners, work)
	Possible restrictions such as travelling abroad
Test procedure and result giving	Positive, negative and indeterminate results
Obtaining informed consent	Written note

Source: Expert Advisory Group on AIDS (2002), Department of Health

Table 14.3 Post-test counselling

Aims	If HIV-positive
• Address immediate concerns	• Address patient's immediate reactions
• Provide support for those who are positive	• Refer for specialist management and treatment
• Provide information on prevention of HIV transmission	• Give details of support service
	• Offer follow-up appointments
	• Ongoing support (legal issues, support for carers and partners etc.)

STIGMA AND DISCRIMINATION

Fear and prejudice regarding HIV infection remain an issue in most societies. There have been incidents of violence towards people with HIV infection and their property, as well as stigmatisation by friends, family, neighbours and colleagues. The Department of Heath (2001) recognised the importance of HIV-related stigma and discrimination as a barrier to prevention, treatment and care services for people with, or at risk from, HIV. Various governmental departments in England have undertaken work in relation to addressing equal access to health care, equality issues around gender, race and sexuality, and homophobic bullying. According to the Department of Health (2007), stigma and discrimination can impede disclosure and deter people from working and using healthcare and social care services, thereby contributing to the social exclusion of people living with HIV. Such prejudice is also sometimes perpetrated by HIV-negative members of minority groups towards others in their communities who *are* HIV-positive. The implementation plan on *Tackling HIV Stigma and Discrimination* (Department of Health 2007) includes funded projects to address the key issues around HIV-related stigma and discrimination and to strengthen cross-government working on stigma involving key non-government organisation stakeholders.

HIV PREVENTION

HIV can be transmitted in three main ways: sexual transmission, transmission through blood and mother-to-child transmission. Sexual behaviour is a major factor determining the transmission of HIV. The prevention of poor sexual health depends on everyone having the information, skills and services that they need in order to make informed choices. Some groups need targeted sexual health information and HIV/STI prevention because they are at higher risk, are particularly vulnerable or have particular access requirements (Department of Health 2007). The 'higher risk' group includes young people (in or out of care), Black and ethnic minority groups, gay and bisexual men, injecting drug misusers, adults and children living with HIV, sex workers and people in prisons and youth offending establishments.

Professionals in health, education, social care and voluntary services can make a significant contribution in HIV prevention by raising awareness of sexual health, helping people to get the health information and services according to their need and applying the strategy of harm reduction. The report by the National Aids Trust (2007) commissioning HIV prevention activities in England recommended that greater investment in effective prevention programmes that target high-risk communities, and in particular gay men and Black African communities, is needed to tackle the growing HIV epidemic in the UK.

TREATMENT OF HIV

Antiretroviral treatment for HIV infection consists of drugs which work against HIV infection itself by slowing down the replication of HIV in the body. Treatment options have had a huge impact on the lives of people with HIV. The treatments for HIV have reduced AIDS-related illnesses, reduced admissions to hospital and death rates, and offered people the chance to stay healthy for much longer. Antiretroviral treatment has also enabled some people to return to full-time employment. The antiretroviral drugs are usually prescribed in combinations of three or more. This is called combination therapy or highly active antiretroviral therapy (HAART). HAART has been proved effective in controlling HIV and delaying the onset of AIDS for many people. However, the treatments are not effective for everyone and can have adverse effects. Some people with HIV have drug resistance to the effects of an antiretroviral drug. In this case, another combination therapy has to be taken but the person will still have HIV in their body. Some people with HIV use complementary therapies either alone or with their antiretroviral treatment. These include vitamin and mineral supplements, herbal remedies, meditation, massage and acupuncture. People undergoing antiretroviral treatment should also abstain from unprotected sex or sharing needles or injecting equipment as the treatment does not stop someone with HIV from being able to pass on the virus.

TUBERCULOSIS

Tuberculosis (TB) is an infection caused by a bacterium (germ) called Mycobacterium tuberculosis. TB usually affects the lungs (pulmonary) but any part of the body can be affected. Only the pulmonary form of TB disease is infectious. Transmission occurs through coughing of infectious droplets, and usually requires prolonged close contact with an infectious case. TB is curable with a combination of specific antibiotics, but treatment must be continued for at least six months. The typical signs of TB are chronic or persistent cough and sputum production, fatigue, lack of appetite, weight loss, night sweats and fever. The Health Protection Agency report (2007) indicates that a total of 8,497 TB cases were reported in the UK as a whole in 2006, which is similar to 2005. TB is common in people with AIDS and is one of the leading causes of death in HIV-infected people.

HIV/AIDS and TB are so closely connected that the term 'co-epidemic' or 'dual epidemic' is often used to describe their relationship. As HIV affects the immune system, this increases the likelihood of people acquiring TB infection. TB occurs earlier in the course of HIV infection than many other opportunistic infections. An estimated one-third of the 40 million people living with HIV/AIDS worldwide are co-infected with TB (WHO 2004). HIV infection is the most potent risk factor for converting latent TB into active TB, while TB bacteria accelerate the progress of AIDS infection in the patient. Many people infected with HIV in developing countries develop TB as the first manifestation of AIDS. The two diseases represent a deadly combination, since they are more destructive together than either disease alone. Furthermore, without proper treatment, approximately 90% of those living with HIV die within months of contracting TB. TB is harder to diagnose, progresses faster in HIV-infected people and is almost certain to be fatal if undiagnosed or left untreated.

HEPATITIS

Hepatitis means inflammation of the liver. It can be caused by a number of factors including alcohol, drugs, immune disorders and infection. The main cause of hepatitis is through blood-borne viruses. At present there are six main types of viral hepatitis: A, B, C, D, E and G. Hepatitis A and E are spread by the faecal oral route whilst the others are spread by blood and body fluids. In the context of drug misuse, hepatitis C, B and A are currently of particular concern. The most common route of infection in England currently is through sharing contaminated needles or injecting equipment by injecting drug users.

HEPATITIS C

The growing importance of hepatitis C as a public health issue in Britain was highlighted in 2002 with the publication of the government's *Hepatitis C Strategy for England* (Department of Health 2002). It brought together existing initiatives to tackle hepatitis C and suggested how prevention, diagnosis and treatment could be improved. This *Action Plan* (Department of Health 2004), which is based on best practice, serves as a broad framework for implementation of the *Hepatitis C Strategy for England*. Many of these infected people do not realise they have the virus as it can take years or even decades for symptoms to appear.

A report from the Health Protection Agency (2007c) shows that the overall hepatitis C prevalence of the general population in England was 43% (1,233 of 2,893) with very marked regional variations. The prevalence of hepatitis C infection among injecting drug users (IDUs) remains high overall. Of the (current and former) IDUs participating, two-fifths (41%, 1,316 of 3,240) had antibodies to hepatitis C, a figure similar to that seen in recent years (2005 42%, 1,325 of 3,175).

Transmission of hepatitis C

Hepatitis C is carried in the blood, and has been detected in other body fluids. The major route of hepatitis C transmission in the UK is by sharing equipment for injecting drug use, mainly via blood-contaminated needles and syringes. Spoons, water and filters may also be vehicles of infection. Mother to baby transmission does occur, either in utero or at the time of birth, but appears to be uncommon. However, it is advisable not to breastfeed. Sexual transmission of hepatitis C is possible but uncommon. There is some evidence that transmission may occur through the sharing of toothbrushes, razors and other personal toiletry items that could be contaminated with blood. Transmission can occur through medical and dental procedures abroad, where infection control may be inadequate. There is a risk from tattooing, ear piercing, body piercing and acupuncture with unsterile equipment. Health and social care workers may be at risk of hepatitis infection from occupational injuries, for example needle stick injuries. Details of guidance for those working with drug users is found in a Department of Health publication (2001b)

Signs and symptoms

Most people who become infected with hepatitis C are unaware of it at the time because it produces no signs or symptoms during its earliest stages. Some people may briefly feel unwell, or may have muscle aches and a high temperature, mild to severe fatigue, nausea, loss of appetite, weight loss, depression or anxiety, pain or discomfort in the liver, jaundice, poor memory or concentration and alcohol intolerance. In many cases, signs and symptoms may not appear for decades, which makes the infection difficult to recognise. Some patients will report quite severe symptoms with no clinical signs of liver disease, while cirrhosis can be present without any obvious symptoms. If hepatitis progresses, its symptoms begin to point to the liver as the source of illness and causes jaundice, foul breath, a bitter taste in the mouth and dark or 'tea-coloured' urine. The signs and symptoms of the early stage and later stage of Hepatitis are presented in Table 14.4. Alcohol consumption and co-infection with HIV or hepatitis B are strongly associated with increased likelihood of progression to severe liver complications.

Testing for hepatitis C

As for HIV testing there are clear guidelines on testing and counselling in hepatitis C infection. There are serious implications in having a hepatitis C test, and there is a need for co-ordinated pre-discussion and post-test counselling. Health professionals should be aware of the implications of hepatitis infection, its routes of transmission, preventative measures and treatment options, so that these can be discussed with clients before testing takes place. The guidelines on HIV test pre-discussion and post-test counselling are applicable for the hepatitis C test.

Prevention and harm-reduction

The goals of prevention are to lower the incidence of acute hepatitis C and reduce the disease burden from chronic hepatitis infection. These are achieved by the education of healthcare professionals and the public at large on the dangers of hepatitis C. There is

Table 14.4 Signs and symptoms of hepatitis C

Early stage	Later stage
• Slight fatigue	• Fatigue
• Nausea	• Lack of appetite
• Poor appetite	• Nausea
• Muscle and joint pains	• Vomiting
• Tenderness (area of the liver)	• Jaundice (yellow skin and eyes)
	• High temperature
	• Weight loss
	• Poor memory
	• Anxiety
	• Depression
	• Alcohol intolerance

also a need to focus on those who are at risk, for example injecting drug users, by the provision of health information, harm-reduction and counselling. In order to reduce or minimise hepatitis C infections, the *Hepatitis C Strategy for England* (Department of Health 2002) recommended the provision of the following services:

- provision of needle, syringe and other injecting equipment exchange services in the community
- safe disposal of used needles and syringes
- provision of outreach and peer education services
- provision of specialist drug treatment services
- provision of information and advice about hepatitis C and other blood-borne viruses and the risks of injecting drugs (including stopping injecting, the risks of sharing injecting equipment and avoiding initiating others)
- provision of disinfecting tablets throughout the prison estate.

In addition, all NHS organisations will need to reduce the risk of hepatitis C transmission within healthcare settings by the adoption of rigorous standard of (universal) infection control precautions, occupational health checks for staff and effective management of occupational blood exposure incidents. If there is a diagnosis of hepatitis C, harm reduction in the following areas needs to be discussed with the client:

- to stop or reduce alcohol consumption
- not to donate blood
- to carry an organ donor card
- never to share any injecting equipment
- to use condoms to minimise this risk of sexual transmission (although rare)
- not to share razors or toothbrushes or any toiletry equipment contaminated with blood
- to avoid body piercing.

The Health Protection Agency (2007c) annual report for 2007 on hepatitis C suggests that the effort to raise awareness of hepatitis C is encouraging more people to be tested, leading to a 10% increase in diagnoses. New prevention initiatives include the national health promotion DVD – *Hepatitis C: Inside and Out* – which has been developed for use within prisons to deliver messages on the prevention, transmission, management and treatment of hepatitis C.

Treatment of hepatitis C

At present there is no vaccination against hepatitis C. Those who are hepatitis C-positive should have their liver function checked on a regular basis to check for liver damage. They should also be advised to stop or reduce their alcohol intake. If there are signs of deteriorating liver function, a liver biopsy may be performed to assess liver changes. The treatment of hepatitis C has improved significantly with the use of two medications. The National Institute for Clinical Excellence (NICE 2000, 2004, 2006) recommends a combination therapy with peginterferon alpha plus ribavirin in the treatment of mild and chronic hepatitis C. The combination therapy is the treatment of choice: it lasts for 6 to 12 months and can eliminate the virus in about 50% of the people infected. There may be some concern about the effectiveness of combination therapy for those who continue to consume alcohol or continue to inject drugs. There is now specific guidance in the relevant NICE technology appraisals that makes clear that those who continue to inject drugs and/or continue to consume or misuse alcohol should not, simply because of those behaviours, be excluded from provision of antiviral treatments for the management of hepatitis C infection.

HEPATITIS B

The World Health Organization estimates that in the UK the prevalence of chronic hepatitis B infection is 0.3%. In the UK, approximately one in a thousand people are thought to have the virus. More than 10% of cases in the UK are thought to result from people travelling to and working in countries where there is increased risk of hepatitis B infection. Hepatitis B is a blood-borne viral infection that can be prevented through vaccination. Transmission of hepatitis B usually occurs by unprotected sexual intercourse; by injecting drug misusers sharing blood-contaminated injecting equipment; receipt of contaminated blood or blood products; from an infected mother to her baby (perinatal); child-to-child contact in household settings; and tattooing and body piercing.

The hepatitis B virus can cause a short-term (acute) infection, which may or may not cause symptoms. Some people may experience sore throat, tiredness, joint pains, nausea and vomiting and a loss of appetite. Acute infection can be severe, causing abdominal discomfort and jaundice. Following an acute infection, a minority of infected adults (but most infected babies) develop a persistent infection called chronic hepatitis B. Many people with chronic hepatitis B remain well but become chronic carriers. They are unaware that they are infected but can still pass on the virus to others. These individuals will remain infectious and will be at risk of developing cirrhosis and primary liver cancer.

The most important measure in the protection against Hepatitis B is by immunisation, which provides protection in up to 90% of recipients. Hepatitis B vaccination should be carried out as soon after initial presentation as possible in all drug users, regardless of the presence of injecting. The vaccine is given as a series of three intramuscular doses. Studies have shown that the vaccine is 95% effective in preventing children and adults from developing chronic infection if they have not yet been infected. Alpha interferon is used to treat patients with chronic hepatitis B infection.

ACTIVITY 14.1

Please choose one correct answer to the following multiple-choice questions

Blood-borne infection is transmitted by
a.   Infected blood or blood-stained body fluids
b.   Saliva
c.   Kissing
d.   None of the above

The main BBVs are
a.   HIV, hepatitis B and hepatitis C
b.   AIDS, hepatitis A and hepatitis D
c.   Hepatitis ABCD
d.   None of the above

Human Immunodeficiency Virus (HIV) is
a.   A bacterial illness treated with antibiotics
b.   A virus which has no cure but can be controlled with medicines
c.   The virus that causes AIDS
d.   Answers b and c

Most HIV transmission occurs through
a.   Blood and blood products
b.   Vaginal secretions
c.   Breast milk
d.   All of the above

Which body fluid CANNOT transmit HIV?
a.   Blood
b.   Semen
c.   Vaginal fluids
d.   Saliva

HIV is a virus that attacks and weakens which body system?
a.   The digestive system
b.   The immune system
c.   The circulatory system
d.   The nervous system

What does it mean to have HIV?
a.   I can never have sex again
b.   I need to give up work
c.   I cannot have children
d.   None of the above

What is the difference between HIV and AIDS?
a.   HIV causes AIDS
b.   There is no difference between HIV and AIDS
c.   There is no cure for AIDS but there is a cure for HIV
d.   HIV is the same as AIDS

You can find out if you have HIV by getting
a.   A blood test
b.   Skin lesions checked
c.   An eye examination
d.   Symptoms

The standard, most common HIV test
a.   Predicts how fast you will develop AIDS
b.   Measures the amount of virus in your blood
c.   Detects antibodies to the virus
d.   None of the above

If you have another sexually transmitted infection, your chance of getting HIV/AIDS through having sex
a.   Is nil
b.   Stays the same
c.   Is higher
d.   Is lower

Sharing a needle and syringe to inject drugs is safe when
a.   You share only with your partner
b.   You only inject crack cocaine
c.   It is never safe
d.   You only inject heroin

Which protects you most against HIV infection?
a.   Contraceptive pills
b.   Spermicidal jelly
c.   Condoms
d.   Condoms and spermicidal jelly

'Drug resistance' means that
a.   HIV changes itself so that the HIV drugs do not work any more
b.   A person with HIV is reluctant to go on medication
c.   A person has no HIV infection
d.   A person does not comply with medication regimes

The best way to prevent HIV infection is
a.   Using latex condoms and not sharing needles
b.   Not worrying because I'm not at risk
c.   Staying away from those with HIV
d.   Not having sexual contact with anyone

HIV affects the immune system; this increases
a.   The likelihood of people acquiring TB infection
b.   The likelihood of people not acquiring TB infection
c.   The likelihood of people acquiring sexually transmitted disease
d.   The likelihood of people not acquiring sexually transmitted disease

Hepatitis means
a.   Inflammation of the liver
b.   Immune disorder
c.   Infections
d.   Blood-borne virus

Hepatitis A and E are spread by
a. The faecal oral route
b. Blood
c. Blood products
d. Body fluids

The major route of hepatitis transmission is by
a. Sharing equipment for injecting drug use
b. Via blood-contaminated needles and syringes
c. Contaminated spoons, water and filters
d. All the above

What are the symptoms if a person becomes infected with hepatitis C?
a. A lot of people get 'flu-like' symptoms
b. No symptoms
c. A rash comes out the following day
d. None of the above

An increased likelihood of progression to severe liver complications may be caused by
a. Alcohol consumption and co-infection with HIV
b. Drug consumption and co-infection
c. Alcohol and drug consumption
d. None of the above

Transmission of hepatitis B usually occurs by
a. Unprotected sexual intercourse
b. Injecting drug misusers
c. Contaminated blood or blood products
d. All of the above

Many people with chronic hepatitis B
a. Are aware that they are infected
b. Remain well but become chronic carriers
c. Cannot pass on the virus to others
d. Do not remain infectious

ACTIVITY 14.2

- Describe current trends in HIV infection
- List the transmission routes of HIV
- Describe the process of HIV pre-discussion and post-test counselling
- Discuss the prevention of HIV
- Discuss the risks of injecting drug use for the transmission of blood-borne viruses

ACTIVITY 14.3

- Describe current trends for hepatitis C and B infections
- List the transmission routes of hepatitis C and B infections
- Describe the effective prevention measures to hepatitis C and B infections
- What current treatment and vaccinations are available for viral infections?

KEY POINTS

- BBVs, especially the human immunodeficiency virus (HIV) and hepatitis viruses B and C (HBV, HCV), pose major risks to the health of people who inject illicit drugs.
- The main BBVs are human immunodeficiency (HIV), hepatitis B and hepatitis C.
- A National Strategy on sexual health and HIV, 'Better prevention, better services, better sexual health', aims to address the rising prevalence of sexually transmitted infections and of HIV.
- HIV stands for Human Immunodeficiency Virus. HIV is the virus that causes AIDS (Acquired Immune Deficiency Syndrome).
- Most HIV transmission occurs through unprotected vaginal or anal intercourse, sharing contaminated needles and syringes, transfusion of contaminated blood and blood products, from mother to baby in utero, at birth or via breast feeding, or transfusion of contaminated blood and blood products.
- There is concern regarding the steady increase in heterosexual HIV transmission especially in the Black ethnic minority and transmission of HIV among injecting drug users.
- Fear and prejudice regarding HIV infection act as a barrier to prevention, treatment and care services for people with, or at risk from, HIV.
- Antiretroviral treatment has had a huge impact on the lives of people with HIV.
- TB is common in people with AIDS and is one of the leading causes of death in HIV-infected people.
- Hepatitis means inflammation of the liver. The main cause of hepatitis is through blood-borne viruses.
- Many people with chronic hepatitis B remain well but become chronic carriers.
- Alpha interferon is used to treat patients with chronic hepatitis B infection.

REFERENCES

Department of Health (2001a) *The National Strategy for Sexual Health and HIV*. London: Department of Health.
Department of Health (2001b) *Hepatitis C – Guidance for Those Working with Drug Users*. London: Department of Health. http://www.dh.gov.uk/assetRoot/04/01/96/49/04019649.pdf.
Department of Health (2002) *Hepatitis C Strategy for England*. London: Department of Health. http://www.publications.doh.gov.uk/cmo/hcvstrategy/hcvstratsum.htm. (accessed 20 July 2007.

Department of Health (2004). *Hepatitis C Action Plan for England*. London: Department of Health.

Department of Health (2007) *Tackling HIV Stigma and Discrimination: Department of Health Implementation Plan*. Department of Health, Electronic Only. http://www.dh.gov.uk/en/ Publicationsandstatistics/Publications/PublicationsPolicyAndGuidance/DH_076423 (accessed 20 July 2007).

Expert Advisory Group on AIDS (EAGA) (2002) *HIV Testing: Guidelines for Pre-test Discussion*. London: Department of Health. http://www.advisorybodies.doh.gov.uk/eaga/guidelineshiv testdiscuss.htm (accessed 21 July 2007).

Health Protection Agency (2007a) *Testing Times – HIV and Other Sexually Transmitted Infections in the United Kingdom 2007 Annual Report*. London: Health Protection Agency. http://www.hpa.org.uk/infections/topics_az/hiv_and_sti/publications/AnnualReport/2007/def ault.htm (accessed 22 July 2007).

Health Protection Agency (2007b) *Tuberculosis in the UK. Annual Report*. London: Health Protection Agency. http://www.hpa.org.uk/infections/topics_az/tb/menu.htm (accessed 22 July 2007).

Health Protection Agency (2007c) *Shooting Up Infections among Injecting Drug Users in the United Kingdom 2006 An Update: October 2007*. London: Department of Health.

National Aids Trust (2005) *Public Attitudes to HIV*. London: NAT Publications. http://www. nat.org.uk.

National Aids Trust (2007) *Updating Our Strategies Report of an Expert Seminar on HIV Testing And Prevention 22 March 2007*. http://www.nat.org.uk (accessed 23 July 2007).

NICE (2000) *Guidance on the Use of Ribavirin and Interferon Alpha for Hepatitis C*. Technology Appraisal Guidance – no. 14. London: National Institute for Clinical Excellence.

NICE (2004) *Interferon Alpha and Ribavirin for the Treatment of Chronic Hepatitis C* – part review of existing guidance no. 14. London: National Institute for Clinical Excellence.

NICE (2006) *Thousands More People with Hepatitis C to Benefit from Latest NICE guidance on Drug Treatments*. 2006/040 Press release 23 August. London: National Institute for Clinical Excellence.

UNAIDS and WHO (2007). *The 2007 AIDS Epidemic Update*. Geneva: World Health Organization.

WHO (2004) *Interim Policy on Collaborative TB/HIV Activities*. Geneva: World Health Organization.

CHAPTER 15

ALCOHOL AND DRUG USE IN WOMEN

OBJECTIVES

- Describe the prevalence of alcohol and drug misuse with women.

- Discuss the psychosocial and environmental issues related to alcohol and drug misuse.

- List the features of foetal alcohol spectrum disorders.

- Discuss the problems associated with illicit drug misuse in pregnancy.

- Discuss the issues of blood-borne viruses in pregnancy.

- Discuss the barriers in preventing women accessing treatment services.

- Discuss the special treatment needs of women with alcohol and drug problems.

Women, like men, use alcohol and other psychoactive substances for a range of reasons including relaxation and pleasure. Women's alcohol and drug misuse needs to be viewed in the context of women's role in contemporary society. For thousands of years, gender-related and religio-social rules have defined what is considered appropriate behaviour for women, including the use of alcohol and drug. Despite the commitment to sexual equality, the expectations of women in society in relation to the notions of carer, motherhood, the occupation of maternity and childbearing remains pervasive. Women are stigmatised for drinking in the home, as this conflicts with an ideology of women and motherhood as being self-denying and nurturing of both men and children

(Waterson 1997). When an alcohol problem is present in women, the feelings of guilt and shame are compounded (Ettore 1997).

In contrast with men, drinking behaviour or drug use in women is considered to be deviant behaviour, and women are more stigmatised, marginalised and labelled. Society has negative attitudes towards women who are intoxicated and are problem drug users or drinkers. However, it has been suggested that it is not the intoxication per se but aggressive or unruly (unfeminine) behaviour associated with intoxication that attracts condemnation (Robbins and Martin 1993). Compared to consumption levels amongst men, women's alcohol consumption, particularly in younger and older women, has been increasing over the last few decades. The number of girls and young women binge drinking has risen dramatically in a decade. British women's binge drinking is clearly defined by their age and education. A study by Jefferis *et al.* (2007) found that educated women binge drink in their 20s, but curb their habits by their 40s. However, the reverse is true of women with little education, whose binge drinking is more likely to take off in their 40s. The prevalence of binge drinking remains substantial into adulthood (31% men and 14% women at 42 years). Highly qualified women were about one-third more likely than women with no or few qualifications to binge drink at the age of 23. This chapter focuses on problems and issues related to women's alcohol and drug misuse.

PREVALENCE

According to data from the Office for National Statistics (ONS), the recent upward trend in heavy drinking among young women may have peaked. The proportion of 16–24-year-old women who had drunk more than six units on at least one day in the previous week increased from 24% to 28% between 1998 and 2002 but then fell to 26% in 2003, to 24% in 2004 and to 22% in 2005 (National Statistics 2006). In 2007, 13% of women drank over the weekly recommendations (14 units for women). In 2006/7 in England and Wales, men reported higher levels of use of 'any illicit drugs' and 'class A drugs' in their lifetime, in the last year and in the past month compared with women. The proportion of women using any illicit drug in the past year decreased between 1998 and 2006/7 from 9% to 7%. In 2006/7, use of class A drugs in the last year was 2% for women had stayed approximately the same for women since 1998 (National Statistics 2007). Overall, there continues to be a higher prevalence of smoking among men than among women. However, among young adults (aged 16–19) more women (26%) smoke than men (23%). Women were less likely to have discussed their drinking with health professionals (only 8% had done so) compared to 14% of male drinkers.

ISSUES OF ALCOHOL AND DRUG USE

There is growing evidence that women are at high risk for the health and social problems caused by alcohol, tobacco and other drugs, compared to men. The physical, psychological and social effects of alcohol are more severe for women than for men. Women develop alcohol-related problems and alcohol dependence faster than men and many die younger than men with similar drinking problems. Women who drink get intoxicated more quickly than men and will attain a higher blood alcohol concentration than a man from the same amount of alcohol consumed. Women have lower levels of the enzyme alcohol dehydrogenase which is responsible for the breakdown (metabolism) of alcohol. In addition, women have on average 10% more fat than men and less body fluid to dilute alcohol in their bodies. The concentrated form of alcohol causes more harm. Compared to men, women have an increased risk of developing alcohol hepatitis, heart disease, liver disease, ulcers, reproductive problems, osteoporosis, pancreatitis, brain damage, breast cancer, memory loss and other illnesses caused by alcohol and drug misuse.

FOETAL ALCOHOL SPECTRUM DISORDERS

Maternal alcohol use during pregnancy contributes to a wide range of disorders in the offspring including social, emotional and cognitive development, learning deficits, hyperactivity and attention problems. The most serious outcome of maternal drinking during pregnancy is foetal alcohol spectrum disorders (FASD). FAS is a term used to describe the full range of mental and physical features seen in some babies who were exposed to alcohol before birth. Children with FASD have a distinctive set of facial anomalies, growth retardation and significant learning and behavioural problems. The signs and symptoms and long-term features of FASD are presented in Table 15.1.

Foetal alcohol spectrum disorders are lifelong conditions and are not always diagnosed at birth. Diagnosis may be made later when the conditions can significantly impact on the life of the individual with learning and behavioural problems. The effects of maternal alcohol consumption are not limited to the range of FASD. Alcohol can

Table 15.1 Foetal alcohol spectrum disorders

Signs at birth	Long-term effects
• Small body size and weight • Facial abnormalities • Small eyes • Small head circumference • Flattened face • Flattened bridge of the nose • Sunken nasal bridge • Small jaw • Opening in roof of mouth • Organ deformities • Heart defects • Genital malformations • Kidney and urinary defects • Mental retardation • Learning disabilities • Short attention span • Irritability in infancy • Hyperactivity in childhood	• Learning difficulties • Delays in normal development • Behavioural problems • Memory problems • Attention deficit hyperactive disorder • Depression • Psychosis • Increased risk of alcohol and drug msisue

adversely impact on the reproductive process in a number of ways, including infertility, higher rates of menstrual disorders, a decreased chance of becoming pregnant, miscarriage, major structural malformations of the foetus, pre-term deliveries and stillbirth (British Medical Association 2007).

The prevention of FASD requires a co-ordinated and multi-faceted approach that incorporates universal prevention strategies aimed at the general population (public awareness and educational campaigns), selective prevention strategies aimed at women of childbearing age, in particular those who are considering a pregnancy (screening for maternal alcohol consumption) and specific prevention strategies aimed at women who are at high risk (referral to specialist alcohol services) (British Medical Association 2007). There is no cure for FASD, and the management of FASD necessitates comprehensive, multi-model approaches based on the needs of the client. Given the current uncertainty regarding the level of risk to the developing foetus, and the lack of clear guidelines, the only safe sensible drinking message is not to drink any alcohol during pregnancy. The World Health Organization recommends that pregnant women should avoid alcohol.

SMOKING DURING PREGNANCY

Tobacco smoking can cause reproductive problems before a woman even becomes pregnant, and a woman who smokes may have more trouble conceiving than non-smokers. However, fertility returns to normal after a woman stops smoking. Smoking during pregnancy not only harms a woman's health but can lead to pregnancy complications and serious health problems in newborns. It is not known for certain which chemicals are harmful to a developing baby but it is believed that both nicotine and carbon monoxide play significant roles in causing adverse pregnancy outcomes. There is a high risk that women who smoke during pregnancy may pass harmful carcinogens on to their baby resulting in babies with lower birth weight (2.5 kg or 5lb 8 oz). There is also an increase in the risk of pre-term delivery. Premature and low-birth weight babies face an increased risk of serious health problems during the newborn period, chronic lifelong disabilities (such as cerebral palsy, mental retardation and learning problems) and even death.

Smoking has been associated with a number of pregnancy complications such as placental problems. These conditions can result in heavy bleeding during delivery that can endanger mother and baby, although a caesarean delivery can prevent most deaths. Placental problems contribute to the slightly increased risk of stillbirth that is associated with smoking. A recent study (Law *et al.* 2003) suggests that babies of mothers who smoke during pregnancy may undergo withdrawal-like symptoms similar to those seen in babies of mothers who use some illicit drugs. For example, babies of smokers appear to be more jittery and difficult to soothe than babies of non-smokers. Babies of women who are regularly exposed to second-hand smoke during pregnancy may also have reduced growth and may be more likely to be born with low birth weight.

The problems of smoking during pregnancy are closely related to health inequalities between those in need and the most advantaged. Women with partners in manual groups are more likely to smoke during pregnancy than those with partners in non-manual groups (Department of Health 1998). Efforts to reduce the proportion of women who smoke during pregnancy were recognised as a priority in the White Paper *Smoking Kills* (Department of Health 1998). This set a target to reduce the proportion of women in England who continued to smoke during pregnancy to 15% by 2010, with a fall to 18% by 2005 (from a baseline of 23%). In 2005, a third (32%) of mothers in England who had recently given birth reported smoking in the 12 months before or during pregnancy (Information Centre 2007a). There is good evidence that helping pregnant women to give up smoking is cost-effective. Of course, many health professionals, particularly midwives and primary care teams, already provide advice to stop smoking to women smokers when they become pregnant.

The National Institute for Clinical Excellence and the National Collaborating Centre for Women's and Children's Health (NICE 2003) have published a guideline for the NHS in England and Wales on the routine care of healthy pregnant women. The guideline includes recommendations on:

- the provision of evidence-based information for pregnant women to support them in making informed decisions
- the number of antenatal appointments and what should happen at each appointment
- the use of ultrasound scanning
- the provision of screening for a range of conditions, including gestational diabetes, HIV and Down's syndrome.

WOMEN AND ILLICIT DRUG MISUSE

Men are more likely to take illicit drugs than women; 13.7 per cent of men compared with 7.4 per cent of women took drugs in the last year. In 2004/5, a larger number of men accessed treatment services than women (114,598 men compared to 45,852 women) (Information Centre 2007b). Existing research evidence shows that between one-quarter and one-third of adult problem drug users in England are women, and that this ratio has remained relatively constant over recent years (Best and Abdulrahim 2005). Research indicates that women with substance use problems are more likely than men to seem to be younger; to have a partner with a substance use problem; to have fewer resources; to have dependent children; to live with a drug using partner; to have more severe problems at the beginning of treatment; to have trauma related to physical and sexual abuse; and to have concurrent psychiatric disorders (UNODC 2004).

PROBLEMS RELATED TO ILLEGAL DRUG MISUSE DURING PREGNANCY

Drugs can be harmful to a developing foetus throughout the pregnancy but the first three months are considered to be the time of highest risk. This is the period when the baby's major organs and limbs are forming. However, some drugs can interfere with functional development of organ systems and the central nervous system in the second and third trimesters and produce serious consequences. During the last 12 weeks of pregnancy, drug use poses the greatest risk for stunting foetal growth and causing pre-term birth. All drugs taken during pregnancy will reach the baby through the placenta. However, there can be great variation in babies' responses to drugs, depending on the type of drug taken, how often the drug is used, how it is used and the amount taken, polydrug use and individual baby's response. A mother taking illegal drugs during pregnancy increases her risk for anaemia, blood and heart infections, skin infections, hepatitis and other infectious diseases.

The World Health Organization (1997) has reported that there is reliable scientific evidence to suggest that cannabis causes any chromosomal or genetic damage. Maternal use of cannabis is associated with reduced birth weight as well as cognitive and memory deficits in offspring (Fergusson *et al*. 2002; Fried *et al*. 2003). Research on whether cannabis use might increase the risk of ectopic pregnancies in women of reproductive ages is cautious regarding chronic cannabis consumption for recreation or pain alleviation (Wang *et al*. 2004). Heroin, cocaine and other psychoactive substances use can cause withdrawal in the newborn as well as growth retardation in the unborn baby.

Cocaine use can lead to premature delivery of the foetus, premature detachment of the placenta, haemorrhage, high blood pressure and stillbirth. Cocaine-exposed babies are more likely than unexposed babies to have health problems during the newborn period, including low birth weight, smaller head circumference, mental disabilities, behavioural disturbances, cerebral palsy, stroke, visual and hearing impairment, heart attack and sometimes sudden infant death syndrome. The chance of dying of sudden infant death syndrome is increased with poor health practices associated with cocaine use. Babies exposed to cocaine before birth sometimes have feeding difficulties and sleep disturbances. Some babies, at birth, go through a process of 'withdrawal effect' including behaviour that is jittery, irritable; they may startle and cry in response to touch and sound. Other symptoms include tremors, sleeplessness, muscle spasms and feeding difficulties. These symptoms start about one to two days after delivery.

These withdrawn or unresponsive babies are very difficult to comfort, and this makes bonding between mother and child very difficult. As yet, little is know of the long-term effects or special problems of babies exposed to cocaine before birth. However, studies of cocaine-exposed school-aged children do suggest subtle effects on intelligence and behaviour and on a child's ability to remain alert and attentive (NIDA 1999). Most

Table 15.2 Maternal, prenatal and postnatal effects of psychoactive substances

Maternal	Prenatal (baby)	Postnatal (mother and baby)
• Insomnia	• Low birth weight	• Withdrawal symptoms
• Poor appetite	• Early delivery	• Sudden Infant Death
• Premature labour	• Miscarriage	Syndrome
• Cognitive functioning affected	• Mental retardation	• Cognitive dysfunction
• Risk of infections (transmitted through sex)	• Death	• Difficulty in bonding with newborn
• Water breaks early		• Meeting needs of newborn
• Sudden haemorrhage		• Depression
• Inability to cope with normal changes in pregnancy		• Psychosis

children who were exposed to cocaine before birth have normal intelligence. A study of four-year-old children who were exposed to cocaine before birth found that they scored just as well on intelligence tests as unexposed children (Singer *et al.* 2004).

There are limited studies on the risks of 'club drugs', such as PCP (angel dust), ketamine (Special K), LSD (acid) and ecstasy. Babies exposed before birth to PCP or ketamine may be at increased risk of learning and behavioural problems and may have withdrawal symptoms with PCP (ACOG 2005). Babies exposed to ecstasy before birth also may face some of the same risks as babies exposed to other types of amphetamines but ecstasy use during pregnancy may be linked to congenital deformities. A study found that babies of women who used methamphetamine during pregnancy were more than three times as likely than unexposed babies to grow poorly before birth (Smith *et al.* 2006). Use of methamphetamine during pregnancy also increases the risk of pregnancy complications, such as premature delivery and placental problems and cases of birth defects (Smith *et al.* 2006). Babies exposed to methamphetamine appear to undergo withdrawal-like symptoms, including jitteriness, drowsiness and breathing problems. The long-term effects of ecstasy and methamphetamines are at present unknown. The use of volatile substances during pregnancy can contribute to miscarriage, slow foetal growth, pre-term birth and birth defects (ACOG 2005). The risks of GHB in pregnancy are similar to those of alcohol. The use of LSD and other hallucinogens appears to be linked to an increased risk of miscarriage, birth complications and a higher incidence of birth defects. If a mother continues to use hallucinogens while breastfeeding, it is possible that the drug will be present in her milk and may have adverse effects on the baby.

Women who use heroin during pregnancy greatly increase their risk of harming an unborn child and have serious pregnancy complications. These risks include low birth weight, poor foetal growth, premature rupture of the membranes, premature delivery and stillbirth. These babies are often born premature, underdeveloped, have breathing problems and infections in the first few weeks of life with increased risk of lifelong disabilities. Babies exposed to heroin before birth also face an increased risk of sudden infant death syndrome. Babies of heroin-dependent mothers can suffer withdrawal symptoms after they are born. The withdrawal symptoms include fever, high-pitched crying, excessive sucking, muscle spasm, sneezing, trembling, irritability, diarrhoea, vomiting and, occasionally, seizures. The sudden withdrawal of heroin of pregnant women may harm the baby and cause poor growth, miscarriage or premature labour. Babies born to mothers taking methadone also have withdrawal symptoms. Injecting heroin increases the risk of becoming infected with HIV infection which may then be passed on to the baby.

BLOOD-BORNE INFECTIONS

The blood-borne viruses such as HIV, hepatitis B and C are transmitted from mother to baby. There is a high risk that an infected mother will transmit HIV on to her unborn baby either during pregnancy or birth or while breastfeeding. Pregnant women who have hepatitis B should have their babies vaccinated with the hepatitis B vaccine and immunoglobulin soon after delivery. This greatly reduces the chance of their babies becoming infected. The risk of a mother passing the hepatitis C virus on to her unborn child during pregnancy and birth is low. Pregnant women should have a blood test if there is any chance they have been exposed to this virus. The risk of passing on hepatitis B or C through breastfeeding is very low as long as the nipples are not cracked or bleeding. Early detection of the blood-borne viruses through testing or vaccinations is recommended.

The Department of Health in England and Wales has recommended that all pregnant women should be offered antenatal screening for blood-borne viruses and antenatal tests. See Immunisation against infectious disease (Department of Health 2008); *Screening of Pregnant Women for Hepatitis B and Immunisation of Babies at Risk* (NHS Executive 1998); and *Hepatitis B in Pregnancy – Information for Midwives* (Department of Health / Royal College of Midwives 2000)

CHILD CARE ISSUES

In relation to pregnant substance misusers, many of the women are reluctant to contact health and social care agencies, fearing that the child or existing children may be taken into care. The overriding feeling among health and social care agencies is that preserving the family is important where at all possible as substance misuse is not always a clear indicator of a parent's lack of commitment to their child. A parent who misuses psychoactive substances should be treated in the same way as other parents whose personal difficulties interfere with or lessen their ability to provide good parenting (ACPC 2006).

The Standing Conference on Drug Abuse (SCODA 1989) has produced useful practical guidelines for professionals working with drug-using parents for assessing risk to children. These guidelines provide a framework for assessing the degree to which parental drug use may be adversely affecting the child, including meeting the physical and safety needs of the child. The following SCODA guidelines should be borne in mind when referral is being considered. Drug use by parents does not automatically indicate child neglect or abuse. Automatic child abuse registration will deter parents from approaching drug dependence clinics or other professionals for help and should be avoided. In families where drug use is a factor, a comprehensive assessment of the relationship between parental drug use and child care is indicated. Each family should be assessed individually.

The establishment of Area Child Protection Committees (ACPC) and the agreement of inter-agency Child Protection Procedures play a key role in ensuring that appropriate procedures, arrangements and training are in place to ensure that children are properly assessed when substance misuse by parents is a possibility. According to the ACPC (2006), a parent's substance misuse problem may mean that their children do not receive the level or quality of care which all children need and which a parent wishes to provide. In such situations, the needs of the child must come first. It is recommended that agencies must ensure that the child's needs, including any need for protection, are thoroughly assessed so that the right services and support can be provided and families can be helped to provide good-quality care (ACPC 2006: 9.67). The recent document *Working Together to Safeguard Children* (DfES 2006) sets out how individuals and organisations should work together to safeguard and promote the welfare of children. When there is concern that neglect or abuse may be occurring or may be a serious possibility, the health professional should take immediate appropriate action according to the local child protection guidelines.

BARRIERS TO TREATMENT

Alcohol and drug treatment have been available to women but the provision of services is seldom based on the special physical, psychological and social needs of women. Most of the alcohol and drug treatment services are male-orientated. Despite the recognition of the need for women-sensitive services for alcohol and drug misusers, the provision of such services is still scant. Fewer women than men access treatment services: this may suggest that, in general, more men than women use drugs or that women face more barriers in their access to treatment than do men (EMCDDA 2006). Women who misuse alcohol or drugs face a variety of barriers including barriers to treatment entry, to engagement in treatment and to long-term rehabilitation.

The most frequently reported barriers for substance misuse treatment entry were responsibilities at home as a mother, wife or partner; reliance on alcohol and other drugs to deal with stresses of daily life in the community; fear that admission of the drug problem would result in loss of custody of their children; shame as a result of their drug problem; inability to stay alcohol- or drug-free after previous treatment episodes; and unavailability of an opening because the treatment programme is full (Allen 1995). The reluctance of women alcohol and drug misusers to seek treatment demonstrates low self-esteem and guilt, social withdrawal, stigmatisation and fear of sexual harassment. Research indicates that women with substance use problems are more likely than men to have a partner with a substance use problem; more severe problems at the beginning of treatment; trauma related to physical and sexual abuse; and concurrent psychiatric disorders (UNDOC 2004). These complex factors give some indications as to why women have been reluctant to engage in treatment programmes.

TREATMENT SERVICES

A detailed analysis of provisional national treatment monitoring data (NTA 2005) indicated that 28% of the residential treatment episodes and 28.7% of those in structured community treatment were women. Nearly one-third of all self-referrals, GP referrals and other referral sources within the treatment system are for women. In the UK, men and women presented to services with different problems and characteristics. Women reported more frequent cocaine use, greater health problems and increased likelihood of having a drug-using partner and responsibility for children (Stewart *et al.* 2003).

The issue on whether women appear to be underrepresented in drug treatment services in England is debatable. A review of women in drug treatment services (Best and Abdulrahim 2005) suggests that, although women enter treatment at different points in their drug-using careers, with different needs and different problems, there is no clear evidence to suggest that women are generally underrepresented in treatment services in England. However, alcohol and drug treatment services are failing to address the special needs of women and the issues that have a significant influence in female alcohol and drug addiction. A survey of treatment agencies by the National Institute on Drug Abuse (NIDA 1993) found that male staff and participants were openly hostile to women clients, employed a confrontational 'therapeutic' style uncomfortable for women, and directed them into gender-stereotyped tasks and training which offered minimal compensation or chance for success after completion of the programme. In addition, the treatment programmes failed to address issues of violence, sexual exploitation and lack of provision for childcare and prenatal medical services.

Addiction services could implement governmental policy recommendations by providing women with day care and treatment services. This may reduce some of the barriers to women seeking help. Because women have many specific needs, a number of components of treatment have been found to be important in attracting and retaining women in treatment. These include the availability of female-oriented services, supportive therapeutic environment and non-coercive treatment approaches. The intervention strategies should include motivational enhancement, cognitive behavioural therapy and brief therapy and treatment for a wide range of medical problems, co-existing disorders and psychosocial problems. Health and social care professionals need to increase their understanding of gender issues and alcohol and drug use, and service provision should be more sensitive to women's needs.

KEY POINTS

- Alcohol and drug misuse by women is considered to be deviant behaviour and women are more stigmatised, marginalised and labelled.
- Women's alcohol consumption, particularly in younger and older women, has been increasing over the last few decades.
- In 2007, 13% of women drank over the weekly recommendations (14 units for women). In 2006/7, 2% of women used class A drugs.
- The physical, psychological and social effects of alcohol are more severe for women than for men.
- Women develop alcohol-related problems and alcohol dependence faster than men and many die younger than men with similar drinking problems.
- The most serious outcome of maternal drinking during pregnancy is foetal alcohol spectrum disorders (FASD).
- Smoking during pregnancy not only harms a woman's health but can lead to pregnancy complications and serious health problems in newborns.
- Premature and low-birth-weight babies face an increased risk of serious health problems during the newborn period, chronic lifelong disabilities and even death.
- All drugs taken during pregnancy will reach the baby through the placenta.
- Alcohol and drug treatment have been available to women but the provision of services is seldom based on the special physical, psychological and social needs of women.
- The blood-borne viruses such as HIV and hepatitis B and C are transmitted from mother to baby.
- Pregnant women who have hepatitis B should have their babies vaccinated with the hepatitis B vaccine and immunoglobulin soon after delivery.

- The Department of Health in England and Wales has recommended that all pregnant women should be offered antenatal screening for blood-borne viruses and antenatal tests.
- Drug use by parents does not automatically indicate child neglect or abuse.
- Women who misuse alcohol or drugs face a variety of barriers including barriers to treatment entry, to engagement in treatment and long-term rehabilitation.
- Women reported more frequent cocaine use, greater health problems, increased likelihood of having a drug-using partner and responsibility for children.
- There is no clear evidence to suggest that women are generally underrepresented in treatment services in England.

ACTIVITY 15.1

There is only one correct answer to the following multiple-choice questions

What are the government's recommended daily alcohol limits for women in the UK?
a.   1 unit per day
b.   1–2 units per day
c.   2–3 units per day
d.   4 units per day

According to recent research, which of the following nations has the highest rate of binge drinking among men?
a.   UK
b.   Finland
c.   Italy
d.   France

Which one of the following is not true?
a.   Although women are less likely than men to abuse alcohol, they are more likely to have alcohol-related health problems, such as liver disease
b.   Women are less likely than men to have problems with prescribed medications
c.   Alcohol and drug misuse in women increases the risk of developing other health problems, such as osteoporosis or depression
d.   Women who misuse alcohol and drugs attempt suicide four times more frequently than non-users

When drinking the same amount, women become
a.   Less intoxicated than men
b.   More intoxicated than men
c.   There is no difference
d.   More depressed than men

The proportion of 16–24-year-old women who had drunk more than six units on at least one day in the previous week was
a.   24%
b.   28%
c.   30%
d.   35%

In 2007, the percentage of women who drank over the weekly recommendations (14 units for women) was
a.   9%
b.   11%
c.   13%
d.   15%

There is growing evidence that
a.   The physical, psychological and social effects of alcohol are more severe for women
b.   The physical, psychological and social effects of alcohol are less severe for women
c.   There is no difference between men and women
d.   The psychological effects are more severe than the physical effects

Women who drink get intoxicated quicker than men because they have
a.   Higher levels of the enzyme alcohol dehydrogenase
b.   Lower levels of the enzyme alcohol dehydrogenase
c.   Lower blood alcohol concentration
d.   More body fluids than men

Compared to men, women have an increased risk of developing
a.   Alcohol hepatitis
b.   Heart disease
c.   Liver disease
d.   All of the above

The most serious outcome of maternal drinking during pregnancy is
a.   Social, emotional and cognitive development
b.   Learning deficits
c.   Growth retardation
d.   Foetal alcohol spectrum disorders

During pregnancy, women
a.   Should avoid alcohol
b.   Can drink 3–4 units a week
c.   Can drink 2–3 units a week to enhance childbirth
d.   Should drink 3–5 units a day

Tobacco smoking can cause reproductive problems such as
a.   Fertility problems
b.   Premature babies

c.   Low-birth weight babies
d.   All of the above

HIV can be transmitted from mother to baby
a.   Prenatally
b.   At birth
c.   By breastfeeding
d.   All of the above

ACTIVITY 15.2

- Describe the prevalence of alcohol and drug misuse with women
- Discuss the psychosocial and environmental issues related to alcohol and drug misuse
- List the features of foetal alcohol spectrum disorders
- List the problems associated with the following drugs during pregnancy:
  a.   Alcohol
  b.   Heroin
  c.   Cocaine
  d.   Metamphetamine
  e.   LSD
- Discuss the issues of blood-borne viruses in pregnancy
- List the barriers in preventing women accessing treatment services
- Discuss the special treatment needs of women with alcohol and drug problems

---

REFERENCES

ACOG (2005) *Your Pregnancy and Birth*, 4th edition. Washington, DC: American College of Obstetricians and Gynecologists.

Allen, K. (1995) Barriers to treatment for addicted African American women. *Journal of the National Medical Association*, 87, 10: 751–6.

Area Child Protection Committees (2006) *Regional Policy and Procedures*. Northern Ireland: Department of Health, Social Services and Public Safety. http://www.dhsspsni.gov.uk/index/hss/child_care/child_protection/child_protection_guidance.htm (accessed 10 August 2007).

Best, D. and Abdulrahim, D. (2005) *Women in Drug Treatment Services*. London: National Treatment Agency.

Braunstein, G.D., Buster, J.E., Soares, J.R. and Gross, S.J. (1983) Pregnancy hormone concentrations in marijuana users. *Life Science*, 33: 195–9.

British Medical Association (2007) *Fetal Alcohol Spectrum Disorders: A Guide for Health Professionals*. London: BMA Board of Science.

Department for Education and Skills (DfES) (2006) *Working Together to Safeguard Children: A Guide to Inter-agency Working to Safeguard and Promote the Welfare of Children*. London: HM Government.

Department of Health (1996) *Immunisation against Infectious Disease.* London: HMSO.

Department of Health (1998) *Smoking Kills: A White Paper on Tobacco.* London: The Stationery Office.

Department of Health (2008) *Immunisation against Infectious Disease 2006.* London: Department of Health.

Department of Health / Royal College of Midwives (2000) *Hepatitis B in Pregnancy: Information for Midwives.* London: Department of Health.

EMCDDA (2006) *Women and Drug Use in Europe: Annual Report.* European Monitoring Centre for Drugs and Drug Addiction, 8 March.

Ettore, E. (1997) *Women and Alcohol: Private Pleasure or a Public Problem?* London: The Women's Press.

Fergusson, D.M., Horwood, L.J. and Northstone, K. (2002) Maternal use of cannabis and pregnancy outcome. *British Journal of Gynaecology*, 109: 21–7.

Fried, P.A., Watkinson, B. and Gray, R. (2003) Differential effects on cognitive functioning in 13- to 16-year-olds prenatally exposed to cigarettes and marihuana. *Neurotoxicology and Teratology*, 25: 427–36.

Information Centre (2007a) *Statistics on Smoking, England 2007.* http://www.ic.nhs.uk/statistics-and-data-collections/health-and-lifestyles/smoking/statistics-on-smoking-england-2007-%5Bns%5D (accessed 15 September 2007).

Information Centre (2007b) *Statistics on Drug Misuse, England, 2007.* www.ic.nhs.uk/statistics (accessed 30 August 2007).

Jefferis, B., Manor, O. and Power, C. (2007) Social gradients in binge drinking and abstaining: trends in a cohort of British adults. *Journal of Epidemiology and Community Health*, 61: 150–5.

Law, K.L., Stroud, L.R., LaGasse, L.L., Niaura, R., Liu, J. and Lester B.M. (2003) Smoking during pregnancy and newborn neurobehavior. *Pediatrics*, 111, 6: 1318–23.

National Institute on Drug Abuse (1993) *National Pregnancy and Health Survey. Drug Use Among Women Delivering Live Births.* 1992, Rockville: NIDA.

National Statistics (2006) *Key Findings from the Survey Drinking: Adults' Behaviour and Knowledge.* National Statistics website: www.statistics.gov.uk (accessed 25 August 2007).

National Statistics (2007) *News Release*, 28 November. National Statistics website: www.statistics.gov.uk.

NHS Executive (1998) *Screening of Pregnant Women for Hepatitis B and Immunisation of Babies at Risk.* London: Department of Health (HSC 1998/127).

NICE (2003) *Antenatal Care: Routine Care for the Healthy Pregnant Woman. Clinical Guideline.* London: National Institute for Health and Clinical Excellence. http://www.nice.org.uk/CG006 (accessed 26 August 2007).

NIDA (1999) *NIDA Studies Clarify Developmental Effects of Prenatal Cocaine Exposure.* NIDA Notes 14, 3. September.

NTA (2005) *National Drug Treatment Monitoring System (NDTMS) Provisional Unpublished Data 2004–05.* London: National Treatment Agency.

Robbins, C.A. and Martin, S.S. cited in Thom, B. (1997) *Women and Alcohol. Issues for Prevention: A Literature Review.* London: Health Education Authority.

Singer, L.T., Minnes, S., Short, E., Arendt, R., Farkas, K., Lewis, B., Klein, N., Russ, S., Min, M.O. and Kirchner, H.L. (2004) Cognitive outcomes of preschool children with prenatal cocaine exposure. *Journal of the American Medical Association*, 291, 20: 2448–56.

Smith, L.M., LaGasee, L.L., Derauf, C., Grant, P., Shah, R., Arria, A., Huestis, M., Haning, W., Strauss, A., Grotta, S.D., Liu, J. and Lester, B.M. (2006) The infant development, environment, and lifestyle study: effects of prenatal methamphetamine exposure, polydrug exposure, and poverty on intrauterine growth. *Pediatrics*, 118, 3: 1149–56.

Standing Conference on Drug Abuse (SCODA) (1989) *Drug Using Parents and Their Children: The Second Report of the National Local Authority Forum on Drug Abuse in Conjunction with SCODA.* London: Association of Metropolitan Authorities.

Stewart, D., Gossop, M., Marsden, J., Kidd, T. and Treacy, S. (2003) Similarities in outcomes for men and women after drug misuse treatment: result of the National Treatment Outcome Research Study (NTORS). *Drug and Alcohol Review*, 22, 1: 35–41.

UNDOC (2004) *Substance Abuse Treatment and Care for Women*. Vienna: United Nations Office on Drugs and Crime. www.UNDOC.org.

Wang, H., Guo, Y., Wang, D., Kingsley, P.J., Marnett, L.J., Das, S.K., DuBois, R.N. and Dey, S.K. (2004) Aberrant cannabinoid signaling impairs oviductal transport of embryos. *Nature Medicine*, 10: 1074–80.

Waterson, M. cited in Thom, B. (1997) *Women and Alcohol Issues for Prevention*. London: Health Education Authority.

WHO (1997) *Cannabis: A Health Perspective and Research Agenda*. Geneva: World Health Organization, Division of Mental Health and Prevention of Substance Abuse.

CHAPTER 16

PSYCHIATRIC DISORDERS AND SUBSTANCE MISUSE (DUAL DIAGNOSIS)

OBJECTIVES

- Explain the meaning of the term 'dual diagnosis'.

- Have an awareness of the prevalence rates nationally and internationally.

- List the associated consequences of having combined mental health and substance use problems.

- Examine the relationship of substance misuse and mental health problems.

- Discuss some of the models of service delivery and treatment.

- Discuss some of the issues and problems relating to the management of patients with psychiatric disorders and substance misuse.

ACTIVITY 16.1

Before reading this chapter, reflect on the following statements

	Agree	Disagree
Drug use is a direct cause of long-term mental health problems		
Individuals with dual diagnosis bring on all their problems because of their substance misuse		
If they stopped using drugs then all their symptoms of mental disorder would remit		

Individuals have to 'hit rock-bottom' before they will change to remain drug-free

It is impossible to work with substance misusers therapeutically

It is important for someone with dual diagnosis to accept that they are an addict before they can benefit from treatment

Small amounts of cannabis will make little difference to someone with schizophrenia

It is not possible to work therapeutically with people who are on prescribed medication for mental health problems

Source: Banerjee *et al.* (2002)

Do you agree or disagree with the above statements? State the reasons why you either agree or disagree. Please read the Royal College of Psychiatrists' Research Unit (2002) *Co-existing Problems of Mental Disorder and Substance Misuse (Dual Diagnosis)*, pages 14–16, for possible explanations of the above statements.

In the United Kingdom, there is broad recognition of the increase in the number of mentally ill patients who misuse psychoactive substances. Alcohol and drug problems are associated with depression, anxiety disorders, schizophrenia and personality disorders amongst other conditions. The combination of substance misuse and mental health problems is associated with a host of serious social, behavioural, psychological and physical problems, resulting in increased demands on mainstream services. Dual diagnosis has gained prominence partly as a result of the closures of long-stay psychiatric institutions, increasing emphasis on care and treatment in the community and the increasing prevalence of alcohol and drug misuse amongst the general population (Rassool 2006). The easy access of psychoactive substances has drawn those individuals with mental health problems into the drug subculture. Some individuals may self-medicate in an effort to treat their psychiatric symptoms, to counteract the effects of their prescribed medications or to alleviate distressing symptoms from chronic illness. It is stated that, with dual diagnosis patients, the psychiatric disorders and the substance misuse are separate, chronic disorders, each with an independent course, yet each able to influence the properties of each other (Carey 1989).

The *National Service Framework for Mental Health* (Department of Health 1999a) clearly identifies dual diagnosis patients as a population with a greater risk of stigmatisation and exclusion from existing service provision. Healthcare professionals may be reluctant to intervene with dual diagnosis patients or those with substance use problems because of either lack of knowledge and expertise regarding substance misuse or negative attitudes towards the substance misusers. Mental health nurses consider those with substance use problems difficult to treat, and addiction nurses feel that they are not prepared to work with psychiatric patients (Allen and Gerace 1996).

CONCEPT, CLASSIFICATION AND THEORIES

However, there is still no consensus or common understanding of what is meant by dual diagnosis. The concept 'dual diagnosis' has been applied to a number of individuals with two co-existing disorders or conditions such as a physical illness and mental health problems, schizophrenia and substance misuse or learning disability and mental health problems. The concepts of 'dual diagnosis' and 'co-morbidity' are now used commonly and interchangeably. The concept of complex or multiple needs is also associated with those having two existing conditions, including medical, psychological, social or legal needs or problems. The term 'dual diagnosis' covers a broad spectrum of mental health and substance misuse problems that an individual might experience concurrently (Department of Health 2002). In the context of this chapter, the concept of dual diagnosis is defined as the co-existence of substance misuse and mental health problems.

The dual-diagnosis individual meets the *Diagnostic and Statistical Manual of Mental Disorders* (DSM-1V) criteria for both substance abuse or dependency and a co-existing psychiatric disorder (American Psychiatric Association 1994). The nature of the relationship between these two conditions is complex. The relationships between substance misuse and mental health problems can manifest itself in various ways, as shown in Table 16.1. There is no single type of dual diagnosis, as there are many patterns of alcohol or drug misuse and different types of psychiatric disorders. In the *Dual Diagnosis Good Practice Guide* (Department of Health 2002), a more manageable and clinically relevant interrelationship between psychiatric disorder and substance misuse has been described. The four possible relationships are:

- a primary psychiatric illness precipitating or leading to substance misuse
- substance misuse worsening or altering the course of a psychiatric illness
- intoxication and/or substance dependence leading to psychological symptoms
- substance misuse and/or withdrawal leading to psychiatric symptoms or illnesses.

Figure 16.1 presents the scope of co-existent psychiatric and substance misuse disorders (Department of Health 2002). The horizontal axis represents severity of mental illness and the vertical axis the severity of substance misuse. Intervention strategies would need to focus on those whose severity falls within the top right and bottom right quadrants.

The aetiology of dual diagnosis is unclear and there is a wide consensus of opinions for co-morbidity to occur. There are a variety of theories that hypothesise why individuals with mental health problems are vulnerable in the misuse of alcohol and drugs. These include the self-medication hypothesis, the alleviation of dysphoria model, the multiple risk factor model and the supersensitivity model. These theories or models are described in Rassool (2006, Chapter 1). The explanations of why substance misuse and psychiatric disorders occur are presented in Table 16.2.

Table 16.1 Substance use and psychiatric syndromes

- Substance use (even single dose) may lead to psychiatric syndromes and/or symptoms
- Harmful use may produce psychiatric syndromes
- Dependence may produce psychological symptoms
- Intoxication from substances may produce psychological symptoms
- Withdrawal from substances may produce psychological symptoms
- Withdrawal from substances may lead to psychiatric syndromes
- Substance use may exacerbate pre-existing psychiatric disorder
- Psychological morbidity not amounting to a disorder may precipitate substance use
- Primary psychiatric disorder may lead to substance use disorder
- Primary psychiatric disorder may precipitate substance disorder, which may, in turn, lead to psychiatric syndromes

---

Source: Based on Crome 1999

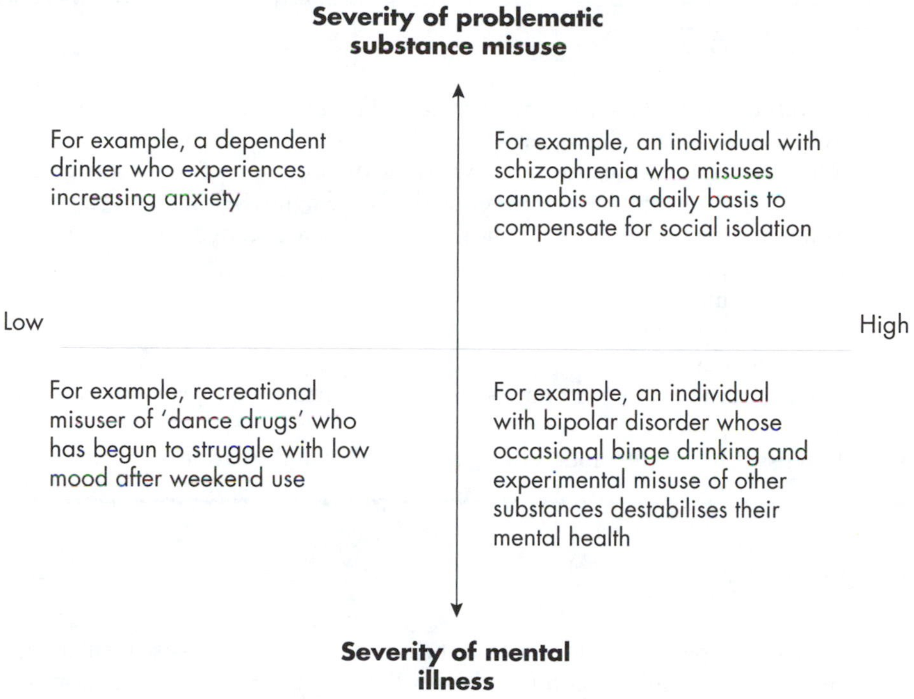

**Severity of problematic
substance misuse**

For example, a dependent
drinker who experiences
increasing anxiety

For example, an individual with
schizophrenia who misuses
cannabis on a daily basis to
compensate for social isolation

Low   High

For example, recreational
misuser of 'dance drugs' who
has begun to struggle with low
mood after weekend use

For example, an individual
with bipolar disorder whose
occasional binge drinking and
experimental misuse of other
substances destabilises their
mental health

**Severity of mental
illness**

FIGURE 16.1 The scope of co-existent psychiatric and substance misuse disorders

Source: Department of Health (2002)

Table 16.2 Why do substance misuse and psychiatric disorders commonly co-occur?

Factors	Explanations
Genetic vulnerabilities	Evidence suggests that common genetic factors may predispose individuals to both psychiatric disorders and addiction or to having a greater risk of the second disorder once the first appears
Environmental triggers	Stress, trauma (for example physical or sexual abuse) and early exposure to drugs are common factors that can lead to addiction and to psychiatric disorders particularly in those with underlying genetic vulnerabilities.
Involvement of similar brain regions	Some areas of the brain are affected by both drug misuse and psychiatric disorders. For example, brain circuits linked to reward processing as well as those implicated in the stress response are affected by abused substances and also show abnormalities in specific psychiatric disorders
Developmental disorders	They often begin in adolescence or even childhood, periods when the brain is undergoing dramatic developmental changes. Early exposure to drugs of addiction can change the brain in ways that increase the risk for mental illness just as early symptoms of a psychiatric disorder may increase vulnerability to alcohol and drug misuse

Source: Adapted from NIDA (2007)

ACTIVITY 16.2

Before reading the next section, try to answer the following questions
- Why is there so much concern about dual diagnosis patients?
- Why do substance misuse and psychiatric disorders commonly co-occur?
- What are the problems associated with dual diagnosis?
- What are the common mental health problems associated with
  a. Alcohol
  b. Stimulants
  c. Hallucinogen
  d. Opiates
- What are the problems and issues faced by healthcare professionals and service providers?
- Discuss some of the models of service delivery and treatment

PREVALENCE

There is now strong research evidence that the rate of substance misuse is substantially higher among the mentally ill compared with the general population. Amongst this severely mentally ill population, use of certain types of drugs, particularly alcohol and cannabis, appears to be quite common. The prevalence rate of substance use disorder among individuals with mental health problems ranges from 35% to 60% (Mueser *et al.* 1995, Menezes *et al.* 1996). The UK study (Menezes *et al.* 1996) of 171 inner-city London patients in contact with psychiatric services found that the one-year prevalence rate among subjects with psychotic illness for any substance misuse problem was 36.3% (31.6% alcohol, 15.8% drugs). The National Treatment Outcome Research Study (NTORS) (Gossop *et al.* 1998) found evidence of psychiatric disorders among individuals with primary substance use disorders. The *National Treatment Outcome and Research Study* (NTORS) found that 10% of substance misuse patients entering treatment had a psychiatric admission (not related to substance dependence) in the previous two years.

In a study of the prevalence and management of co-morbidity amongst adult substance misuse and mental health treatment populations (Weaver *et al.* 2002), the findings showed that some 74.5% of users of drug services and 85.5% of users of alcohol services experienced mental health problems. Most had affective disorders (depression) and anxiety disorders and psychosis. Almost 30% of the drug treatment population and over 50% of those in treatment for alcohol problems experienced 'multiple' morbidity (co-occurrence of a number of psychiatric disorders or substance misuse problems). Some 38.5% of drug users with a psychiatric disorder were receiving no treatment for their mental health problem. Some 44% of mental health service users reported drug use and/or were assessed to have used alcohol at hazardous or harmful levels in the past year.

In a study of the prevalence of co-morbid psychiatric illness and substance misuse in primary care in England and Wales (Frisher *et al.* 2004), the rate of mental illness combined with drug misuse was shown to have climbed more than 60% in five years.

The data were taken from 230 general practices (equivalent to over 3% of the population) of England and Wales between 1993 and 1998. Drug misuse excluded alcohol and tobacco, but included prescription and illegal psychoactive substances. The findings suggest that the number of people with mental illness and drug misuse problems rose from 23,624 in 1993 to 37,361 in 1998. The problem was greatest in certain types of mental health problems. The rate of psychosis and drug misuse soared by 147% in five years, while that of paranoia and drug misuse rose by 144%. Rates of schizophrenia combined with drug misuse rose 128%. In relation to the use of drug and alcohol misuse among inpatients with psychotic illness, a study by Phillips and Johnson (2003) showed that 83% of the patients had used at least once on current admission. In addition, 4% reported to have had their first ever experience of drug use on a ward with other patients.

A study by Frisher *et al*. (2005) showed that patients exposed to substance misuse were 1.54 times more likely to develop psychiatric illness than those not exposed to substance misuse. Patients exposed to psychiatric illness were 2.09 times more likely to develop substance misuse than those not exposed to psychiatric illness. The authors suggest that problematic substance misuse does not make an important contribution to the population burden of psychiatric illness. Only a comparatively small proportion of psychiatric illness seems possibly attributable to substance use whereas a more substantial proportion of substance use seems possibly attributable to psychiatric illness.

A UK study (Barnett *et al*. 2007) found that the majority of patients presenting with first episode psychosis reported substance use. Reported substance use in this population was twice that of the general population. Cannabis and alcohol were the two most frequently reported forms of substance use or abuse, 51% of the sample meeting standard criteria for cannabis abuse or dependence and 43% meeting the criteria for alcohol abuse or dependence at some point in their life. Despite certain methodological difficulties and given the nature of the problem, it is likely that the prevalence figures underrepresent the actual level of substance misuse and psychiatric disorders.

MULTIPLE AND COMPLEX NEEDS

Individuals with substance misuse and psychiatric disorders are a vulnerable group of people with complex needs and problems. A variety of problems are possible as a result of a dual diagnosis: the withdrawal from alcohol or drug can mimic or give the appearance of some psychiatric disorders; psychiatric symptoms may be covered up or masked by alcohol or drug use; untreated alcohol and drug dependence can contribute to a reoccurrence of psychiatric symptoms; and untreated psychiatric disorders can contribute to an alcohol or drug lapse or relapse. Individuals with this combination of problems often have a lot of additional difficulties which are not purely medical, psychological or psychiatric. They are more likely to have worse prognosis with high levels of service use including emergency clinic and inpatient admissions (McCrone *et al*. 2000) and problems related to social, legal, housing, welfare and 'lifestyle' matters. In summary, the major problems associated with individuals with dual diagnosis are presented in Table 16.3.

In addition, individuals from Black and ethnic minority groups with dual diagnosis face compounded pressure of stigma, prejudice, institutional racism and ethnocentric

Table 16.3 Problems associated with dual diagnosis

- Increased likelihood of self-harm
- Increased risk of HIV infection
- Increased use of institutional services
- Poor compliance with medication or treatment
- Homelessness
- Increased risk of violence
- Increased risk of victimisation or exploitation
- Higher recidivism
- Contact with the criminal justice system
- Family problems
- Poor social outcomes including impact on carers and family
- Denial of substance misuse
- Negative attitudes of healthcare professionals
- Social exclusion

intervention strategies. These complex needs cannot be dealt with by a single approach and would require a more holistic approach from several different agencies or services in order to meet the medical, psychological, social, spiritual and legal needs of the individual. It is acknowledged that, as a group, dual diagnosis patients are more difficult to manage and treat in view of their complex needs. Dual diagnosis patients tend to place a heavy demand on service provision and have been associated with poor outcomes on most measures – housing status, employment status, social functioning and family relationships (Department of Health 1999b).

ALCOHOL AND MENTAL HEALTH

Alcohol and mental health problems are often linked, and 85.5% of users of alcohol services experienced mental health problems (Weaver *et al.* 2002). Most had affective disorders (depression), anxiety disorders and psychosis. Common links with alcohol and mental health include depression, suicidal behaviour, anxiety, obsessive-compulsive disorders, bipolar disorders, schizophrenia and personality disorders (Institute of Alcohol Studies 2004). Just over 50% of those in treatment for alcohol problems experienced 'multiple' morbidity (co-occurrence of a number of psychiatric disorders or substance misuse problems). The alcohol strategy for England (Prime Minister's Strategy Unit 2004) clearly states that mental health and alcohol problems are of high concern, particularly in relation to suicide, vulnerability, homelessness and physical and mental health problems. Jenkins *et al.* (1997) reported that, in any week, 16% of the UK population aged 16–64 met criteria for an ICD-10 anxiety or depressive disorder, and that, in any year, 4.7% had alcohol dependence and 2.2% drug dependence.

The links between alcohol and mental health can be extremely complex; however there are four broad characteristics used in dual diagnosis to explain relationships (Abdulrahim 2001).

- Alcohol is used to medicate psychological distress or symptoms (self-medication).
- Alcohol use causes psychological distress or symptoms (side effect).

- Alcohol is used with no causal or preventative mechanism for psychological distress or symptoms.
- Underlying trauma results in alcohol use and mood disorders.

RELATIONSHIP OF ALCOHOL AND ANXIETY DISORDERS

Anxiety disorders are among the most common mental health problems, affecting 10% of the population. The number of UK hospital admissions with a primary or secondary diagnosis of mental and behavioural disorders due to alcohol rose from 71,900 in 1995/6 to over 90,000 in 2002/3 (Department of Health 2004). At least two-thirds of alcohol-dependent individuals entering treatment show evidence of anxiety, sadness, depression and/or manic-like symptoms (Crawford 2001). The *Diagnostic and Statistical Manual of Mental Disorders* (DSM-IV) defines a diagnosis of substance-induced anxiety disorder as present when there is evidence that persistent anxiety symptoms, including panic attacks, obsessions, or compulsions have arisen out of use of or withdrawal from either prescribed or recreational drug use (including alcohol) (APA 1994).

Evidence from research studies has shown substantial co-occurrence between anxiety disorders and alcohol problems, and indicates that alcohol misusers are at two to three times the risk of suffering from an anxiety disorder (Ross *et al.* 1988). Anxiety disorders may be a risk factor for the development of substance misuse, and anxiety symptoms are likely to be present during chronic intoxication and withdrawal. There is evidence to suggest that people with high anxiety sensitivity may be at risk for alcohol misuse (MacDonald *et al.* 2000). Those who experience symptoms such as 'butterflies', rapid breathing or an increased heart rate in the face of a stressful situation are described as having high anxiety sensitivity according to the study, and they are more likely to 'soothe' their anxiety by drinking. Additionally, alcohol misuse may result from increased dosing of alcohol, which appears to provide increased relief from anxiety sensitivity. Scientists have identified a brain mechanism in rats that may play a central role in regulating anxiety and alcohol-drinking (Pandey *et al.* 2005). The finding could provide important clues about the neurobiology of alcohol-drinking behaviours in humans.

The feelings of anxiety may be temporarily relieved by alcohol consumption but prolonged alcohol misuse often heightens anxiety. It is reported that alcohol can increase clinical anxiety, especially after prolonged drinking and during withdrawal, and thus anxiety disorders such as panic disorder and generalised anxiety disorder may be related to these situations rather than be a primary psychiatric disorder in these individuals (Harrison and Abou-Saleh 2001). For this reason, alcohol may be consumed in increasing quantities by people with a drinking problem, involving them in a vicious cycle: drinking to self-medicate their anxiety but, in so doing, furthering their anxiety in the long term (Lingford-Hughes *et al.* 2002). Agoraphobia, social phobias, panic disorder and generalised anxiety are all more commonly reported by heavy drinkers than by the general population (Stockwell 1995). The self-medication hypothesis has been popular, and in many studies patients describe using alcohol to control their phobic fears and anxiety (Bibb and Chambless 1986). The relationship between alcohol and anxiety may differ between genders. One study of hospitalised male and female depressive patients found that there was a strong association between anxiety and alcohol misuse for women and a weaker association for men (Fischer and Goethe 1998).

RELATIONSHIP OF ALCOHOL AND DEPRESSION

Alcohol consumption may be either a cause or a consequence of depression. There is evidence to suggest that alcohol-use disorders are linked to depressive symptoms, and that alcohol dependence and depressive disorders co-occur to a larger degree than expected by chance (Mental Health Foundation 2006). Depressive symptoms have been found to be most common in heavy drinkers (over 50 units a week for men and 35 units a week for women) (Mehrabian 2001, Alcohol Concern 2004). However, it is not clear whether depression precedes or causes alcohol problems, whether the alcohol consumption or alcohol problems cause depression. It is likely that alcohol problems and depression interact with a number of other factors that maintain or worsen depressive symptoms and that risk factors for poor mental health are also risk factors for alcohol misuse (Mental Health Foundation 2006).

Some people use alcohol when they experience moderate to high levels of shyness or fear or fail to cope with social anxiety. The findings of a survey (Mental Health Foundation 2006) were that approximately one-third of the sample reported that drinking made them feel less anxious (40%), less depressed (26%) and more able to forget problems (30%). This is consistent with the theory that people use alcohol to medicate low levels of stress, anxiety and depression. As stated above, self-medication has been proposed as an explanation for alcohol consumption in people with anxiety. The same self-perpetuating and vicious cycle can also offer an explanation for people with depression. The increase of tolerance of alcohol leads to increased drinking to achieve the same desired effect. The pharmacological actions of alcohol can also interact with an individual's pre-existing mood or personality and the drinker's beliefs and expectations about the effect of the alcohol and the context in which it is being consumed (Institute of Alcohol Studies 2004). Alcohol acts as a reinforcing agent exacerbating the cyclical pattern of more alcohol consumption to reduce the feelings of depression. In addition, there is some evidence that abstaining from alcohol consumption significantly reduces depressive symptoms in individuals who are dependent on alcohol within a short time frame (Schuckit and Monteiro 1988).

Research shows that people with alcohol dependence are more at risk of suicide, and as many as 65% of suicides have been linked to excessive drinking (Department of Health 1993). It is estimated that the risk of suicide of problem drinkers is eight times greater than in the absence of current alcohol misuse or dependence (Institute of Alcohol Studies 2005). Amongst men with a chronic alcohol problem, about 40% try to kill themselves and as many as 70% of those who succeed have drunk alcohol before doing so (Royal College of Psychiatrists 2004). Excessive alcohol consumption in women has also been found to be significantly associated with attempted suicide by drug overdose (Watson et al. 1991). Young people are also particularly vulnerable and it is estimated that one-third of suicides amongst young people are committed whilst the young person is intoxicated (NHS Advisory Service 1994).

DRUGS AND MENTAL HEALTH

Drug misusers may show symptoms such as mania, psychosis, depression, anxiety and personality disorder symptoms. This is dependent on the type of drug used, the quantity consumed and the route of administration. Psychiatric symptoms occur more commonly in drug-related problems and it is difficult to distinguish between the psychiatric symptoms and dual diagnosis.

In relation to stimulants, up to 80% of regular cocaine users experience symptoms such as euphoria, grandiosity, impulsiveness, impaired judgement and marked psycho-motor activity, usually subsiding within half an hour and which are indistinguishable from hypomania (Harrison and Abou-Saleh 2001). Hallucinations, both visual and auditory, similar to those seen in schizophrenia, and tactile hallucinations are experienced by the cocaine user. A condition known as a toxic psychosis results from prolonged or high-dose use of cocaine but may be indistinguishable from acute psychosis of other causes. However, the condition usually subsides within 24 hours. In a study examining the relationship between social phobia and cocaine dependence, Myrick and Brady (1997) found a lifetime prevalence of social phobia in these cocaine dependent individuals to be 13.9%. They also found that the social phobic individuals were more likely to have additional psychopathology and use multiple psychoactive substances, and were more likely to develop alcohol misuse at an earlier age. Amphetamines may produce similar toxic reactions: the psychosis may last longer than that produced by cocaine, but will usually resolve within a few days (Connell 1958). This condition usually occurs in long-term users, but may start a day or two after use and consists of disordered thinking, hallucinations and paranoid ideas and repetitive behaviour such as involuntary picking and scratching at the skin.

The consumption of cannabis can lead to the development anxiety and panic attacks. Symptoms are usually brief in duration and may include restlessness, depersonalisation, derealisation, paranoia and transient mood disorders (Thomas 1993). Acute toxic confusional states can be developed as a result of high doses or prolonged consumption of cannabis and are indistinguishable from schizophrenia. It is difficult to differentiate whether these illnesses are in fact relapses in previously psychotic patients who use cannabis, precipitated in patients who are vulnerable, or actual reactions produced by ingestion of cannabis (Harrison and Abou-Saleh 2001). There is no conclusive evidence that cannabis can cause long-term psychiatric disorders or is an independent risk factor for schizophrenia.

A summary of the negative effects of specific psychoactive substance is presented in Table 16.4.

RELATIONSHIP OF ALCOHOL, DRUGS AND PERSONALITY DISORDERS

Individuals receiving treatment for alcohol dependence are often also diagnosed with a personality disorder. The estimation of prevalence rate varies from 44% among alcohol patients to 79% among opiate users, and many of these individuals may have more than one type of personality disorder (Harrison and Abou-Saleh 2001). In a study

Table 16.4 Substance misuse and psychiatric disorders

Category of substance	Type of substance	Common mental health problems
	Alcohol	• Alcoholic hallucinosis (persecutory auditory hallucinations) • Depression and suicidal ideation • Social phobia • Pathological jealousy • Delirium tremens • Wernike's encephalopathy • Korsakoff's 'psychosis' • Personality disorder
Stimulant	Amphetamine	• Disordered thinking • Hallucinations • Paranoid ideas • Production of random, pointless, repetitive behaviour (such as involuntary picking and scratching at the skin) • Restlessness • Sleep disturbances
Stimulant	Cocaine	• Experience of hallucinations (visual, auditory and tactile) • Paranoid feelings • Irritability • Toxic psychosis with persecutory delusions and hallucinations • Loss of insight (condition which usually subsides within 24 hours) • Depression • Sleep disturbances
Hallucinogen	Cannabis	• Anxiety and panic attacks • Restlessness • Depersonalisation • Derealisation • Paranoia • Transient mood disorders • Acute toxic confusional state
	LSD	• Hallucinations • Panic reactions • Flashback (recurrence of symptoms)
Opiate	Heroin	• Anxiety • Depression • Suicide • Overdose • Personality disorder

of the prevalence of personality disorders among patients with a current alcohol use disorder, 28.6% had at least one personality disorder, and 47.7% of those with a current drug use disorder had at least one personality disorder (Grant *et al.* 2004). The findings also showed that individuals with alcohol use disorders were almost five times as likely to have antisocial personality disorder and were three times as likely to have a dependent personality. Individuals with drug-use disorders were 11 times more likely to have antisocial personality disorder. The researchers also found that associations between obsessive-compulsive, histrionic, schizoid, and antisocial personality disorders and specific alcohol and drug use disorders were significantly stronger among women than men, whereas the association between personality disorder and drug dependence was significantly greater among men than women. A recent study found that 44.3% of the alcohol-dependent patients showed at least one personality disorder (Echeburua *et al.* 2007). Bernstein and Handelsman (1995) have proposed three mechanisms to try to explain the high levels of co-morbidity:

- Substance misuse often takes place in the context of a deviant peer group, and antisocial behaviours are shaped and reinforced by social group norms.
- Psychoactive substances have the potential to alter behaviour through their effects as reinforcers or conditioning agents, linking environmental and internal cues to substance use.
- Chronic substance use may alter personality through its direct effects on brain chemistry.

People with antisocial personality disorder are more susceptible to alcohol's aggression-related effects than people without the disorder. Several studies have demonstrated that aggressive personality traits are associated with an increase in aggression after drinking alcohol (Moeller and Dougherty 2001). Personality disorders have been found to be related to poor treatment response and outcome in patients with substance misuse and psychiatric problems. Several studies suggest that impaired coping, social functioning and low motivation or readiness to change are associated with higher rates of low attrition caused by the treatment (Ball *et al.* 2006). Motivational, interpersonal, and perceptional problems need to be considered as core features in the treatment of dually diagnosed patients, thus maximising the effectiveness of treatment and outcome.

RELATIONSHIP OF ALCOHOL, DRUGS AND SCHIZOPHRENIA

Some individuals who misuse drugs show symptoms similar to those of schizophrenia, and people with schizophrenia may be mistaken for people who are high on drugs. It is estimated that up to 50% of people with psychiatric disorders misuse alcohol and drugs (Selzer and Lieberman 1993). However, substance use may exacerbate schizophrenic symptoms and produce psychotic symptoms in their own right, with the impact of the substance use varying depending on the class of drug used, the quantity consumed, the route of administration and the state of use (Harrison and Abou-Saleh 2001). Patients with schizophrenia have a preference for activating drugs such as amphetamines, cocaine, cannabis and hallucinogens (Ries *et al.* 2000).

Schizophrenic patients who misuse alcohol may be more likely to exhibit hostile behaviour, paranoid thoughts and depression than non-alcohol-using patients (Harrison and Abou-Saleh 2001). There is evidence to suggest that drug misuse in schizophrenia is correlated significantly with negative and positive symptoms but, in the case of alcohol use, it was not unless it reached the point of alcohol treatment (Swofford *et al.* 2000). Substance misuse can also reduce the effectiveness of treatment for schizophrenia and also makes it more likely that individuals will not follow their treatment programme. The most common form of substance misuse in individuals with schizophrenia is an addiction to nicotine. Quitting smoking may be especially difficult for people with schizophrenia since nicotine withdrawal may cause their psychotic symptoms to temporarily get worse.

MODELS OF CARE

Models of Care sets a national framework for promoting evidence-based practice and good practice guidelines. The care and management of patients with substance misuse and psychiatric disorders require a multidisciplinary approach. While there is some evidence on the various models of treatment, the complex nature of this patient group would suggest the need to work towards an integrated approach by all the relevant services, with one lead service co-ordinating the comprehensive care package (National Treatment Agency 2002). However, the document fails to address important issues relating to social care, the resource implications of this major service development and the interface between mainstream mental health services and addiction services, as well as implications for the future and the scope of addiction services (Abou Saleh 2004).

The involvement of service users, families and carers is central in the care planning and treatment process and must not be tokenistic or superficial. The involvement should takes place at all stages: in treatment, in the planning, delivery and development of existing services and in the planning and commissioning of future services (Rethink and Turning Point 2004). Attention also needs to be focused on special populations in relation to dual diagnosis such as Black and ethnic minority groups, homeless and older people (alcohol and tranquillisers), young people and women (Health Advisory Service 2001).

Generally, four models of service provision have been described for the treatment of substance misuse and psychiatric disorders: the serial model, the parallel model, the integrated treatment model and the joint liaison/collaborative approach (see Rassool 2002). The four models of service delivery potential problems and difficulties of each model are presented in Table 16.5. However, there is no clear evidence supporting the advantage of any model in preference over others (Health Advisory Service 2001, Ley *et al.* 2001). Service configurations for dual diagnosis patients need to be based on local needs assessment.

PROBLEMS AND ISSUES FOR HEALTHCARE PROFESSIONALS

The term 'dual diagnosis' is often used to describe this co-existence, and these patients tend to be more problematic to treat and manage in view of higher rates of non-compliance, violence, homelessness and suicide. The relationship between substance misuse and mental health problems is complex. Intoxication and withdrawal from drugs and alcohol can produce psychiatric symptoms while on the other hand some individuals with psychiatric disorders such as antisocial personality disorders and schizophrenia are more susceptible to substance misuse (Rassool 2006).

Table 16.5 Models of treatment and potential difficulties

Model of treatment	Description	Problems or difficulties
Serial treatment	Treatment programmes are provided consecutively by the mental health services and substance-misuse services depending on the presenting problem	• Limited communication between the services • Health problems treated as separate entities • Patients are shunted between the two services
Parallel treatment	The care of the patient is provided by both services concurrently, facilitated by communication between the two services	• Patients are shunted between the two services • Health problems are treated as separate entities • Medical responsibility not clearly defined
Integrated treatment	The care of the patient is jointly managed by both services (designated service)	• Isolated from mainstream services • Views dual diagnosis as a static condition • Expensive service provision
Joint liaison/ collaborative approach	The care of the patient is jointly managed by both services	• Joint working between mental health and substance misuse services • Joint responsibility • Ensures the skills and expertise of both spheres of healthcare are utilised

Source: NTA 2002

The mental state of the individual may act as a barrier to recognition, as some patients may not be able to understand the nature of the symptoms they experience or adequately describe them in a way that enables clinical staff to make an accurate assessment. The task of assessing their needs is compounded by the fact that some patients are not capable of understanding or describing the nature of the symptoms they experience. This is further complicated by the fact that individuals may use a combination of psychoactive substances. Even when substance misuse is identified, it is often difficult to distinguish between symptoms that are related to substance misuse or a psychiatric disorder. Failure to recognise and treat substance misuse at an early stage will not only lead to ineffective management and treatment outcomes but may also result in a deterioration of the patient's symptomatology. Furthermore, it is difficult to get individuals with a dual diagnosis to follow or comply with the treatment regimes. Compliance with taking prescribed medication has been shown to be poor in mentally ill clients with substance misuse problems (Pristach and Smith 1990).

There is also the need to address the training and continuing professional development of staff to working with the co-existence of substance misuse and psychiatric disorders. There is evidence to suggest that mental health service workers lacked the knowledge and skills for assessment and treatment of substance misuse and were insufficiently aware of the available resources and how to access substance misuse services (Maslin *et al*. 2001). Dual diagnosis, similar to substance misuse, is not the sole responsibility of one discipline or specialist. It requires a multidimensional approach and involving inter-agency collaboration in the ownership of common goals in meeting the complex physical or medical, social psychological and spiritual needs of the individual (Rassool 2006).

KEY POINTS

- The term 'dual diagnosis' covers a broad spectrum of mental health and substance misuse problems that an individual might experience concurrently.
- There is no single type of dual diagnosis as there are many patterns of alcohol or drug misuse and different types of psychiatric disorders.
- Intoxication and/or substance dependence can lead to psychological symptoms.
- Substance misuse and/or withdrawal can lead to psychiatric symptoms or illnesses.
- There are a variety of theories that hypothesise why individuals with mental health problems are vulnerable in the misuse of alcohol and drug.
- The prevalence rate of substance-use disorder among individuals with mental health problems ranges from 35% to 60%.
- Most users of substance-misuse services had affective disorders (depression) and anxiety disorders and psychosis.
- Patients exposed to psychiatric illness were 2.09 times more likely to develop substance misuse than those not exposed to psychiatric illness.
- Individuals with substance-misuse and psychiatric disorders are a vulnerable group of people with complex needs and problems.
- Alcohol misusers had affective disorders (depression), anxiety disorders and psychosis.
- Just over 50% of those in treatment for alcohol problems experienced 'multiple' morbidity (co-occurrence of a number of psychiatric disorders or substance-misuse problems).
- The Alcohol Strategy for England clearly states that mental health and alcohol problems are of high concern, particularly in relation to suicide, vulnerability, homelessness and physical and mental health problems
- Evidence from research studies has shown substantial co-occurrence between anxiety disorders and alcohol problems.
- Drug misusers may show symptoms such as mania, psychosis, depression, anxiety and personality disorder symptoms.
- Individuals receiving treatment for alcohol-dependence are often also diagnosed with a personality disorder.
- It is estimated that up to 50% of people with psychiatric disorders misuse alcohol and drugs.
- The mental state of the patient may act as a barrier to recognition as some patients may not be able to understand the nature of the symptoms they experience or adequately describe them in a way that enables clinical staff to make an accurate assessment.
- The assessment is compounded by the fact that some patients are not capable of understanding or describing the nature of the symptoms they experience.
- Dual diagnosis, like substance misuse, requires a multi-dimensional approach involving inter-agency collaboration.

REFERENCES

Abdulrahim, D. (2001) *Substance Misuse and Mental Health Co-morbidity (Dual Diagnosis)*. London: The Health Advisory Service.

Abou-Saleh, M.T. (2004) Dual diagnosis: management within a psychosocial context. *Advances in Psychiatric Treatment*, 10: 352–60.

Alcohol Concern (2004) *Factsheet 17: Alcohol and Mental Health*. London: Alcohol Concern.

Allen, K.M. and Gerace, L.M. (1996) Psychiatric nursing. In K.M. Allen (ed.) *Nursing Care of the Addicted Client*. Philadelphia: Lippincott.

American Psychiatric Association (APA) (1994) *Diagnostic and Statistical Manual of Mental Disorders*, 4th edition. Washington, DC: American Psychiatric Press.

Ball, S.A., Carroll, K.M., Canning-Ball, M. and Rounsaville, B.J. (2006) Reasons for dropout from drug abuse treatment: symptoms, personality, and motivation. *Addictive Behaviours*, 31: 320–30.

Banerjee, S., Clancy, C. and Crome, I. (2002) *Co-existing Problems of Mental Disorder and Substance Misuse (Dual Diagnosis)*. London: Royal College of Psychiatrists' Research Unit. www.rcpsych.ac.uk/cru.

Barnett, J.H., Werners, U., Secher, S.M., Hill, K.E., Brazil, R., Masson, K., Pernet, D.E., Kirkbridge, J.B., Murray, G.K., Bullmore, E.T. and Jones, P.B. (2007) Substance use in a population-based clinic sample of people with first-episode psychosis. *British Journal of Psychiatry*, 190: 515–20.

Bernstein, D.P. and Handelsman, L. (1995) *The Neurobiology of Substance Abuse and Personality Disorders: Neuropsychiatry of Personality Disorders*. Oxford: Blackwell Science.

Bibb, D.L. and Chambless, D.L. (1986) Alcohol use and abuse amongst diagnosed agoraphobics, *Behaviour Research Therapy*, 24: 49–58.

Carey, K.B. (1989) Emerging treatment guidelines for mentally ill chemical abusers. *Hospital and Community Psychiatry*, 42: 721–4.

Connell, P.H. (1958) *Amphetamine Psychosis*, Maudsley Monograph no. 5. London: Oxford University Press.

Crawford, V. (2001) *Co-existing Problems of Mental Health and Substance Misuse ('Dual Diagnosis'): A Review of Relevant Literature*. London: Royal College of Psychiatrists, College Research Unit.

Crome, I.B. (1999) Substance misuse and psychiatric comorbidity: towards improved service provision. *Drugs: Education, Prevention and Policy*. 6: 151–74.

Department of Health (1993) *Health of the Nation Key Area Handbook, Mental Health*. London: HMSO.

Department of Health (1999a) *National Service Framework for Mental Health*. London: HMSO.

Department of Health (1999b) *Effective Care Co-ordination in Mental Health Services: Modernising the Care Programme Approach – A Policy Document*. London: Department of Health.

Department of Health (2002) *Mental Health Policy Implementation Guide. Dual Diagnosis Good Practice Guide*. London: DOH Publications. www.doh.gov.uk/mentalhealth.

Department of Health, Office for National Statistics (2004) *Statistics on Alcohol: England 2004*. London: The Stationery Office.

Echeburua, E., De Medina, R.B. and Aizpiri, J. (2007) Comorbidity of alcohol dependence and personality disorders: a comparative study. *Alcohol and Alcoholism*, 42, 6: 618–22.

Fischer, E.H. and Goethe, J.W. (1998) Anxiety and alcohol abuse in patients in treatment for depression. *American Journal of Alcohol Abuse*, 24, 3: 453–63.

Frisher, M., Collins, J., Millson, D., Crome, I. and Croft, P. (2004) Prevalence of comorbid psychiatric illness and substance misuse in primary care in England and Wales. *Journal of Epidemiology & Community Health*, 58: 1036–41.

Frisher, M., Crome, I., Macleod, J., Millson, D. and Croft, P. (2005) Substance misuse and psychiatric illness: prospective observational study using the general practice research database. *Journal of Epidemiology & Community Health*, 59: 847–50.

Gossop, M., Mardsen, J. and Steward, D. (1998) *NTORS at One Year: The National Treatment Outcome and Research Study*. London: Department of Health.

Grant, B.F., Stinson, F.S., Dawson, D.A., Chou, S.P., Ruan, W.J. and Pickering, R.P. (2004) Co-occurrence of 12-month alcohol and drug use disorders and personality disorders in the United States. *Archives of General Psychiatry*, 61: 361–8.

Harrison, C.A. and Abou-Saleh, M.T. (2001) Psychiatric disorders and substance misuse: psychopathology. In G. Hussein Rassool (ed.) *Dual Diagnosis: Substance Misuse and Psychiatric Disorders*. Oxford: Blackwell Publications.

Health Advisory Service (2001) *Substance Misuse and Mental Health Co-morbidity (Dual Diagnosis): Standards for Mental Health Services*. London: Health Advisory Service.

Institute of Alcohol Studies (2004) *Alcohol and Mental Health*. St Ives, Cambridgeshire: Institute of Alcohol Studies.

Institute of Alcohol Studies (2005) *Alcohol Policies*. St Ives, Cambridgeshire: Institute of Alcohol Studies.

Jenkins, R., Lewis, G., Bebbington, P., Brugha, T., Farrell, M., Gill, B. and Meltzer, H. (1997) The national psychiatric morbidity surveys of great Britain – initial findings from the household survey. *Psychological Medicine*, 27: 775–89.

Ley, A., Jeffery, D., McLaren, S. and Siegfried, N. (2001) *Treatment Programmes for People with both Severe Mental Illness and Substance Misuse*. Cochrane Review Issue 3. The Cochrane Library.

Lingford-Hughes A., Potokar, J. and Nutt, D. (2002) Treating anxiety complicated by substance misuse. *Advances in Psychiatric Treatment*, 8: 107–16.

McCrone, P., Menezes, P.R., Johnson, S. Scott S., Thornicroft, H. and Marshall, J. (2000) Service use and costs of people with dual diagnosis in South London. *Acta Psychiatrica Scandinavia*, 101: 464–72.

MacDonald, A.B., Baker, J.M., Stewart, S.H. and Skinner, M. (2000) Effects of alcohol on the response to hyperventilation of participants high and low in anxiety sensitivity. *Alcoholism: Clinical and Experimental Research*, 24, 11: 1656–65.

Maslin, J., Graham, H.L., Cawley, M.A.C., Birchwood, M., Georgiou, G., McGovern, D., Mueser, K. and Orford J. (2001) Combined severe mental health and substance use problems: what are the training and support needs of staff working with this client group? *Journal of Mental Health*, 10, 2: 131–40.

Mehrabian, A. (2001) General relations among drug use, alcohol use, and major indexes of psychopathology. *Journal of Psychology*, 35, 1: 71–86.

Menezes, P., Johnson, S., Thornicroft, G., Marshall, J., Prosser, D., Bebbington, P. and Kuipers, E. (1996) Drug and alcohol problems among individuals with severe mental illnesses in South London. *British Journal of Psychiatry*, 168: 612–19.

Mental Health Foundation (2006) *Cheers? Understanding the Relationship between Alcohol and Mental Health*. London: Mental Health Foundation.

Moeller, F.G. and Dougherty, D.M. (2001) Antisocial personality disorder, alcohol, and aggression. *Alcohol Research & Health, Alcohol and Violence*, 25, 1: 5–11.

Mueser, K., Bennett, M. and Kushner, M. (1995) *Epidemiology of Substance Use Disorders among Persons with Chronic Mental Illness*. In A. Lehman and L. Dixon (eds) *Double Jeopardy: Chronic Mental Illness and Substance Use Disorders*. Switzerland: Harwood Academic.

Myrick, H. and Brady, K. (1997) *Comorbid Social Phobia and Cocaine Dependence*. American Psychiatric Association New Research Abstracts.

NHS Advisory Service (1994) *Suicide Prevention: The Challenge Confronted*. London: HMSO.

NIDA (2007) *Comorbid Drug Abuse and Mental Illness: A Research Update from the National Institute on Drug Abuse*. Topics in Brief, NIDA. www.drugabuse.gov.

NTA (2002) *Models of Care for Treatment of Adult Drug Users*. London: National Treatment Agency.

Pandey, S.C., Zhang, H., Roy, A. and Xu, T. (2005) Deficits in amygdaloid Camp responsive element-binding protein signaling play a role in genetic predisposition to anxiety and alcoholism. *Journal of Clinical Investigations*, 115: 2762–73.

Phillips, P. and Johnson, S. (2003) Drug and alcohol misuse among in-patients with psychotic illness in three inner London psychiatric units. *Psychiatric Bulletin*, 27: 217–20.

Prime Minister's Strategy Unit (2004). *Alcohol Harm Reduction Strategy for England*. London: Cabinet Office.

Pristach, C.A. and Smith, C.M. (1990) Medication compliance and substance abuse among schizophrenic patients. *Hospital and Community Psychiatry*, 41: 1345–8.

Pristach, C.A. and Smith, C.M. (1996) Self-reported effects of alcohol use on symptoms of schizophrenia. *Psychiatric Services*, 47: 421–3.

Rassool G. Hussein (2002) *Dual Diagnosis: Substance Misuse and Psychiatric Disorders*. Oxford: Blackwell Publishing.

Rassool G. Hussein (2006) Understanding dual diagnosis: an overview. In G. Hussein Rassool (ed.) *Dual Diagnosis Nursing*. Oxford: Blackwell Publishing.

Rethink and Turning Point (2004) *Dual Diagnosis Toolkit, Mental Health and Substance Misuse*. London: Rethink and Turning Point.

Ries, R.K., Russo, J., Wingerson, D., Snowden, M., Comtois, K.A., Srebnik, D. and Roy-Byrne, P. (2000) Shorter hospital stays and more rapid improvement among patients with schizophrenia and substance use disorders. *Psychiatric Services*, 51: 210–15.

Ross, H.E., Glaser, F.B. and Germanson, T. (1988) The prevelance of psychiatric disorders in patients with alcohol and other drug problems. *Archives of General Psychiatry*, 45: 1023–31.

Royal College of Psychiatrists (2004) *Alcohol and Depression – Help Is at Hand*. London: The Royal College of Psychiatrists.

Schuckit, M.A. and Monteiro, M.G. (1988) Alcoholism, anxiety and depression. *British Journal of Addiction*, 83, 12: 1373–80.

Selzer, J.A. and Lieberman, J.A. (1993) Schizophrenia and substance abuse. *Psychiatric Clinic of North America*, 16: 401–12.

Stockwell, T. (1995) Anxiety and stress management. In R. Hester and W. Miller (eds) *Handbook of Alcoholism Treatment Approaches: Effective Alternatives*, Needham Heights, MA: Allyn and Bacon. pp. 242–50.

Swofford, C.D., Scheller-Gilkey, G., Miller, A.H., Woolwine, B. and Mance, R. (2000) Double jeopardy: schizophrenia and substance. *American Journal of Drug and Alcohol Abuse*, 26, 3: 343–53.

Thomas, H. (1993) Psychiatric symptoms in cannabis users. *British Journal of Psychiatry*, 163: 141–9.

Watson, H.E., Kershaw, P.W. and Davies, J.B. (1991) Alcohol problems among women in a general hospital ward. *British Journal of Addiction*, 86, 7: 889–94.

Weaver, T, Charles, V., Madden, P. and Renton A. (2002) *Co-morbidity of Substance Misuse and Mental Illness Collaborative Study (COSMIC)*. London: National Treatment Agency.

ALCOHOL AND DRUG MISUSE IN BLACK AND ETHNIC MINORITY COMMUNITIES

OBJECTIVES

■ Have awareness that Black and ethnic minority communities in the UK are a heterogeneous group.

■ Provide an overview of the policy and strategy in relation to Black and ethnic minority communities.

■ Describe the nature and patterns of substance misuse in Black and ethnic minority communities.

■ Have an awareness of the nature and extent of HIV in Black and ethnic minority communities.

■ Discuss the failure of service provision in meeting the needs of Black and ethnic minority communities.

■ Discuss the barriers to service utilisation by Black and ethnic minority communities.

The socio-political, economic and health perspectives of a nation are instrinsically linked to the issues of race, culture, ethnicity and substance misuse. The 1920s saw the 'birth of the British drug underground' and are associated with the popular myth that characterised 'the Chinese population as drug dealers and sexual deviants who preyed upon vulnerable young white women' (Kohn 1992). Nevertheless, these beliefs and stereotypes, with racial undertones, have remained in the popular or collective consciousness of the nation and mask the full understanding of the state of knowledge regarding the patterns of use, perceptions and health beliefs of Black and minority groups towards the use of psychoactive substances (Rassool 1997). Historically, Black and ethnic minority communities (BEM) have been the victims of negative stereotypes, social exclusions, health inequalities, disparate treatment and racism, and these factors have continued to contribute to the epidemiologic healthcare gap between Black and ethnic minority communities and whites (Rassool 2006).

The United Kingdom is a multicultural society with approximately 7.9% of the total population (4.6 million people) representing Black and ethnic minority communities (OPCS 2001). In England people from ethnic minority groups made up 9% of the total population in 2001/2 compared with only 2% in both Scotland and Wales. Nearly half (48%) of the total ethnic minority population are established in metropolitan geographical areas and reside predominantly in the London region, where they comprised 29% of all residents, and in the West Midlands, West Yorkshire and Greater Manchester (OPCS 2001). The largest Black and ethnic minority groups are Indians (1.8%), followed by Pakistanis (1.3%), Black Caribbeans (1.0%), Black Africans (0.8%), Bangladeshis (0.5%) and Chinese (0.4%). There are around 2.3 million ethnic minority women and 2.3 million ethnic minority men in the UK, and they are on average younger than the white population. The Black and ethnic minority communities are concentrated in some of the most deprived inner-city areas and continue to experience high levels of poverty, deprivation, educational disadvantage and discrimination in the labour market.

Black and ethnic minority groups in the UK are a heterogeneous group with varying values, attitudes, religious beliefs and customs that affect the patterns of mental health and substance misuse. This cultural diversity, with a wide variation in lifestyle, health behaviour, religion and language, has profound effects on their perception and recognition of health problems and ill-health constructed within the paradigm of western medicine and healthcare system (Rassool 1995). This growing diversity has strong implications for the provision of healthcare in substance-misuse services. Nurses and other healthcare professionals need to be aware of the existence of ethnic minorities within the community they serve. The practitioners should be able to assess the healthcare needs of the ethnic groups and develop services which take account of linguistic, religious and cultural differences. In order to provide equitable and fair access to healthcare provisions, practitioners should be able to assess the healthcare needs of ethnic groups. The provision and the delivery of services should take account of linguistic, religious and cultural differences.

The focus of the chapter is to provide an overview of alcohol and drug misuse in Black and ethnic minority communities and to examine the issues and problems faced by Black and ethnic minority groups.

DRUG MISUSE: POLICY INITIATIVES AND STRATEGY FOR BLACK AND ETHNIC MINORITY COMMUNITIES

It was during the 1990s that the UK government finally responded to the problems associated with alcohol and drug misuse in Black and ethnic minority communities. It has been notable that recent national drug policies in the UK have failed to address the health status and health care needs of Black and ethnic minority communities (Lord President of the Council 1998). The needs of Black and ethnic minority groups were highlighted in the Task Force review of services for drug misusers (Department of Health 1996), which focused briefly on the services to respond to the needs of Black and ethnic minority groups and the inclusion of staff from these groups. The Advisory Council on the Misuse of Drugs stated that 'Ethnic differences in patterns of drug misuse suggest that the needs of some minority ethnic groups are marginalized by existing services, which tend to focus on injecting rather than smoking' (ACMD 1998: 52).

Much of the impetus for current government policy that impacts on Black and ethnic minority communities comes from the need to provide accessible substance misuse services. The current UK drug policy, *Tackling Drugs to Build a Better Britain* (Department of Health 1998), and the *Updated Drug Strategy* (Department of Health 2002a) recognised the failure of Black and ethnic minority drug users to utilise the range of available treatment services and provided guidance for those involved in the purchasing and provision of drug services to tackle race equality, accessibility and practice. In addition, the strategy encouraged drug action teams (DATs) to undertake healthcare needs assessment and consider cultural diversity in service provision and delivery. The National Treatment Agency for Substance Misuse (NTA) has identified diversity as one of its key strategic objectives, recognising the need to ensure equal access to service provision regardless of age, gender, sexuality, disability and ethnicity.

In *Models of Care* (NTA 2002 Part 2), a framework for the commissioning and delivery of drug services in the UK, the treatment needs of Black and ethnic minority substance misusers are recognised throughout the document. In addition, there is a specific section on Black and ethnic minority communities (pp. 130–8) focusing on service accessibility and service utilisation, the barriers to drug treatment services, service appropriateness, professional guidance and legal framework, care pathways, needs assessment and treatment. The document identifies individuals from Black and ethnic minority communities experiencing drug and alcohol problems as a special group. It emphasises the need to locate drug use among Black and ethnic minority users within a wider context of social exclusion, deprivation and discrimination. It also reiterates that service provisions need to be sensitive to the needs of these groups, to be aware of legislation relating to race and racial discrimination, and to employ approaches that maximise treatment engagement and retention of these groups. The document comments on the underrepresentation of Black and ethnic minority substance misusers in treatment services in the majority of the country and that service provision for drug users often fails to retain Black and ethnic minority clients in treatment with high attrition rates.

The Mental Health Policy Implementation Guidance: Dual Diagnosis Good Practice Guide (Department of Health 2002b) contained a section on people from Black and ethnic minority communities claiming that, although there were no definitive studies on the influence of culture and ethnicity upon individuals with a dual diagnosis, it is known that severe mental illness and substance misuse present differently across cultures and ethnic groups. The guide pointed out, for example, that ethnicity is associated with poor access to services and with different meanings and values attributed to drugs and alcohol. Service provision must therefore be congruent with and sensitive to the needs of each minority ethnic group.

The Race Relations (Amendment) Act 2000 (Home Office 2000) is another piece of legislation which is relevant to the above policy initiatives. The Act places a general duty on specified public authorities to work towards institutional racism and the elimination of unlawful discrimination and to promote race equality of opportunity. In relation to substance-misuse services, the Act requires the services not to discriminate on the grounds of race in employment, policies, service provision and delivery. The codes of practice are enforceable by the Commission for Racial Equality (Commission for Racial Equality 2001). Taken all together, the implementation of policies and guidance in substance misuse should enable the appropriate services to remedy their institutional failings in meeting the needs of Black and ethnic minority groups.

DRUG MISUSE: PATTERNS AND PREVALENCE

A comprehensive literature review on drug use and related service provision is provided elsewhere (National Treatment Agency 2003). Most of the studies on alcohol and drug misuse amongst Black and ethnic minority communities are contained in so-called grey literature. However, the lack of academic rigour is overcome by the consistency of the local reports on the prevalence of drug misuse among this population. It is reported that there is far more information on drug use amongst South Asian populations (Bangladeshis, Indians and Pakistanis) than amongst other Black and minority groups especially from refugees' and asylum seekers' groups (National Treatment Agency 2003: 7).

The psychoactive substances misused by Black and ethnic minority groups are not clearly different from those used by the white population but there seem to be preferences for a certain class or classes of substances and mode of consumption by different ethnic groups which are linked with the historical and cultural characteristics of each ethnic group (Oyefeso et al. 2000). It is argued that compulsory hospital admissions distort the statistics of problematic drug use amongst Black Caribbean and African males as a result of the use of 'stop and search' tactics and of the diagnosis 'cannabis psychosis' (Harrison et al. 1997).

Key findings from the 2001/2 British Crime Survey (Aust and Smith 2003) indicate that the rate of prevalence of drug misuse within the Black and ethnic minority groups, particularly among South Asians and Black Africans, is lower than that of the white population but with increasing trends. The level of use among Black Caribbeans is similar to that of the white majority population, although this similar level is primarily driven by cannabis. There are indications that problematic drug use among this group may centre on crack cocaine. The British Crime Survey 2001/2 also indicates higher levels of drug use among people defining themselves as mixed background compared to any other ethnic group (including white).

However, there are clear indications that drug misuse is increasingly being reported amongst young Black and ethnic minority women (National Treatment Agency 2003: 13). The Black and Minority Ethnic Drug Misuse Needs Assessment Project (Bashford et al. 2003) involved 47 Black and ethnic minority community groups, constituting the largest sample of Black and ethnic minority drug users in the UK. The findings showed that 18% of the sample of community respondents (2,078) reported using a wide variety of drugs. Nearly one in five reported use of cocaine and one in ten had used heroin. The findings also showed that 18% reported use of khat and others reported using a wide range of traditional substances about which little is known. One in three of those reporting drug uses are women and the largest concentration of female respondents reporting drug use is South Asian (29%). The motivations for using drugs include peer influence, experimentation and pleasure seeking (74% of respondents), and 30% cite their reasons for drug use as being to avoid or help deal with problems. Only 10% of respondents have experience of using drug treatment services and of these most report that their experience was negative. The waiting time is often reported as a key barrier to accessing services.

In the Needs Assessment Project (Bashford *et al.* 2003), cannabis is the most widely reported drug used (51%), followed by cocaine (19%) and khat (18%). Heroin use is reported by 10%. Cannabis is the most widely used illicit drug amongst the younger members of Black and ethnic minority communities, and presentations to drug services by Black Caribbeans are more likely to focus on crack cocaine than other ethnic groups (including white groups) (Sangster *et al.* 2002). Heroin is the drug of choice amongst young South Asians in some areas of England, particularly Pakistani and Bangladeshi males. In some cases, heroin is also the first drug used (Patel *et al.* 2001) and reported to be used by South Asian, Iranian, Vietnamese and Chinese people (Sangster *et al.* 2002). South Asian reported drug use is more characterised by use of heroin (43% of all users) than crack (29%) (Bashford *et al.* 2003). Cocaine was reported as a main drug of use by Black Caribbean, African and 'other' than either South Asian or white drug users (Perera *et al.* 1993). Comparative differences between Black African and the combined Black Caribbean and Black African group may indicate that Black Caribbean drug use is characterised by crack, amphetamine and ecstasy (Bashford *et al.* 2003). Crack cocaine has been reported to be used by young Bangladeshis and Kashmiris (Sheikh *et al.* 2001). These observations suggest that the widely held assumptions of the substance-specific cultural stereotypes that Asians do not use opiates and cocaine are gradually becoming less tenable.

There is also the contention that injecting drug use behaviour is very uncommon among Black and ethnic minority groups. Injecting by Black and ethnic minority drug users is generally reported to be less prevalent than amongst white drug users, largely because of the lack of BEM drug users' presentations at needle exchanges (Sangster *et al.* 2002) and the marginalisation from services adopting harm reduction approaches that focus on injecting behaviour. However, South Asians have been reported to be injecting heroin by Patel *et al.* (2001), Sangster *et al.* (2002) and Sheikh *et al.* (2001). Studies have also reported young South Asian males injecting steroids (Sheikh *et al.* 2001). Sangster *et al.* (2002) report injecting amongst Black Caribbean heroin users in London, suggesting that this may be linked to the tendency for drug users to switch to heroin whilst in prison. Although there is generally a low uptake of needle exchanges by South Asian drug injectors, South Asian males have been shown to access injecting equipment via white friends or white girlfriends (Sheikh *et al.* 2001). There is great concern that dangerous injecting practices are occurring, particularly amongst South Asian female drug-injecting sex workers (Hall 1999).

Evidence of the use of 'club' drugs (ecstasy, amphetamine and LSD) by young members of Black and ethnic minority communities is rather limited. South Asians are reported to use ecstasy and LSD (Bashford *et al.* 2003). However, stimulants, ecstasy, hallucinogens, LSD and ice (a smokable form of amphetamine) have been reported to be used by Indians at Bhangra (clubbing) events (Bola and Walpole 1999). Khat was found to be used by the Somali community (Fountain *et al.* 2002), Yemeni communities (Mohammed 2000), Ethiopians (Fountain *et al.* 2002), and amongst Arabs from the Middle East (Iran, Iraq, Lebanon and Yemen) (Fountain *et al.* 2002).

ALCOHOL MISUSE

In the UK the high levels of alcohol consumption in Black and ethnic minority communities, especially Irish and Sikh groups, have resulted in higher rates of morbidity and mortality than the general population (Douds *et al.* 2003).The report on the health of minority ethnic groups (National Centre for Social Research 2001) found that, in England, men and women from all Black and ethnic minority groups (except white Irish) were less likely to drink alcohol than the general population and consumed smaller amounts. Overall, the findings show that 7% of men from the general population were non-drinkers, compared with 5% of Irish men, 13% of Black Caribbean men, 30% of Chinese men, 33% of Indian men, 91% of Pakistani men and 96% of Bangladeshi men. Higher proportions of women than men were non-drinkers, both in the general population and among ethnic minority groups. Of the general population, 12% of women reported being non-drinkers compared with 10% of Irish women, 18% of Black Caribbean women, 41% of Chinese women, 64% of Indian women, 97% of Pakistani women and 99% of Bangladeshi women.

On the heaviest drinking day in the last week 59% of the general population drank over 4 units compared to 74% of Irish drinkers, 50% of Indian, 43% of Black Caribbean and 21% of Chinese (no figures were available for Pakistani and Bangladeshi men as so few drank in the past week). For women the proportion of women drinking over 3 units was 47% for the general population, 56% for Irish women, 36% Indian women, 35% Black Caribbean women and 30% Chinese women. In common with the general population, weekly levels of alcohol consumption decrease with age with the exception of Black Caribbean and Indian men. However, these figures also show that a significant proportion of people from the Indian and Black Caribbean communities exceed weekly limits and, among those who do drink, both men and women report exceeding the daily limits.

A survey (Alcohol Concern 2001) conducted among 1,684 second or subsequent generation men and women in the Midlands from Black (African), African-Caribbean, Black (British), Indian Hindu, Indian Sikh and Bengali and Pakistani communities in Birmingham and Leicester (England) found relatively high levels of drinking amongst Black communities and male Sikhs. Whilst most Pakistani and Bengali men and women, and Sikh and Hindu women, were non-drinkers, among African-Caribbean men and women and Sikh men, alcohol was used by most people. A study of 16–25-year-olds from Pakistani, Indian and Chinese communities in Glasgow, Scotland (Bakshi *et al.* 2002), shows that higher proportions of the younger members of Asian communities do drink, with 19% of Pakistanis saying they drink, as do 49% of Indians and 73% of Chinese. Interestingly this study also shows that, although young Pakistanis are less likely to drink, those who do drink consume the highest number of alcohol units on average (13.8 units per week compared to 7.94 for young Indians and 4.76 for young Chinese. Subhra and Chauhan (1999) point to the fact that, although certain groups of the ethnic communities place restrictions on the use of alcohol (for religious or cultural reasons), there already exist complex patterns of alcohol use within these communities.

The Health Survey of ethnic minority groups for England 2004 (Information Centre 2004) reported that Pakistani adults (89% of men and 95% of women) and Bangladeshi adults (97% of men and 98% of women) were the most likely to be non-drinkers. The survey also found that 45% of men and 30% of women in the general population had exceeded the recommended daily limit (for example, had drunk at least 4 units for men or 3 for women). Amongst Black and ethnic minority communities, those exceeding the daily recommended limit were Irish (56% of men, 36% of women), but intake was lower for all other ethnic groups: Black Caribbean (28% of men, 18% of women), Indian (22% men, 8% women), Chinese (19% men, 12% women), Black African (17% men, 7% women), Pakistani (4% men, <1% women) and was lowest amongst Bangladeshi participants (1% of male and <1% of female drinkers). Except for the Irish (32% of men, 16% of women), the proportion of men and women who were binge drinking was lower for all the other minority ethnic groups than in the general population, ranging from 0.5% for Bangladeshi men to 12% for Black Caribbean men, and from <1% of both Pakistani and Bangladeshi women to 6% of Black Caribbean women.

Taken together, the evidence from quantitative surveys strongly indicates that the prevalence of alcohol misuse within the Black and minority groups is increasing especially among the Indian and Black Caribbean communities. This has significant implications for service provision. For a more comprehensive literature on alcohol in Black and ethnic minority groups see Alcohol Concern (2001).

TOBACCO

Smoking patterns have been shown to vary between different Black and ethnic minority groups according to the data from the 1999 Health Survey for England (National Centre for Social Research 2001). When compared to the national prevalence rate of 24% in men, the rates are particularly high in the Bangladeshi (40%), Irish (30%), Pakistani (29%), Black Caribbean (25%), Black African and Chinese (21%), and Indian (20%) populations (Information Centre 2004). Self-reported smoking prevalence was higher among women in the general population (23%) than most minority ethnic groups, except Irish (26%) and Black Caribbean women (24%). The figures for the other groups were 10% Black African, 8% Chinese, and 5% Indian and Pakistani, and 2% in Bangladeshi women.

Among ethnic minority groups, many types of smokeless tobacco are used, particularly among the South Asian population. The survey (Information Centre 2004) found that Bangladeshis (both men and women) were more likely than other South Asian groups to report chewing tobacco. Nine percent of Bangladeshi men and 16% of Bangladeshi women reported chewing tobacco. The chewing tobacco was most prevalent among those aged 35 and over among Bangladeshi women (26%). Among men, there was no difference in use of chewing tobacco by age. Saliva cotinine samples suggest that prevalence of tobacco use is greater than self-reported estimates.

Tobacco is often consumed in combination with other products. Use of paan (a leaf preparation stuffed with betel nut and/or with tobacco or other ingredients), believed to be a risk factor in oral cancer, is high among some South Asian ethnic groups. Ready-made mixtures of snuff, known as gutka or paan masala, are chewed either on their own or in betel quid. They are prepared by baking and curing a mixture comprising areca nut, lime, spices and tobacco (Pearson and Patel 1998, Champion *et al.* 2001).

HIV AND BLACK AND ETHNIC MINORITY COMMUNITIES

Black and ethnic minority communities in the UK, especially Black Africans and Afro-Caribbeans, are disproportionately affected by HIV. The rate of new HIV diagnoses amongst the African community in the UK continues to rise, and is one of the most serious challenges posed by the HIV/AIDS epidemic in Britain.

There were an estimated 24,800 persons born in sub-Saharan Africa who were living with HIV in the UK in 2006, of whom an estimated 36% of men and 23% of women aged 15–59 were unaware of their infection (Health Protection Agency 2007). The document *Testing Times – HIV and Other Sexually Transmitted Infections in the United Kingdom* (Health Protection Agency 2007) reports that almost half of all new HIV diagnoses in 2006 were among Black Africans and 3.2% were among Black Caribbeans. An increasing number of Black Africans and Black Caribbeans are being infected heterosexually in the UK. In England in 2006, 2,968 per 100,000 (3.0%) of black Africans and 246 per 100,000 (0.25%) of black Caribbeans were living with diagnosed HIV. There is high uptake of HIV testing among sub-Saharan-born persons attending genito-urinary medicine clinics and women attending antenatal care. Late diagnosis of HIV among Black African and Black Caribbean communities is a persisting problem, with 40% of HIV-infected Black Africans and Black Caribbeans being diagnosed late.

The HIV/AIDS epidemic has compounded the stigmatisation, discrimination and racism faced by Black and ethnic minority communities, and this has a direct impact on equal access to health services. HIV/AIDS-related stigma and discrimination linked to race and ethnicity increases vulnerability to HIV infection in the following ways (ukblackout 2005). Those who are HIV-positive are more vulnerable to the effects of HIV/AIDS because they are less likely to access treatment and health services, or choose not to seek treatment for fear of being stigmatised and discriminated against, and those who are not yet infected run a higher risk of acquiring HIV because HIV/AIDS stigma can prevent people from accessing information and education about HIV transmission. HIV infection is the strongest risk factor known for tuberculosis and tuberculosis accounted for 27% of initial diagnoses of AIDS in Black Africans in London compared with 5% in non-Africans (Del Amo *et al.* 1996)

SERVICE PROVISION AND BARRIERS TO SERVICE UTILISATION

The Report 'Inside Out' (Sashidaran 2002) acknowledged the problems faced by Black and ethnic minority groups in mental health care, saying that there is an over-emphasis on institutional and coercive models of care, professional and organisational requirements are given priority over individual needs and rights, and institutional racism exists within mental health care. This statement is equally applicable to substance service provision and delivery. The marginality and social exclusion experienced by Black and ethnic minority groups compounded with racial discrimination and institutional racism are likely to be significant in understanding the experiences in these communities and their access to substance-misuse services (Rassool 2006).

There is evidence to suggest that Black and ethnic minority substance misusers are underrepresented in treatment services and especially those from South Asian communities and women (Advisory Council on the Misuse of Drugs 1998, NTA 2002).

The Advisory Council for the Misuse of Drugs (ACMD 1998: 41) commented that 'The under-representation of Black people among populations of drug users known to agencies might, for example, be a consequence of the failure of agencies to make themselves accessible and meaningful to all members of a multi-cultural society'. The development of service provision for Black and ethnic minority drug users is ad hoc, patchy and unco-ordinated, and the less well-established Black and ethnic minority groups are even more marginalised in terms of drug services (Sangster *et al.* 2002).

Potential barriers occurred at three different levels: patient level, provider level and system level (Schepperd *et al.* 2006). The patient level related to the patient characteristics: demographic variables (age, gender, ethnicity), social structure variables, health beliefs and attitudes, personal enabling resources, community enabling resources, perceived illness and personal health practices. The barriers at provider level were related to the provider characteristics: skills and attitudes. The barriers at system level were related to the system characteristics: the organisation of the healthcare system. The low rates of presentation to alcohol and drug services by ethno-cultural groups may be due to a multitude of factors that include acculturation, systems of cultural values, cultural dissonance, education and literacy, previous experience of persecution, communication difficulties, religio-cultural prescriptions, discrimination, the lack of understanding of Black and ethnic minority cultures, ethnicity of staff, denial of substance misuse by Black and ethnic minority communities and lack of understanding of Black and ethnic minority culture (Rassool 1995, Alcohol Concern 2003). Many agencies are mainstream and ethnocentric in their services to culturally diverse communities, resulting in poor delivery of service in meeting the health needs of these groups (Rassool 2006).There are a myriad of potential barriers that may inhibit Black and ethnic minority communities from utilisation of alcohol and drug services. Some of the barriers are presented in Table 17.1. In order to overcome some of the personal, provider and organisational barriers, the recommendations of the Black and Minority Ethnic Drug Misuse Needs Assessment Project (Bashford *et al.* 2003) are presented in Table 17.2.

Table 17.1 Barriers to service utilisation

- Unawareness of local services
- Experience of racism
- Language barrier
- Lack of skills of staff
- Problems with access to translated health information
- Problems with access to trained interpreters
- Opiate focus of drug treatment
- Inadequate services
- Stigma
- Family honour
- Services remote
- Immigration status and displacement
- Previous negative experiences

Table 17.2 Recommendations for drug service provision for Black and ethnic minority community groups

- Employment of Black and ethnic minority workers
- Training for drug service staff in diversity and cultural sensitivity
- Better access to interpreters who are trained in drug misuse
- Community-orientated telephone helplines
- Ensuring refugee and asylum seekers are aware of services
- Community partnerships between groups and agencies
- Health education on risks related to blood-borne diseases
- Targeting of services for crack and cocaine use within communities
- Increased representation of Black and ethnic minority communities on DATs and related forums
- Ensuring services are inclusive, and able to work effectively with diversity
- Recording of client demography and ethnic monitoring
- Developing services for family members and carers
- Separate service provision for women that is located sensitively
- Increased shared care with general practitioners

Source: Bashford *et al.* 2003

In relation to the utilisation of alcohol services, it is reported that there are low levels of uptake by Black and ethnic minority groups. Despite the levels of alcohol use among second-generation migrant populations there remain low levels of awareness, perceived accessibility or sources of advice relating to drinking (Orford *et al.* 2004). Some of the barriers in the utilisation of drug services are also relevant to the utilisation of alcohol services by Black and ethnic minority communities. The findings of the study on alcohol use and the South Asian and African Caribbean communities (Johnson *et al.* 2006) suggest that, in order to ensure greater sensitivity and availability of alcohol services, some of the following key areas need to be implemented: socio-cultural and religious awareness, adequate provision of training of staff, matching clients to staff, regular consultation with users, working with families and offering complementary therapies. Services from health information to rehabilitation and after-care need to be culturally sensitive and linguistically appropriate. However, alcohol services appear to be failing to meet their obligations under the Race Relations Amendment Act, and are certainly not reaching and delivering services to people from BEM communities who need them (AERC 2007). There need to be more explicit and overt organisational commitment to diversity and more resources dedicated to meeting the needs of people from ethnic and culturally diverse communities.

In summary, research on Black and ethnic minority drug users suggests a number of institutional failings: the failure to provide equitable and accessible services; poor responses in identifying and respond to the distinct patterns of drug and alcohol misuse; and an inability to respond to cultural and diverse needs.

KEY POINTS

- Black and ethnic minority communities in the UK are a heterogeneous group.
- Historically, Black and minority ethnic communities have been the victims of negative stereotypes, social exclusions, health inequalities, disparate treatment and racism.

- The largest Black and ethnic minority groups are Indian followed by Pakistanis, Black Caribbeans, Black Africans, Bangladeshis and Chinese.
- It was during the 1990s that the UK government finally responded to the problems associated with alcohol and drug misuse in Black and ethnic minority communities.
- There is recognition of the failure of Black and ethnic minority drug users to utilise the range of available treatment services.
- Cannabis is the most widely used illicit drug amongst the younger members of Black and ethnic minority communities.
- Cocaine was reported as a main drug of use by Black Caribbean, African and 'other' users more than by either South Asian or white drug users.
- There is also the contention that injecting drug use behaviour is largely uncommon among Black and ethnic minority groups.
- There is some evidence of the use of 'club' drugs (ecstasy, amphetamine and LSD) by young members of Black and ethnic minority communities.
- Amongst Black and ethnic minority communities, those exceeding the daily recommended limit of alcohol were Irish.
- Higher proportions of women than men were non-drinkers, both in the general population and among ethnic minority groups.
- Self-reported smoking prevalence was higher among women in the general population than in most minority ethnic groups, except Irish and Black Caribbean women.
- Among ethnic minority groups, many types of smokeless tobacco are used, particularly among the South Asian population.
- Black Africans and Afro-Caribbeans are disproportionately affected by HIV.
- Almost half of all new HIV diagnoses in 2006 were among Black Africans and 3.2% were among Black Caribbeans.
- In England in 2006, 2,968 per 100,000 (3.0%) of Black Africans and 246 per 100,000 (0.25%) of Black Caribbeans were living with diagnosed HIV.
- Late diagnosis of HIV among Black African and Black Caribbean communities is a persisting problem.
- There is evidence to suggest that Black and ethnic minority substance misusers are underrepresented in treatment services and especially those from South Asian communities and women.
- The development of service provision for Black and ethnic minority drug users is ad hoc, patchy and unco-ordinated.
- There are a myriad of potential barriers that may inhibit Black and ethnic minority communities from utilisation of alcohol and drug services.

ACTIVITY 17.1

State whether the statements are true or false

	True	False
The socio-political, economic and health perspectives of a nation are intrinsically linked to the issues of race, culture, ethnicity and substance misuse		

Black and ethnic minority communities have been the victims of negative stereotypes, social exclusions, health inequalities etc.

In England people from ethnic minority groups make up 9% of the total population

The largest Black and ethnic minority groups are Pakistanis and Bangladeshis

Black and minority ethnic groups in the UK are a homogeneous group

There is no difference in linguistic, religious and cultural aspects amongst ethnic communities

Recent national drug policies in the UK have failed to address the health status and healthcare needs of Black and ethnic minorities

Much of the impetus for current government policy is the provision of accessible substance-misuse services

The Race Relations Act 2000 focuses on the elimination of unlawful discrimination and the promotion of race equality of opportunity

The psychoactive substances misused by Black and ethnic minority groups are different from those used by the white population

Drug misuse is increasingly being reported amongst young Black and ethnic minority women

South Asians do not use opiates and cocaine

Injecting drug use behaviour is largely uncommon among Black and ethnic minority groups

There is generally a low uptake of needle exchanges

An increasing number of black Africans and black Caribbeans are being infected heterosexually with HIV in the UK

There is low uptake of HIV testing among sub-Saharan-born persons attending genito-urinary medicine clinics

ACTIVITY 17.2

Please choose one correct answer for the following multiple-choice questions

The rate of prevalence of drug misuse within the Black and ethnic minority groups is
a.   Lower than that of the white population
b.   Higher than that of the white population
c.   Same as the white population
d.   Different from that of the white population

The level of drug use among Black Caribbeans is
a.   Similar to that of the white majority population
b.   Not similar to that of the white majority population
c.   Higher than those with mixed background
d.   Problematic compared to the white population

Problematic drug use among Black Caribbeans is centred on
a.   Heroin
b.   LSD
c.   Crack cocaine
d.   Amphetamines

The largest concentration of females reporting drug use is in
a.   The South African community
b.   The South Asian community
c.   The South Indian community
d.   The South Pakistani community

The most widely reported drug used by ethnic minorities is
a.   Cocaine
b.   Cannabis
c.   Heroin
d.   Ecstasy

Heroin is the drug of choice amongst
a.   South Africans
b.   South Asians
c.   South Indians
d.   South Americans

Khat use is common amongst
a.   The Somali community
b.   The Yemeni community
c.   Ethiopians
d.   All of the above

A high level of alcohol consumption in found in
a.   Black and ethnic minority groups
b.   Irish and Sikh groups
c.   Pakistani and Bangladeshi groups
d.   Black African groups

The most likely Black and ethnic minority communities to be non-drinkers are
a.   South Africans and South Asians
b.   Black Africans and Black Caribbeans
c.   Indians and Pakistanis
d.   Pakistanis and Bangladeshis

The proportion of men and women who were binge drinking was higher amongst
a.   The Bangladeshi community
b.   The Indian community
c.   The Pakistani community
d.   The Irish community

Smoking patterns have been shown to be high in

a.   The Bangladeshi community
b.   The Pakistani community
c.   The Black Caribbean community
d.   The Black African community

Smokeless tobacco is used particularly among

a.   The Bangladeshi community
b.   The Pakistani community
c.   The Black Caribbean community
d.   The Black African community

The rate of new HIV diagnoses amongst the African community in the UK continues

a.   To lower
b.   To rise
c.   No difference
d.   Same as before

ACTIVITY 17.3

- List the potential barriers in the utilisation of services by Black and ethnic minority communities

REFERENCES

Advisory Council on the Misuse of Drugs (ACMD) (1998) *Drug Misuse and the Environment.* London: The Stationery Office.

Alcohol Concern (2001) *Alcohol Survey: Black and Ethnic Minorities.* London: Alcohol Concern.

Alcohol Concern (2003) *Alcohol Drinking among Black and Minority Ethnic Communities (BME) in the United Kingdom.* London: Acquire.

Alcohol Education and Research Council (AERC) (2007) *Alcohol Services and the Needs of Black and Minority Ethnic Groups.* Alcohol Insight No. 29. Leicester: Mary Seacole Research Centre, De Montfort University.

Aust, R. and Smith, N. (2003) *Ethnicity and Drug Use: Key Findings from the 2001/2002 British Crime Survey.* London: Home Office.

Bakshi, N., Ross, R. and Heim, D. (2002) *Drug and Alcohol Issues Affecting Pakistani, Indian and Chinese Young People and Their Communities.* Glasgow: Greater Glasgow NHS Board.

Bashford, J., Buffin, J. and Patel, K. (2003) *The Department of Health's Black and Minority Ethnic Drug Misuse Needs Assessment Project. Part 2 The Findings.* Preston: The Centre for Ethnicity and Health, Faculty of Health, University of Central Lancashire. http://www.uclan.ac.uk/facs/health/ethnicity/reports/documents/rep2comeng2.pdf.

Bola, M. and Walpole, T. (1999) *Drugs Information and Communication Needs among South Asians in Crawley.* Executive summary. Crawley: Youth Action Crawley.

Champion, J., Bedi, B. and Anees, K. (2001) *Transcultural Tobacco Programme*. Educational programme for trading standards and Customs and Excise officers. London: National Centre for Transcultural Oral Health.

Commission for Racial Equality (2001) *Statutory Code of Practice on the Duty to Promote Race Equality: A Guide for Public Authorities*. London: Commission for Racial Equality. www.cre.gov.uk.

Del Amo, J., Petruckevitch, A., Phillips, A., Johnson, A.M., Stephenson, J.M., Desmond, N., *et al*. (1996) Spectrum of disease in Africans with AIDS in London. *AIDS*, 10: 1563–9.

Department of Health (1996) *The Task Force to Review Services for Drug Misusers: Report of an Independent Review of Drug Treatment Services in England*. London: Department of Health.

Department of Health (1998) *Tackling Drugs to Build a Better Britain*. London: Department of Health.

Department of Health (2002a) *Updated Drug Strategy*. London: Department of Health.

Department of Health (2002b) *The Mental Health Policy Implementation Guidance: Dual Diagnosis Good Practice Guide*. London: Department of Health.

Douds, A.C., Cox, M.A., Iqbal, T.H. and Cooper, B.T. (2003) Ethnic differences in cirrhosis of the liver in a British city: alcoholic cirrhosis in South Asian men. *Alcohol & Alcoholism*, 38: 148–50.

Fountain, J., Bashford, J., Underwood, S., Khurana, J., Winters, M., Patel, K. and Carpentier, C. (2002) *Update and Complete the Analysis of Drug Use, Consequences and Correlates amongst Minorities*. Cited in: National Treatment Agency (2003) *Black and Minority Ethnic Communities: A Review of the Literature on Drug Use and Related Service Provision*. London: NTA.

Hall, C. (1999) *Drug Use and HIV Infection in South Asian and Middle Eastern Communities in the UK: A Literature Review*. London: NAT Project.

Harrison, L., Sutton, M. and Gardiner, E. (1997) Ethnic differences in substance use and alcohol use-related mortality among first generation migrants to England and Wales. *Substance Use and Misuse*, 32, 7/8: 849–76.

Health Protection Agency (2007) *Testing Times – HIV and Other Sexually Transmitted Infections in the United Kingdom, 2007 Annual Report*. London: Health Protection Agency. http://www.hpa.org.uk/infections/topics_az/hiv_and_sti/publications/AnnualReport/2007/default.htm.

Home Office (2000) *Race Relations (Amendment) Act 2000*. London: The Stationery Office. www.homeoffice.gov.uk.

Information Centre (2004) *Health Survey for England 2004: The Health of Minority Ethnic Groups*. Leeds: The Information Centre.

Johnson, M.R.D., Banton, P.M., Dhillon, H., Subhra, G. and Hough, J. (2006) *Alcohol Issues and the South Asian & African Caribbean Communities*. London: The Alcohol Education and Research Council.

Kohn, M. (1992) *Dope Girls: The Birth of the British Drug Underground*. London: Lawrence and Wishart.

Lord President of the Council (1998) *Tackling Drugs to Build a Better Britain: The Government's Ten Year Strategy for Tackling Drug Misuse*. CM 3945. London: The Stationery Office.

Mohammed, S. (2000) *A Gob Full of Khat: A Study of Contemporary Khat Use in Toxteth*. London: Liverpool Avaanca Publications.

National Centre for Social Research and Dept of Epidemiology and Public Health at the Royal Free and University College Medical School (2001) *The Health of Minority Ethnic Groups '99* (Health Survey for England). London: Office for National Statistics.

NTA (2002) *Models of Care for Treatment of Adult Drug Misusers*. London: National Treatment Agency. www.nta.nhs.uk.

NTA (2003) *Black and Minority Ethnic Communities: A Review of the Literature on Drug Use and Related Service Provision*. London: National Treatment Agency. www.nta.nhs.uk.

OPCS (2001) *The 2001 Census of Population – Ethnicity and Religion in England and Wales.* CM4253. London: The Stationery Office.

Orford, J., Johnson, M.R.D. and Purser, R. (2004) Drinking in second generation Black and Asian communities in the English Midlands. *Addiction Research and Theory*, 12, 1: 11–30.

Oyefeso, A., Ghodse, H., Keating, A., Annan, J., Phillips, T., Pollard, M. and Nash, P. (2000) *Drug Treatment Needs of Black and Minority Ethnic Residents of the London Borough of Merton.* Addictions Resource Agency for Commissioners (ARAC) Monograph Series on Ethnic Minority Issues. London: ARAC.

Patel, K., Wardle, I., Bashford, J. and Winters, M. (2001) *The Evaluation of Nafas – a Bangladeshi Drug Service.* Ethnicity and Health Unit, Faculty of Health. Preston: University of Central Lancashire.

Pearson, G. and Patel, K. (1998) Drugs, deprivation, and ethnicity: outreach among Asian drug users in a northern English city. *Journal of Drug Issues*, 28, 1: 199–224.

Perera, J., Power, R. and Gibson, N. (1993) *Assessing the Needs of Black Drug Users in North Westminster.* London: Hungerford Drug Project / Centre for Research in Drugs and Health Behaviour.

Rassool, G. Hussein (1995) The health status and health care of ethno-cultural minorities in the United Kingdom: an agenda for action. *Journal of Advanced Nursing*, 21: 199–201.

Rassool, G. Hussein (1997) Ethnic minorities and substance misuse. In G. Hussein Rassool and M. Gafoor (eds) *Addiction Nursing: Perspectives on Professional and Clinical Practice.* Cheltenham: Stanley Nelson.

Rassool, G. Hussein (2006) Black and ethnic minority communities: substance misuse and mental health: whose problem anyway? In G. Hussein Rassool (ed.) *Dual Diagnosis Nursing.* Oxford: Blackwell Publications.

Sangster, D., Shiner, M., Sheikh. N. and Patel, K. (2002) *Delivering Drug Services to Black and Minority Ethnic Communities.* DPAS/P16. London: Home Office Drug Prevention and Advisory Service (DPAS). Also available on www.drugs.gov.uk.

Sashidaran, S.P. (2002) *Inside Out: Improving Mental Health Services for Black and Minority Ethnic Communities in England.* London: Department of Health.

Schepperd, E., Van Dongen, E., Dekker, J. Geertzen, J. and Dekker J. (2006) Potential barriers to the use of health services among ethnic minorities: a review. *Family Practice*, 23, 3: 325–48.

Sheikh, N., Fountain, J., Bashford, J. and Patel, K. (2001) *A Review of Current Drug Service provision for Black and Minority Ethnic Communities in Bedfordshire.* Final report to Bedfordshire Drug Action Team, August 2001. Preston: Centre for Ethnicity and Health, Faculty of Health, University of Central Lancashire.

Subhra, G. and Chauhan, V. (1999) *Developing Black Services: An Evaluation of the African, Caribbean and Asian Services.* London: Alcohol Concern.

ukblackout (2005) http://www.ukblackout.com/health/are-you-hiv-prejudiced.html (accessed 5 January 2008).

CHAPTER 18

VULNERABLE PEOPLE: ELDERLY AND HOMELESS PEOPLE AND ALCOHOL AND DRUG MISUSE

OBJECTIVES

- Describe the prevalence and pattern of substance misuse amongst the elderly.

- List the signs and symptoms associated with alcohol misuse.

- Identify the type of illicit and prescribed psychoactive substances used.

- Describe the nature and pattern of substance misuse among the homeless.

- List the factors which contribute to becoming homeless.

- Discuss the relationship between homelessness and substance misuse.

ALCOHOL, DRUGS AND THE ELDERLY

Owing to longer life expectancy and the ageing of the population there are more elderly people in the UK. Alcohol and drug misuse in elderly people is a common but underrecognised problem with significant negative impact on the physical and psychological health and quality of life. Recent surveys show that older people do indeed experience significant alcohol and drug problems which may be largely under-diagnosed and undertreated (Crome and Day 1999). There is limited data on the prevalence of illicit substance misuse in the elderly despite the likely imminent emergence of a cohort of recreational addicts (Patterson and Jeste 1999). Many physical or psychological conditions in the elderly may mimic drug and alcohol misuse. Classic features of dependence, such as craving, may be absent and the older person may be in denial with not much information being offered upon direct questioning (McGrath *et al.* 2005)

ALCOHOL

The over-55s in Britain are more likely than their continental European counterparts to be regular drinkers (20%), and Britain is the only country in Europe to have a statistically significant number of over-55s drinking more than 6 units per day (1%) (Alcohol Concern 2007). Older people were more likely to drink regularly: 28% of men and 18% of women aged 45–64 drank on five or more days in the week prior to interview compared to 10% of men and 5% of women aged 16–24 (Information Office 2007). Younger people were more likely to drink heavily, with 42% of men and 36% of women aged 16–24 drinking above the daily recommendations, compared to 16% of men and 4% of women aged 65 and over (National Statistics 2006a). The prevalence of mild alcohol dependence in the 65–9 age groups was 17 per 1,000 population and in the 70–4 age group it was 9 per 1,000 population (Coulthard *et al.* 2002). Levels of alcohol dependence in elderly vary according to setting: 6–11% elderly patients admitted to general hospitals; 20% admissions to psychiatric wards; 14% elderly patients in A&E settings; and up to 49% in nursing homes (Marshall 2006).

Three groups of older alcohol misusers have been identified: early-onset drinkers or 'survivors', late-onset drinkers or 'reactors' and intermittent or binge drinkers. Early-onset alcohol misusers account for about 70% of older alcoholics; a family history of alcoholism is more prevalent in this group (McGrath *et al.* 2005). In addition, they have had a lifelong pattern of problem drinking, have probably been alcoholics for most of their lives and have psychiatric illness, cirrhosis and organic brain syndromes (Menninger 2002). The chances of reaching old age are reduced early amongst this group of elderly problem drinkers. One estimate is that the life span of a problem drinker may be shortened by on average ten to fifteen years as a result of the health risks connected to heavy drinking and dependence on alcohol (Institute of Alcohol Studies 2007). Late-onset drinkers or 'reactors' begin problematic drinking later in life, often in response to traumatic life events such as the death of a loved one, loneliness, pain, insomnia, retirement etc. (Institute of Alcohol Studies 2007). Intermittent or binge drinkers use alcohol occasionally and sometimes drink to excess, which may cause them problems. It is thought that both the late-onset drinkers and the intermittent or binge drinkers have a high chance of managing their alcohol problem if they have access to appropriate treatment such as counselling and general support (Institute of Alcohol Studies 2007). The risk factors associated with alcohol problems in the elderly are presented in Table 18.1.

Table 18.1 Risk factors for alcohol problems in elderly people

Psychosocial problems	Medical problems	Practical problems
• Bereavement • Decreased social activity • Loss of friends • Loss of social status • Loss of occupational role • Impaired ability • Family conflict • Reduced self-esteem • Reduced self-efficacy • Depression	• Physical disabilities • Chronic pain • Insomnia • Sensory deficits • Reduced mobility • Cognitive impairment	• Impaired self-care • Reduced coping skills • Altered financial circumstances

Source: Adapted from Dar (2006)

ALCOHOL-RELATED PROBLEMS

Alcohol-use disorders in elderly people can cause a wide range of physical and psychosocial problems. There is a risk of accidents, and alcohol has been identified as one of the three main reasons for falls, which are a significant cause of mortality and ill-health in older people (Wright and Whyley 1994). Elderly people are less tolerant of the adverse effects of alcohol owing to a fall in the ratio of body water to fat, a decreased hepatic blood flow, inefficiency of liver enzymes and reduced renal clearance (Dunne and Schipperheijn 1989). Problem drinkers are at greater risk of developing serious liver problems, including cirrhosis, and have increased incidence of cancer of the liver, oesophagus, nasopharynx and colon (Smith 1995). The signs and symptoms of alcohol misuse in the elderly are presented in Table 18.2.

CO-EXISTING DISORDERS

There is limited research on the co-existence of alcohol misuse and psychiatric disorders in late life. Older people are more likely to have the triple diagnosis of alcoholism,

Table 18.2 Signs and symptoms of alcohol misuse in elderly people

Physical	Psychological
• Falls • Bruises • Incontinence • Increased tolerance to alcohol • Poor hygiene • Poor nutrition • Seizures • Gastro-intestinal complaints • Hypertension	• Anxiety • Acute confusional state • Withdrawn • Depression • Blackouts • Disorientation • Memory loss • Difficulty in decision-making

depression and personality disorder, whereas younger people are more likely to have the single diagnosis of schizophrenia (Speer and Bates 1992). There is evidence to suggest that 13% of people over the age of 65 years with a lifetime diagnosis of depression also meet criteria for lifetime alcohol abuse (Grant and Harford 1995) and older alcoholics with depression have an increased risk of suicide (Waern 2005). More rarely, other psychiatric disorders such as schizophrenia may co-exist with alcohol problems and complicate the treatment of both (Dar 2006). It has been reported that there is increased occurrence of all types of dementia except Alzheimer's disease in elderly people with alcohol use disorders (Thomas and Rockwood 2001). There is also concern that elderly people are taking prescribed medication or over-the-counter drugs in conjunction with alcohol, which can cause adverse side effects. Alcohol is contraindicated for use with many of the drugs taken by older people.

ILLICIT PSYCHOACTIVE SUBSTANCES

The reported prevalence and patterns of drug misuse in older people are lower than in the younger population (Beckett *et al.* 2005). The lifetime prevalence rates for illicit drug dependence are less than 1% for the over-60 group. The prevalence of drug dependence in Great Britain was 4 per 1,000 population for tranquillisers within the 65–9 age group, and in the 70–4 age group 4 per 1,000 population for cannabis, and one per 1,000 for tranquillisers (McGrath *et al.* 2005). However, addiction to psychoactive substances amongst the elderly is due to 'iatrogenic dependence', that is the inappropriate prescribing of psychoactive substances by medical practitioners. Older people receive more prescribed medications, and the prevalence of drug misuse is four times greater in women than in men. The risk of dependence is increased if the women happen to be widowed, less educated, of lower income, in poor health, and with reduced social support (King *et al.* 1994). The prevalence of use of hypnotic drugs, mainly benzodiazepines, among persons aged 65 years or older in a nationally representative British sample was 16% (Morgan *et al.* 1988). A study by Whitcup and Miller (1987) found that 21% of patients aged 65 years or older who were admitted to a psychiatric unit had a diagnosis of drug dependence with a majority of drug-dependent patients who had a diagnosis of benzodiazepine dependence. However, not all patients who are taking benzodiazepines for long periods become dependent. Benzodiazepine dependence in general can be more problematic among elderly persons, because tolerance to alcohol and benzodiazepine decreases with age (Bogunovic and Greenfield 2004).

NICOTINE ADDICTION

Tobacco is the most commonly used psychoactive substance amongst the elderly. It is estimated that 19% of men and 23% of women between 65 and 74 years of age smoke and that 10% of men and 9% of women over the age of 75 smoke (Department of Health 1998). The over-60s are more likely than younger people to have smoked at some time in their lives. However, they are more likely than younger people to have given up, and only 14% smoked in 2004/5, the smallest proportion for any age group (National

Statistics 2006b). The consequences of tobacco smoking occur later in life and many elderly people have chronic disease including cardiovascular diseases, lung cancer, bladder cancer and chronic obstructive pulmonary disease.

The nature and pattern of alcohol and drug misuse in older people and the associated psychological and physical co-morbidity are different from those seen in younger populations. The development of substance misuse is more likely to be associated with alcohol and prescribed and over-the-counter medications. However, older people are not exempt on the misuse of illicit psychoactive substances. General practitioners are usually the first point of contact for elderly people, but many fail to recognise and diagnose alcohol or drug misuse. Routine questions on the use of alcohol and drugs should be asked. In view of the complexity of the health and social issues involved, appropriate care, management and treatment should be tailored to meet the specific needs of this vulnerable group.

HOMELESSNESS AND SUBSTANCE MISUSE

Homelessness is an increasing problem in the United Kingdom. A study by the Office of the Deputy Prime Minister (Homelessness Directorate 2002) found that three-quarters of homeless people have a history of problematic substance misuse. Drug misusers are seven times more likely to be homeless than the general population (Kemp et al. 2006) and more than two-fifths of homeless people cite drug use as the main reason for homelessness (Fountain et al. 2002). In a study of 154 homeless people in Northern Ireland (Deloitte MCS Ltd 2004), the findings showed that 69% drank alcohol on a monthly or more frequent basis; 69% had used drugs at some stage in their lives; 50% drank alcohol and had used drugs; and 13% had never used drugs and did not currently drink. In addition, 58% were recent users (had used drugs in the past year), and 54% were current users of one or more substance. Men were more likely than women to have used drugs irrespective of prevalence and were more than twice as likely to be currently using drugs. Cannabis was the most commonly used drug among all types of users, with 67% of the sample having used the substance at some stage. The three drugs most commonly used by lifetime users were cannabis, ecstasy and amphetamines. However, among recent and current users, this changed to cannabis, tranquillisers and ecstasy. It is estimated that 95% of homeless young people had used drugs, and their experimentation with illicit psychoactive substances started as early as 14 years of age (Wincup et al. 2003). Levels of use of cannabis, amphetamine and ecstasy were particularly high, but a substantial minority had used heroin and crack cocaine.

Factors which contribute to becoming homeless include unemployment and financial problems, mental health problems, alcohol or drug misuse, or physical disability. Lack of availability of affordable accommodation and aspects of regulation of Social Security benefits also contribute to the incidence of homelessness. In some cases a growing involvement with drug use or heavy drinking causes a rift with family and friends and may have led to job loss, which in turn may have caused a drift towards the company of other drug users or problem drinkers.

The relationship of homelessness and substance misuse is complex as trends in homelessness are clearly affected by changing social, political and economic factors. Homelessness, particularly sleeping rough, appeared to have a detrimental effect on physical and psychological health. Generally these people suffer many health problems related to their substance misuse in combination with poor diet, lack of regular healthcare and poor living conditions. Health complications associated with alcohol misuse may consist of gastric or digestive problems, gastrointestinal bleeding, skin ulcers and sores, hypertension, cardiac problems, memory loss, accidental injury, epileptic fits linked with heavy drinking or temporary unavailability of alcohol due to shortage of money, loss of consciousness and alcohol-related psychosis.

In a Home Office study, 70% of homeless people had been diagnosed with depression or other mental health problem, or had concerns about their mental health (Wincup *et al.* 2003). Some homeless people rely on alcohol or drugs as a means of coping with the inevitable stress of being without a stable home. Being homeless can induce feelings of worthlessness, reduced self-esteem and rejection. Some may use alcohol or drugs as a means of self-medication for a range of mental health problems, such as chronic depression or schizophrenia. Risky behaviours such as polydrug use and unsafe injecting are common practices. The lack of secure housing can exacerbate the health problems associated with injecting drug use. The lack of hygiene, security and personal organisation that is part of a transient lifestyle increases the tendency towards, and exposure to, risky drug use behaviours with implications for both the drug user and the wider community (Rowe 2005). Recently, there has been a rise in the incidence of tuberculosis (TB), and this is magnified in the homeless as a result of poor living conditions and diet. The presence of such an infection may go undetected for a considerable period of time and a homeless person may present at an accident and emergency department with a chronic cough, fever and haemoptysis (coughing up blood) and perhaps weight loss.

The majority of homeless alcohol and substance misusers do not use traditional primary healthcare services, but are more likely to use accident and emergency services at times of crisis or difficulty. The willingness of a homeless person to engage with health services will depend to a large degree on how distant or alienated they feel from the rest of society. Many alcohol or drug misusers find themselves barred from rehabilitation facilities and may be refused shelter in some hostels if intoxicated. It is notoriously difficult for someone who is entirely homeless or is frequently homeless to gain access to or to benefit from rehabilitation and treatment facilities. In some areas outreach teams or specialist services which are nurse-led have been established in an attempt to access this hard-to-reach group. Health workers need be sensitive in the style and manner in which they approach these vulnerable people, and endeavour to gain their trust and make suggestions for health improvement which are least alienating in nature.

KEY POINTS

- Alcohol and drug misuse in elderly people is common but may be largely under-diagnosed and undertreated.
- Alcohol use disorders in elderly people can cause a wide range of physical and psychosocial problems.
- Three groups of older alcohol misusers have been identified: early-onset drinkers or 'survivors', late-onset drinkers or 'reactors' and intermittent or binge drinkers.

- Alcohol is contraindicated for use with many of the drugs taken by older people.
- The reported prevalence and patterns of drug misuse in older people are lower than in the younger population.
- Tobacco is the most commonly used psychoactive substance amongst the elderly.
- The nature and pattern of alcohol and drug misuse in older people and the associated psychological and physical co-morbidity are different from those seen in younger populations.
- Drug misusers are seven times more likely to be homeless than the general population.
- It is estimated that 95% of homeless young people had used drugs, and their experimentation with illicit psychoactive substances started as early as 14 years of age.

ACTIVITY 18.1

There is only one correct answer to the following multiple-choice questions

Substance misuse in elderly people
a.   Is not a common problem
b.   Is under-diagnosed and untreated
c.   Can present as self-neglect
d.   Is more common in women

Many physical or psychological conditions in the elderly
a.   May mimic drug and alcohol misuse
b.   May show signs of craving
c.   May be present
d.   Shows denial

Early-onset drinkers
a.   Are also known as 'reactors'
b.   Have no family history of alcohol problems
c.   Have a lifelong pattern of problem drinking
d.   Account for about 20% of older alcoholics

Late-onset drinkers
a.   Are also known as 'survivors'
b.   Begin problematic drinking later in life
c.   Have a lifelong pattern of problem drinking
d.   Have limited chance of managing alcohol problems

Intermittent drinkers
1.   Are also known as 'Binge Drinkers'
2.   Begin problematic drinking later in life
3.   Have a lifelong pattern of problem drinking
4.   Have limited chance of managing alcohol problems

Elderly people have

a.   More tolerance to the adverse effects of alcohol
b.   Less tolerance to the adverse effects of alcohol
c.   An increase in body water
d.   Increased hepatic blood flow

Alcohol-related health problems in elderly people include

a.   Decreased risk of coronary heart disease
b.   Decreased risk of falls
c.   Decreased risk of Alzheimer's disease
d.   Decreased risk of prescribed drug interactions

The reported prevalence and patterns of drug misuse in older people

a.   Are higher than the younger population
b.   Are lower than the younger population
c.   Are the same
d.   Are higher than 10%

Older people receive

a.   Less prescribed benzodiazepine medication
b.   More prescribed benzodiazepine medication
c.   The same as other age groups
d.   More major tranquilliser medication

In elderly people

a.   There are no clear recommended sensible drinking limits
b.   There is greater vulnerability to the harmful effects of alcohol
c.   Routine screening for alcohol problems is not useful
d.   Alcohol and drug problems are the same

Drug misusers are

a.   10 times more likely to be homeless than the general population
b.   15 times more likely to be homeless than the general population
c.   7 times more likely to be homeless than the general population
d.   There is no significant difference

Amongst homeless people the type of drug most commonly used is

a.   Heroin
b.   Cocaine
c.   LSD
d.   Cannabis

ACTIVITY 18.2

- List the signs and symptoms of alcohol misuse in older people
- Identify the types of illicit and prescribed psychoactive substances used
- Describe the nature and pattern of substance misuse among homeless people
- List the factors which contribute to becoming homeless
- Discuss the relationship between homelessness and substance misuse

REFERENCES

Alcohol Concern (2007) *Alcohol and the Elderly*, Fact Sheet London: Alcohol Concern.

Beckett, J., Kouimtsidis, C., Reynolds, M. and Ghodse, H. (2005) Substance misuse in elderly general hospital in-patients. *International Journal of Geriatric Psychiatry*, 17, 2: 193–4.

Bogunovic, O.J. and Greenfield, S.F. (2004) Practical geriatrics: use of benzodiazepines among elderly patients. *Psychiatric Services*, 55: 233–5.

Coulthard, M., Farrell, M., Singleton, N. and Meltzer, H. (2002) *Tobacco, Alcohol and Drug Use and Mental Health*. London: TSO.

Crome, I.B. and Day, E. (1999) Substance misuse and dependence, older people deserve better services. *Review in Clinical Gerontology*, 9: 327–42.

Dar, K. (2006) Alcohol use disorders in elderly people: fact or fiction? *Advances in Psychiatric Treatment*, 12: 173–81.

Deloitte MCS Ltd (2004) *Research into Homelessness and Substance Misuse*. Drug and Alcohol Information and Research Unit, Department of Health, Social Services and Public Safety on behalf of Northern Ireland Drugs and Alcohol Campaign.

Department of Health (1998) *Smoking Kills – A White Paper on Tobacco*. London: The Stationery Office. CM4177.

Dunne, F.J. and Schipperheijn, J.A.M. (1989) Alcohol and the elderly: need for greater awareness. *British Medical Journal*, 298: 1660–1.

Fountain, J., Howes, S., Marsden, J. and Strang, J. (2002) Who uses services for homeless people: an investigation amongst people sleeping rough in London. *Journal of Community and Applied Social Psychology*, 12: 71–5.

Grant, B.F. and Harford, T.C. (1995) Comorbidity between DSM-IV alcohol use disorders and major depression: results of a national survey. *Drug and Alcohol Dependence*, 39: 197–206.

Homelessness Directorate (2002) *Drug Services for Homeless People*. London: Office of the Deputy Prime Minister.

Information Centre (2007) *Statistics on Alcohol 2007*. http://www.ic.nhs.uk/statistics-and-data-collections/healthand-lifestyles/alcohol/statistics-on-alcohol:-england-2007-%5Bns%5D.

Institute of Alcohol Studies (2007) *Alcohol and the Elderly*. St Ives, Cambridgeshire: Institute of Alcohol Studies.

Kemp, P., Neale J. and Robertson, M. (2006) Homelessness amongst problem drug users: prevalence, risk factors and trigger events. *Health and Social Care in the Community*, 14, 4: 319–28.

King, C.J., Van Hasselt, V.B., Segal, D.L. and Hersen M. (1994) Diagnosis and assessment of substance abuse in older adults, current strategies and issues. *Addictive Behaviours*, 19: 41–5.

McGrath, A., Crome, P. and Crome, I.B. (2005) Substance misuse in the older population. *Postgraduate Medical Journal*, 81: 228–31.

Marshall, J. (2006) *Alcohol and Drug Use Disorders in Older People: National Trends and Associations*. 23 November 2006. www.uea.ac.uk/swk/mha/presentations/Jane%20Marshall.pdf (accessed 26 September 2007).

Menninger, J.A. (2002) Assessment and treatment of alcoholism and substance related disorders in the elderly. *Bulletin of the Menninger Clinic*, 66: 166–84.

Morgan, K., Dallosso, H., Ebrahim, S., Arie, T. and Fentem, P.H. (1988) Prevalence, frequency, and duration of hypnotic drug use among the elderly living at home. *British Medical Journal Clinical Research*, 27: 296, 601–2.

National Statistics (2006a) *Smoking and Drinking among Adults 2005 and Drinking: Adults' Behaviour and Knowledge*. www.statistics.gov.uk (accessed 25 September 2007).

National Statistics (2006b) *Smoking Habits in Great Britain*. www.statistics.gov.uk (accessed 25 September 2007).

Patterson, T.L. and Jeste, D.V. (1999) The potential impact of the baby-boom generation on substance abuse among elderly persons. *Psychiatric Services*, 50, 9: 1184–8.

Rowe, J. (2005) Laying the foundations: addressing heroin use among the 'street homeless'. *Drugs: Education, Prevention and Policy*, 12, 1: 47–59.

Smith, J.W. (1995) Medical manifestations of alcoholism in the elderly. *International Journal of Addictions*, 30: 1749–98.

Speer, D.C. and Bates, K. (1992) Comorbid mental and substance disorders among older psychiatric patients. *Journal of the American Geriatric Society*, 40: 886–90.

Thomas, V.S. and Rockwood, K.J. (2001) Alcohol abuse, cognitive impairment and mortality among older people. *Journal of the American Geriatric Society*, 49: 415–20.

Waern, M. (2005) Alcohol dependence and misuse in elderly suicides. *Postgraduate Medical Journal*, 81: 228–31.

Whitcup, S.M. and Miller, F. (1987) Unrecognized drug dependence in psychiatrically hospitalized elderly patients. *Journal of the American Geriatric Society*, 35: 297–301.

Wincup, E., Buckland, G. and Bayliss, R. (2003) *Youth Homelessness and Substance Use*, Report to the Drugs and Alcohol Research Unit, Home Office Research Study 258. London: Home Office Research, Development and Statistics Directorate.

Wright, F. and Whyley, C. (1994) *Accident Prevention and Risk-taking by Elderly People: The Need for Advice*. London: Age Concern Institute of Gerontology.

CHAPTER 19

YOUNG PEOPLE: ALCOHOL AND DRUG MISUSE

OBJECTIVES

- Discuss the prevalence of substance misuse in young people.

- Identify the factors that contribute to the initiation and continuation of adolescent alcohol and drug misuse.

- Discuss the factors and motivations for not using drugs.

- List the presenting physical, psychological and social features of young substance misusers.

Substance misuse in young people ranges from readily available and legal substances such as tobacco, alcohol and volatile substances to more uncommon and illegal substances such as ecstasy, cannabis, cocaine or heroin. The widespread use of illicit drugs and their associations with physical and psychological morbidity, mortality and social disabilities has made substance misuse among young people a significant public health problem (Pudney 2002). Substance misuse in young people should be considered in the context of 'normal' adolescent risk-taking behaviours and experimentation. Many young people will experiment with alcohol and/or illegal drugs and most of them will probably suffer no long-term physical, psychological and social harm. However, for a small minority of young people, the use of alcohol and/or illegal drugs will escalate into addiction. Although the use of heroin and cocaine gives rise to more public concern, there is little doubt that tobacco smoking and alcohol consumption can have a far more deleterious effect on the health of young people. Stimulant drugs such as crack, cocaine, amphetamines and ecstasy are currently popular amongst the younger age groups and are integral to the ethos of the 'club scene'.

A central aim of the government's *Updated National Drug Strategy* is to reduce drug use by young people, particularly the most vulnerable. A key aim of the report *Every Child Matters: Young People and Drug* (DfES 2005) is to encourage young people to choose not to take illegal drugs. It is recommended that a holistic multi-agency outcomes-focused approach should be undertaken to enhance the prevention of substance misuse by children and young people. Following a government review, the NTA has been asked from April 2008 to take on a leadership role for young people's substance-misuse treatment, championing high-quality provision and assuring local delivery of services.

PREVALENCE OF SUBSTANCE MISUSE

The 2005/6 British Crime Survey (Home Office 2006) estimates that there are over two and three-quarter million people aged 16 to 24 in England and Wales who have used illicit drugs at some point in their lives. Cannabis is the drug most likely to be used, with 21.4% of 16- to 24-year-olds using cannabis in the last year. Cocaine is the next most commonly used drug with 5.9%, followed by ecstasy at 4.3%. Amyl nitrite use is estimated at 3.9%, use of hallucinogens at 3.4% and use of amphetamines at 3.3%. It is estimated that just over 350,000 young people took cocaine powder and just over 250,000 took ecstasy. The biggest increase in the use of cocaine powder occurred between 1998 and 2000 but since 2000 cocaine powder use has been stable. The findings for 2005/6 showed a decrease in the use of cannabis and an increase in the use of LSD amongst 16- to 24-year-olds. Currently, 20,000 young people are receiving specialist substance misuse treatment. Five per cent are experiencing problems with dependency on class A drugs, 90% are experiencing problems with cannabis and/or alcohol use (NTA 2007).

There are five vulnerable groups of young people identifiable in the *Crime and Justice Survey* (Home Office 2005):

• those who have ever been in care
• those who have ever been homeless
• those who have ever been homeless truants
• those excluded from school
• those who are serious or frequent offenders.

The findings from the survey (Home Office 2005) of vulnerable young people suggested that only 4% of those who were not vulnerable used class A drugs in the last year, while 16% of those in vulnerable groups used class A drugs during the same period. When comparing individual vulnerable groups, those who had been in care or homeless had the lowest levels of drug use while serious or frequent offenders and truants showed the highest levels of drug use. For example, class A drug use in the last year was 5% for those who had been in care or homeless, 13% for serious or frequent offenders and 16% for truants.

The findings of a study (Mutale 2003) showed that nearly 40% of young people referred to the adolescent psychiatric service had reported substance misuse in the past year and that the most popular illicit drugs were cannabis followed by alcohol and volatile solvents. Just over 50% of those who had reported substance misuse admitted to polydrug use. Data also showed that, of the 54 young people reporting substance misuse, at least 70% had at least one diagnosable psychiatric disorder and that boys had a significantly higher rate of co-morbidity than girls. However, the findings suggested that depression was the category least likely to be associated with substance misuse and that substance misuse probably played a significant role in the aetiology and self-medication of anxiety disorders and some cases of depression or psychosis.

ADJUSTMENT AND RISK-TAKING BEHAVIOUR

Adolescence is naturally a time of experiment, adventure, risk-taking and challenging authority. It is also a time when young people are particularly impressionable and vulnerable to many environmental factors (Fullerton and Ursano 1994) that influence their lifestyle and behaviours. It is also a time when identity is being formed and peer-group membership and approval is all-important, while at the same time there is a move away from family and parental ties. Peer influence may bear increased influence in situations where a young person lacks support or understanding or lacks the affection of parental figures and family.

There is not a single factor that predisposes young people to substance misuse; rather there are multiple risk factors which act together on any one individual and contribute to their decision to use alcohol or drugs. A study by the Home Office (2007) exploring the risk, protective factors and resilience to drug use in young people found that there are relatively well established associations between several risk and protective factors and problematic drug use among young people but these associations are not necessarily causal. There is evidence to suggest that the number of risk factors that a person is exposed to is a predictor of drug use, regardless of what those particular risk factors are; the more risk factors there are, the greater the likelihood of drug use (Home Office 2007).

Many factors contribute to the initiation and continuation of adolescent alcohol and drug misuse. Several groups of young people vulnerable to problematic drug use have been identified from a review of the literature on risk factors. These groups are: truants, those excluded from school, the homeless, those 'looked after' by local authorities or in foster care, young offenders, those involved in prostitution, children from families with substance-abusing parents or siblings and young people with conduct or depressive disorders (Lloyd 1998). Early introduction to substance abuse (for example, in early teens) is commonly regarded as a risk factor as well as alcohol or other substance problems in parents and family members, school difficulties, early onset of smoking, peer influence, media influence, family dynamics, social isolation, poor self-esteem, unemployment, criminal behaviour and genetic influences. Both positive and negative parental views may increase a young person's risks of substance misuse. Young people who are trying to cope with the divorce of parents or a breakup of their family for other reasons may be particularly vulnerable to the possibilities of substance misuse as a means of dealing with their sadness, distress or feelings of rejection. Many adjustments are called for in a young person's life, such as coming to terms with sexual relationships which may be transient or turbulent, awareness and coming to terms with sexuality and individual sexual orientation, the transition from school to work or university or perhaps the prospect of unemployment. In addition, sexual exploitation and disinhibited sexual behaviour may be regarded as risky contexts.

Most people manage the transition from adolescence to adulthood satisfactorily, despite exposure to risky contexts, through the process of resilience. Resilience is defined as those behaviours and methods that young people utilise in making their decisions not to use drugs, despite being exposed to drugs and other risk factors (Dillon *et al.* 2006). Some of the factors for using and motivations for not using drugs are presented in Table 19.1. Since only a minority of substance misusers actually start their drug use in adulthood, it is vital that the prevention and management of adolescence substance misuse is given high priority.

PRESENTING FEATURES OF SUBSTANCE MISUSE OF YOUNG PEOPLE

The presentation of features of substance misuse of young people may be divided into physical, psychological and social features but the patient will usually present with a mixture of these (see Table 19.2). Substance misuse can contribute to and compound physical and mental health problems, and the impact of these is covered in previous chapters.

Table 19.1 Reasons for using and motivations for not using drugs

Reasons for using drugs	Motivations not to use drugs
• Escape from problems • Alleviate boredom • For the 'buzz' • Feel for confidence • Ease physical pain • Look 'hard'	Relating to lifestyle aspirations and relationships • Other people's disapproval • Legal consequences • Role as parent • Career aspirations Relating to the practicalities of being a user • Availability of time • Financial cost Relating to the physical and psychological effects of drugs • Personal experiences with drugs • Current health conditions or difficulties • Fear of effect on health • Fear of addiction • Fear of losing control Relating to some of the perceived benefits of using drugs • Sources of 'buzz' • Sources of support or coping mechanisms

Source: Home Office (2007)

Table 19.2 Presenting features of substance misuse in young people: physical, social and psychological

Physical	Social	Psychological
• Respiratory symptoms caused by smoking • Peri-oral and peri-nasal lesions caused by inhalation or snorting • Physical injuries incurred during intoxication • Agitation after polydrug or prolonged use • Needle tracks, thrombosis or abscesses owing to intravenous use • Withdrawal syndromes	• Deteriorating educational performance • Family conflict • Crime: petty associated with intoxication; theft to provide funds; 'dealing' as part of more serious association with drug culture	• Mood changes • Confusion • Depression on withdrawal of stimulants • Irritability as part of withdrawal syndrome • Deliberate self-harm or suicide attempt • Psychosis

Source: World Health Organization (2003–4)

CONCLUSION

This task of recognition and accurate diagnosis of alcohol and drug misuse in young people is made more difficult because of the increasing trend towards the use of combinations of substances, rather than the sole use of a single psychoactive substance. Although substance misuse is a significant and growing problem, it is rare for adolescents to be referred to psychiatric or specialist agencies because of their smoking or drinking habits (Hoare 1993). So far there have been no specialist substance-misuse services developed specifically for young people, but instead they tend to be seen either by child psychiatry services or by adult substance-misuse services, neither of which is ideally suited to their complex needs. However, this is changing, owing to the commissioning of young people's substance-misuse treatment and the provision of local delivery of services. Swadi and Zeitlin (1987) argue that adolescent substance experimenters and users should be considered vulnerable and as a potential source of future social difficulty with major implications for health service planning. This is why it is so important that general and primary healthcare services, accident and emergency units, teachers, probation officers and school healthcare professionals are prepared to identify and respond to substance-misuse problems in young people, as well as being involved with health education and preventative initiatives.

Young vulnerable people who use substances, whether drugs and/or alcohol, are heterogeneous and it would be excluding to ignore their diversity (Epling and McGregor 2006). Preventative and educational programmes are of the utmost importance (see Chapter 21), as well as skills of identification or assessment strategies, brief intervention techniques (see Chapters 24 and 26), family work and social skills training – for example, helping young people, through discussion and role play, to make informed choices and to be assertive when confronted with offers of drugs or peer pressure.

KEY POINTS

- Substance misuse in young people ranges from readily available and legal substances such as tobacco, alcohol and volatile substances to more uncommon and illegal substances such as ecstasy, cannabis, cocaine or heroin.
- The widespread use of illicit drugs and their association with physical and psychological morbidity, mortality and social disabilities have made substance misuse among young people a significant public health problem.
- Substance misuse in young people should be considered in the context of 'normal' adolescent risk-taking behaviours and experimentation.
- A central aim of the government's *Updated National Drug Strategy* is to reduce drug use by young people, particularly the most vulnerable.
- A key aim of the report *Every Child Matters: Young People and Drugs* is to encourage young people to choose not to take illegal drugs.
- Currently, 20,000 young people are receiving specialist substance-misuse treatment.
- There is not a single factor that predisposes young people to substance misuse; rather there are multiple risk factors which act together on any one individual and contribute to their decision to use alcohol or drugs.
- There are relatively well established associations between several risk and protective factors and problematic drug use among young people.
- Many factors contribute to the initiation and continuation of adolescent alcohol and drug misuse.
- Several groups of young people vulnerable to problematic drug use have been identified from a review of the literature on risk factors.
- A holistic multi-agency outcomes-focused approach should be undertaken to enhance the prevention of substance misuse by children and young people.

ACTIVITY 19.1

Please choose one correct answer to the following multiple-choice questions

Substance misuse in young people should be considered
a.   As 'normal' adolescent risk-taking behaviour
b.   As abnormal adolescent development
c.   As part of the pathology of addiction
d.   As a reaction to adult culture

Many young people will
a.   Not experiment with alcohol and/or illegal drugs
b.   Experiment with alcohol and/or illegal drugs
c.   Experiment with prescribed medications
d.   Not experiment with prescribed medication

The number of people in the UK aged 16–24 who have used illicit drugs is
a.   5 million
b.   3.5 million
c.   2.75 million
d.   1 million

The drug most commonly used by 16–24-year-olds is
a.   Heroin
b.   Cocaine
c.   LSD
d.   Cannabis

Vulnerable young people compared to non-vulnerable people are
a.   Less likely to use illicit drugs
b.   More likely to use illicit drugs
c.   More likely to be in secure accommodation
d.   Less likely to be in care

Young people are predisposed to substance misuse because of
a.   A single risk factor
b.   Multiple risk factors
c.   Protective factors
d.   Resilience

ACTIVITY 19.2

•   Discuss the prevalence of substance misuse in young people
•   List the factors that contribute to the initiation and continuation of adolescent alcohol and drug misuse
•   Discuss the factors and motivations for not using drugs
•   The presentation of features of substance misuse of young people may be divided into physical, psychological and social features. List the features

REFERENCES

DfES (2005) *Every Child Matters: Young People and Drugs*. Nottingham: Department for Education and Skills, DfES Publications. www.everychildmatters.gov.uk.

Dillon, L., Chivite-Matthews, N., Grewal, I., Brown, R., Webster, S., Weddell, E., Brown, G. and Smith, N. (2006) *Risk, Protective Factors and Resilience to Drug Use: Identifying Resilient Young People and Learning from their Experience*. London: Home Office.

Epling, M. and McGregor, J. (2006) Vulnerable young people and substance misuse. In G. Hussein Rassool (ed.) *Dual Diagnosis Nursing*. Oxford: Blackwell Publications.

Fullerton, C.S. and Ursano, R.J. (1994) Preadolescent peer friendships: a critical contribution to adult social relatedness. *Journal of Youth and Adolescence*, 23: 43–64.

Home Office (2005) *Drug Use among Vulnerable Groups of Young People: Findings from the 2003 Crime and Justice Survey*. Findings 254. The Research, Development and Statistics Directorate, London: Home Office. www.homeoffice.gov.uk/rds/pubintro1.html.

Home Office (2006) *Drug Misuse Declared: Findings from the 2005/06 British Crime Survey England and Wales*. The Research, Development and Statistics Directorate. London: Home Office. www.homeoffice.gov.uk/rds/index.htm.

Home Office (2007) *Identifying and Exploring Young People's Experiences of Risk, Protective Factors and Resilience to Drug Use*. Home Office Development and Practice Reports. London: Home Office.

Hoare, P. (1993) *Essential Child Psychiatry*. London: Churchill Livingstone.

Lloyd, C. (1998) Risk factors for problem drug use: identifying vulnerable groups. *Drugs: Education, Prevention and Policy*, 5, 3: 217–32.

Mutale, T. (2003) Substance misuse among young people referred to a UK psychiatric service. *British Journal of Forensic Practice*, November. FindArticles.com. 02 Jan. 2008. http://find articles.com/p/articles/mi_qa4121/is_200311/ai_n9303273 (accessed 25 September 2007).

NTA (2007) *New Era for Young People's Substance Misuse Treatment*. Media release, 31 July. London: National Treatment Agency.

Pudney, S. (2002) *The Road to Ruin? Sequences of Initiation into Drug Use and Offending by Young People in Britain*. Home Office Research Study 253. London: Research, Development and Statistics Directorate.

Swadi, H. and Zeitlin, H. (1987) Drug education to school children: does it really work? *British Journal of Addiction*, 82: 741–6.

WHO (2003–4) *Substance Misuse in Young People*. World Health Organization – UK Collaborating Centre www.iop.kcl.ac.uk/who. NHS National Library for Health (accessed 25 September 2007).

PART 4

ROLE, PREVENTION AND STRATEGIES FOR CHANGE

CHAPTER 20

GENERIC ROLE IN RESPONSE
TO ALCOHOL AND DRUG MISUSE

OBJECTIVES

◾ Discuss the rationale for working with substance misusers.

◾ Describe some of the roles and interventions of health, social care and
criminal justice system professionals in working with substance misusers.

ACTIVITY 20.1

- Have you come into contact with alcohol and drug misusers or have you
  alcohol and drug misusers in your caseload?
- Identify the number of contacts you have made during the past month
- If contact was made, how many were alcohol or drug misusers or both?
- Reflect on your own roles, whether generic or specialist, in working with
  substance misusers
- What are the challenges in working with substance misusers?

ACTIVITY 20.2

Addiction Intervention Confidence Skills Questionnaire (AICSQ-16)
Please indicate your level of confidence (high, moderate or low level of confidence)
by putting a tick where appropriate for each statement

	Low	Moderate	High

Alcohol

Providing alcohol-use education and prevention information

Recognising signs and symptoms of alcohol problems

Talking to patients about risks of alcohol misuse

Taking an alcohol history

Referring patients for alcohol treatment

Providing care for patients with alcohol problems

Drugs

Providing drug-use education and prevention information

Recognising signs and symptoms of drug problems

Talking to patients about risks of drug misuse

Taking a drug history

Referring patients for drug treatment

Providing care for patients with drug problems

Giving health risk information on prescribed medication

Informing smokers about health risks of smoking

Providing tobacco smoking education and prevention information

Knowledge of drug and alcohol services

Health and social care professionals in both primary healthcare and residential settings are usually the first point of contact for clients who have potential or early alcohol and drug problems. The initial management of those with the early stage of use is not the sole responsibility of specialist workers and addiction specialists (Rassool and Marshall 2001). An active involvement of the different cadres of health and social care workers is indispensable in the early prevention, recognition, screening and brief interventions of alcohol and drug misusers. This chapter will examine the generic role of health and social care professionals in hospital and primary healthcare settings in relation to intervention and management of alcohol and drug misuse and the rationale for working with substance misusers.

RATIONALE FOR WORKING WITH SUBSTANCE MISUSERS

Given this increasing prevalence of alcohol and drug misuse and the normalisation of psychoactive substances in society, only a minority of drug and alcohol misusers are likely to come into contact with specialist drug and alcohol agencies. Most of them will have first contact with primary care services, medical and psychiatric services, social services and voluntary agencies and the criminal justice system.

The Advisory Council's Report (ACMD 1982) on treatment and rehabilitation stressed the need for a comprehensive approach to drug misuse with the emphasis and focus on a multidisciplinary response from generic, specialist and non-specialist agencies. In the context of substance misuse, some of the particular areas identified as threats to the nation's health are smoking, alcohol-related diseases, drugs and HIV disease (Department of Health 1992). All the key areas for health education and harm reduction targets are invariably related to the misuse of psychoactive substance.

The *Updated Drug Strategy* (Home Office 2002), the *Alcohol Harm Reduction Strategy for England* (Prime Minister's Strategy Unit 2004) and *Choosing Health: Making Healthy Choices Easier* (Department of Health 2004) build on the foundations laid and lessons learned from previous substance strategies and set out a range of policies and interventions to prevent drug misuse and to encourage stabilisation in treatment and support for abstinence. The policies also focus on reducing alcohol-related harm and the encouragement of sensible drinking. The government's wider national drugs strategy is also to reduce drug-related death due to overdose and blood-borne viruses. The policies recognise the need for co-ordination of services and commits to working within the Models of Care framework on integrated care pathways.

The extent and nature of the substantial health and social problems associated with substance misuse highlight the pressing need for members of the primary healthcare team, nurses, social workers and those working in the criminal justice system to respond to the needs of substance misusers. Intervention in the lifestyle and behaviours of substance misusers at an early stage helps to limit the associated health, social and familial harms. Early intervention strategies from health and social care professionals can have dramatic impact on preventing substance misuse becoming a long-term problem.

GENERIC ROLE IN RESPONSE TO ALCOHOL AND DRUG MISUSE

This section outlines the particular setting and specialty of healthcare professionals and aspects of generic interventions. The nature and extent of substance abuse require a multi-professional approach. Liaison with other health and social care agencies and specialist substance-misuse services are desirable. A wide variety of roles exist in the substance-misuse field and include not only specialist workers but also professionals whose work brings them into contact with drug and alcohol misuse. It is fundamental that the central role of health, social care professionals and those in the criminal justice system, in hospital or community settings, should focus on the early recognition and the provision of effective care, prevention and health education. It is recognised that the generic roles and skills of the health, social and criminal justice professionals could be easily adapted to meet the needs of the problem drug user and problem drinker as well as the 'non-using' population. Roles in the substance-misuse field are characterised by the level and frequency of contact with substance misuse and substance misusers. The workforce is best imagined as a continuum from specialist to generic, falling across all sectors.

The competence of the workforce has the most crucial relationship to the achievement of the aims of the Drug Strategy. A broad range of workers have a key role to play in addressing substance misuse, and the reduction of substance misuse should be regarded as core business for many services. Every role in the drug and alcohol field requires a particular set of competences. Some of these will be generic, others more specific to the substance-misuse field, and the required competences will vary from one role to another (Home Office 2005). Examples of the types of role that might fall within each category are presented in Table 20.1.

Table 20.1 Working with substance misusers

Generic workers with occasional substance-misuse portfolio	Generic workers with a substance-misuse portfolio	Specialist workers
• Nurse	• Mental health nurse	• Addiction nurses
• Hospital pharmacist	• Ambulance staff	• Alcohol and drug worker
• Teacher/lecturer	• Connexions worker	• Young people's substance
• Early years worker	• Youth worker	misuse worker
• Citizens' Advice Bureau worker	• Pupil Referral Unit teacher	• Drugs and employment
• Social worker	• Housing officer	co-ordinator
• Prison visitor	• Care Leavers Team social worker	• Drugs unit police officer
• Magistrate	• Homelessness worker	• Custody suite-based drug
• HM Customs worker	• Probation officer	worker
• Solicitor	• Prison officer	• Progress2work adviser
	• Psychologist	• Substance misuse
	• Community Support Officer	commissioner
		• Drug Action Team
		co-ordinator
		• CARAT worker
		• Education drug adviser

Source: Home Office (2005)

NURSES

Nurses must assume a multitude of roles which focus on the provision of effective care, prevention and education (Rassool 1993). The roles of the nurse in relation to substance misuse have been articulated in a document from the World Health Organization / International Council of Nurses (WHO/ICN 1991). These roles are: Provider of care; Educator/resource; Counsellor/therapist; Advocate; Promoter of health; Researcher; Supervisor/leader; and Consultant. A brief description of the roles is shown in Table 20.2.

Table 20.2 Nursing roles in relation to substance misuse

Provider of Care	Caring for those who misuse or affected by psychoactive substances
Counsellor/therapist	Focusing on the needs of the individuals, their families and colleagues
Educator/resource	Providing health information to community groups, schools, families, individuals and to professional and non-professional groups
Advocate	Lobbying for change and improved care
Health promoter	Campaigning for policy and legislation to reduce demands of abused drugs
Researcher	Determining the most effective method of helping, caring and preventing substance misuse
Supervisor/leader	Guiding professionals and non-professionals
Consultant	Providing consultancy to professionals in this speciality

Source: WHO/ICN (1991)

NURSES IN MEDICAL AND SURGICAL UNITS

Patients who misuse psychoactive substances may be admitted to a general or surgical ward but the health problems may or may not be associated with substance misuse. Hospital-based surveys indicate that 30% of acute medical admissions to hospitals have alcohol problems and that up to one-third of men admitted to medical and surgical wards have alcohol-related problems (Tomlinson Report 1992, UK Alcohol Forum 1997). Patients attending hospital with alcohol-related problems fall into two broad categories: those with less severe drinking problems who may be amenable to brief interventions; and patients with features of alcohol dependence, requiring detoxification and ongoing treatment (Owen *et al.* 2005). The appropriate referral and management of both types of patients in specialist services secondary care are important. According to Maxwell (1990), the ranges of acute medical problems nurses are likely to encounter are shown in Table 20.3.

Aspects of interventions include the provision of total nursing care, screening or taking a drug and alcohol history, brief interventions and counselling, harm-reduction approach, dealing with withdrawal symptoms and intoxication, and referral to specialist agencies. However, a survey by Owen *et al.* (2005), on how NHS general hospitals in England deal with patients with alcohol-related problems reported that only a minority

Table 20.3 Range of medical and surgical problems

Medical units	*Surgical units*
• Unexplained fever	• Abscess
• Acute or chronic infections of skins and joints	• Acute abdominal pain
• Unexplained cardiac murmurs	• Intestinal obstruction (body packers)
• Endocarditis	• Vascular problems
• Venous and arterial thrombosis	• Trauma (such as road traffic accidents or burns)
• Jaundice	• Rhinitis
• Abnormal liver function	• Rhinorrhoea
• Lymphadenopathy	
• Features of immunosupression	
• Munchausen syndrome	

Source: Adapted from Maxwell (1990)

of the hospitals had guidelines for the screening and detection of alcohol-related problems and there was a lack of care pathways for the pharmacological and non-pharmacological management of patients with alcohol withdrawal.

During the past decade, there has been a significant increase in the number of dedicated alcohol nurse specialists in the hospitals (Owen *et al.* 2005). Such workers are highly effective in different health care settings (Ockene *et al.* 1999) and can adopt a multidimensional role ranging from providing advice on detoxification, screening for alcohol-related problems and optimising medical management through providing ongoing support, and information for referral for specialist alcohol treatment (Hillman *et al.* 2001). Alcohol specialist nurses may represent a highly cost-effective mechanism for achieving the targets set out in the *Choosing Health* White Paper from the Department of Health (2004) (Owen *et al.* 2005).

PSYCHIATRIC NURSES

Substance misuse is common among people with mental health problems, and such dual needs are to be met by mainstream services with the support of specialist advice (Department of Health 2002). Problems associated with alcohol or drug use are more common in mental health services, particularly acute admission services. *From Values to Action: The Chief Nursing Officer's Review of Mental Health Nursing* (Department of Health 2006) recommends that mental health nurses in all settings will be able to respond to the needs of the people with mental health and substance misuse problems. Many psychiatric patients use psychoactive substances as a means of self-medication in order to relieve anxiety, depression and other psychopathological conditions. Some individuals are admitted to acute psychiatric settings as a result of drug-induced psychiatric reactions from stimulants and hallucinogens. Some of the health-related problems include:

- drug-induced psychosis (stimulants and alcohol)
- drug-withdrawal psychosis (hypnosedatives)
- alcohol psychosis
- suicidal behaviour and depression as a result of substance misuse
- withdrawal symptoms
- dual diagnosis (mental illness co-existing with substance misuse).

The areas of interventions include assessment of drug and alcohol misuse, risk behaviours, brief interventions, cognitive therapy, relapse prevention and management of patients with dual diagnosis and drug-induced psychotic reactions. Health education and harm reduction should be included in the intervention strategies.

COMMUNITY MENTAL HEALTH NURSES

Community mental health nurses are exposed to a wide range of clients with varying degrees of psychiatric disorders. Part of their caseload will include individuals with substance-use problems, both illicit and prescribed medications. More community mental health nurses are now in services and have undertaken courses in addiction nursing and addictive behaviour. These community nurses face the ethical dilemma of encouraging their clients to adhere to medication compliance and at the same time discouraging and rationalising their alcohol or other drug use (Rassool 1998). This may play a part in the ambivalence that nurses experience, resulting in the resistance to use specialist services in a consultative capacity, preferring to refer clients to them for 'treatment and management' (Kennedy and Faugier 1989). There are also inherent problems in treatment philosophies and goal between those with substance misuse and those with psychiatric disorders. Gafoor and Rassool (1998) stated that workers may be reluctant to intervene because of feelings of frustration, inadequacy, or lack of confidence in their ability to effect change; they often hold negative views about treatment outcomes and may demonstrate opposition to what they perceive as overtly self-abusive behaviour.

Community drug and alcohol teams may include community psychiatric nurses. Their work may cover the recognition of substance misusers, liaison with primary health care workers, for example general practitioners, in detoxification, motivational and relapse prevention, counselling, alcohol, drug and HIV education and other harm minimisation work (Royal College of Psychiatrists 1997). The health-related problems in relation to alcohol and drug misuse include dual diagnosis, problems related to withdrawal from alcohol or benzodiazepines, or opiates, blood-borne infections and amphetamine or cocaine psychosis. Aspects of intervention include the assessment of mental health or substance-misuse problems, counselling, harm reduction, relapse prevention, cognitive therapy, health education, alternative therapies in the rational use of psychoactive substances, alternative to drug-prescribing, home detoxification and prevention of substance misuse.

ACCIDENT AND EMERGENCY NURSES

Alcohol and drug misusers may present to the accident and emergency department as a result of physical or psychological complications of substance misuse. For many drug misusers, accident and emergency (A&E) departments may be the first or only point of contact with health services, most often because of accidental overdoses and other crises (Gossop *et al.* 1995). The results of a recent survey (Patton *et al.* 2006) suggest that English A&E departments may be willing to address hazardous alcohol consumption as part of their package of clinical care. However, there is cause for concern about the low numbers of departments utilising formal screening tools, suggesting that patients who may benefit from help or advice remain undetected.

There has been a marked increase in the number of patients attending A&E departments following binge drinking and drug misuse. An increase of overnight alcohol-related emergency to A&E after the introduction of new UK alcohol licensing legislation has also been reported (Newton *et al.* 2007). It is estimated that alcohol places a major burden on A&E departments.

Alcohol misuse is responsible for 10% or more of A&E attendances in general, and a higher percentage of those with head and facial injuries and trauma requiring orthopaedic admission (Royal College of Physicians 2001). In addition, attendances to A&E by substance misusers result from complications from the pharmacological action of the drug, hazards related to administration, factors related to the patient's lifestyle (Royal College of Psychiatrists and British Association of Accident and Emergency Medicine 2004), intoxication or withdrawal, self-harm and psychiatric disturbances. It is estimated that up to 5% of patients attending A&E departments present with primary psychiatric problems, whilst another 20–30% have psychiatric symptoms in addition to physical disorders (Ramirez and House 1997). The most common presenting psychiatric problem in most A&E departments is self-harm, typically constituting one-third of the total. About 170,000 cases of self-harm present to A&E departments in the UK each year (Bolton 2006).

The *Models of Care* (NTA 2002) recommend that for staff at A&E departments intervention strategies should include screening, provision of drug-related information and advice and referral to specialised alcohol or drug agencies. In summary, A&E staff will need to intervene in cases of overdose or coma, management of intoxicated clients and disruptive behaviour, management of withdrawal behaviour (for example, to prevent opiate withdrawal in a pregnant woman), alcohol or drug-related accidents, respiratory failure (common after opiate overdose), self-harm and drug-induced psychosis or other mental health problems. A&E has a vital role to play in reducing drug-related deaths. The key points of reducing drug-related deaths by A&E staff are presented in Table 20.4.

Table 20.4 Key points in reducing drug-related deaths

• Injectors should be given injecting equipment	If needle exchange services are closed and they need injecting equipment
• Encourage drug users to seek treatment	Reduce overdose and blood-borne infections
• Hepatitis B immunisation for injectors who attend A&E	Should be a routine procedure
• Risk of overdose due to loss of tolerance	Loss of tolerance after detoxification, rehabilitation or prison. Homeless injectors are a high-risk group
• Long-term users and polydrug users are at high risk of overdose	The greater the overdose, the greater the risk of one of the overdoses being fatal
• Provision of health information literature	Overdose prevention Viral transmission Local drug or alcohol services
• Linking with local drug or alcohol agencies	Establish relationship with substance misuse services
• Encourage drug or alcohol users to attend A&E	Non-judgemental and non-hostile attitude would be a positive experience for substance misusers and their friends or families

Source: Adapted from NTA (2004)

PRACTICE NURSES

With the new NHS system focusing in identifying the need for local services and on primary prevention with health improvement programmes, practice nurses are ideally placed to screen for drug misuse and for those at-risk alcohol consumption and to deliver health information and brief interventions. There is some evidence suggesting that 13% of men and 2.5% of women having an alcohol-use disorder consult their general practice (McMenamin 1997). It is reported that an average of 3.1 patients per month with potential alcohol problems are seen in general practice (Deehan *et al.* 1998).

There is growing evidence to support the effectiveness of nurse-led brief interventions in primary care settings. In a study by Owen *et al.* (2000), the findings showed that practice nurses are happy to give advice regarding sensible drinking and routinely and appropriately take a history of alcohol intake, usually within well-woman and well-man clinics. However, fewer nurses took alcohol histories in other clinics, such as hypertension or diabetic clinics. The authors suggested that this may reflect a lack of understanding of the role of alcohol in diseases such as hypertension. A particular concern was that one in two women and one in three men are not receiving correct advice on sensible limits of alcohol consumption, this despite the fact that alcohol histories are taken. Nurses have also been found to provide a brief intervention to patients in a more consistent manner than general practitioners although they screened fewer patients overall (Lock and Kaner 2004).

The practice nurse has a valuable role to play in the prevention of alcohol and drug-related problems. Aspects of interventions include the early identification and recognition of substance misuse, screening for drug and alcohol as part of the wellness approach, brief interventions with clients with early drinking problem or drug taking and health education and counselling.

NURSES WORKING IN SEXUAL HEALTH

The past few years have seen nurse-led clinics in genito-urinary medicine (GUM) to co-ordinate first-line comprehensive care of patients presenting with sexual health conditions and issues. Substance misusers will come into contact with genito-urinary medicine services as a result of concern relating to their HIV status or sexually transmitted infections. Injecting drug users have high-risk behaviours which may lead to unsafe sexual behaviour and practice whilst under the influence of drugs or alcohol. Substance misusers with HIV-positive status will require care and management in relation to their substance-use problems and HIV-related disease. Close working relationship with substance-misuse and general services are needed. Areas of intervention include taking a drug and alcohol history and sexual history, pre- and post-test counselling, general counselling, health education and harm reduction.

MIDWIVES OR OBSTETRIC NURSE

Midwives are hospital or community-based, providing support to women, their babies, their partners and families, from conception to the first phase of post-natal care. The number of women misusing alcohol and drug has increased considerably in the past 30 years, and many misusers are of childbearing age. It is common for midwives and obstetric nurses to come into contact with and manage pregnant substance misusers. It is acknowledged that for some women this may be the only contact with the statutory health services. However, pregnant substance misusers may not come into contact with general health services until late into pregnancy, resulting in increasing the health risks for both mother and baby. Late booking for antenatal care by women with problem drug and/or alcohol use is variously attributed either to lack of awareness of pregnancy owing to the menstrual disturbances and amenorrhoea that are common features of drug use or else simply to lack of motivation (Hepburn 2004).

The report *Confidential Enquiry into Maternal Deaths* (Department of Health 1998) recommended that women with a substance-misuse problem should receive especially close supervision during pregnancy and be managed using evidence-based guidelines by maternity services that are part of a wider multi-agency or multi-disciplinary network. The specialist substance-misuse midwifery team is now firmly established: this involves shared care with the drug and alcohol treatment services.

Midwives can play an important role in nudging a woman who is misusing substances to make a positive change to their substance-misusing behaviour. Aspects of intervention include promotion of harm reduction, encouragement of screening for cervical cytology (antenatal care) and observation of babies undergoing withdrawal symptoms for those born with a high degree of dependence on opiates. Health education should be related to maternal health, antenatal screening (hepatitis C, B and HIV), antenatal counselling and health information, smoking cessation, prevention of HIV infections, management of abstinence syndrome, antenatal care, aftercare and support to mother and child and liaison with specialist services. There are a growing number of examples of good practice where midwives are taking the lead in cessation of smoking programmes, in which pregnant women are given advice and support based on effective health promotion methods (Department of Health 1998).

HEALTH VISITORS

Health visitors will encounter a large client group, with family and significant others misusing alcohol, tobacco and prescribed and illicit drugs. Although they are responsible for child health up to the age of five, they are mainly concerned with preventative health education. Aspects of intervention include advice, counselling, health education and health promotion, and harm reduction.

A number of primary health care trusts have appointed specialist health visitors for substance misuse. However, those specialist health visitors have a specific role to supplement existing health visitor services with families and the drug counselling service but with a remit of working with all age groups. The roles of the specialist vary but may include identifying the risks to those living with substance users, assessment of needs and plan care for the family and working with homeless substance users and socially excluded drug users. In addition, they will be linking with the area child protection committee, social services, midwifery services, general healthcare services, school nurses (if there are schoolchildren in the family) and specialist alcohol and drug teams.

DISTRICT NURSE

District nurses usually encounter patients at different stages in their illness and are responsible for the provision of total nursing care. District nurses care for people in a variety of non-hospital settings including patients' homes, GP surgeries and residential care homes. They too have a role to play in prevention and harm reduction in relation to substance misuse. Aspects of interventions include the early identification and recognition of substance misuse, health education and the generic assessment of substance-use health-related problems. A study (Peckover and Chidlaw 2007) of the accounts by district nurses encountering and providing care to substance misusers highlighted the limited knowledge and experience of working with this client group. The authors suggested that some of the challenges and tensions of district nurses involve 'prejudice' and 'risk' which served to shape service provision for substance misusers resulting in the provision of suboptimal care.

SCHOOL NURSES

The use of tobacco, alcohol and illicit drugs by young people and schoolchildren is the source of much public concern. One of the key areas of the government strategy is to reduce the acceptability and availability of drugs to young people in schools. It is estimated that between 780,000 and 1.3 million children are affected by parental alcohol problems (Prime Minister's Strategy Unit 2004). The resulting problems for the child can be grouped under three main headings – antisocial behaviour (increased risk of aggressive behaviour towards others, hyperactivity and other forms of conduct disorder), emotional problems (a wider range of psychosomatic problems from asthma to bedwetting, negative attitudes to their parents and themselves, high levels of self-blame, withdrawal and depression) and within the school environment (learning difficulties, reading retardation, loss of concentration, generally poor school per-formance, aggression and truancy) (Alcohol Concern 2006).

School nurses are often asked to play a role in delivering health education or promotion (drug and sex education) under the personal, social and health education curriculum (PHSE). Aspects of intervention include the provision of advice, information and health counselling to parents and children, health promotion and referral to other specialist or non-specialist agencies if appropriate. The school nurse should be in the core personnel in contributing to the school policy on substance use. A toolkit for school nurses (Alcohol Concern 2006) has been developed to provide information about the effects of parental alcohol misuse on children and what can be done to support these children, both individually and within the wider school context.

OCCUPATIONAL HEALTH NURSES

The misuse of psychoactive substances in the workplace is one of the major concerns of management, professional organisation, and occupational health staff. The use and misuse of psychoactive substances such as tobacco and alcohol among workers have resulted in absenteeism, accidents and loss of efficiency of the workforce. Occupational health services, provided at the workplace to address the healthcare needs of working populations, have been identified as an important component of the public health strategy. These services can also make a significant contribution to other government initiatives, such as reducing health inequalities, reducing social exclusion and sickness absence, and protecting and promoting the health of the working population (WHO 2001).

The Health and Safety Executive has recommended that the responsibility of all organisations to ensure a health and safe working environment should include recognition of the need for a substance-misuse policy. There is evidence to suggest that a policy on tobacco smoking or alcohol use can lead to reduced absenteeism, improved safety performances, lower maintenance costs, lower air-conditioning and ventilation costs, increased productivity, improved morale among non-smokers, fewer accidents and a lowered risk of losing skilled employees through premature retirement or death (McEwen 1991). The occupational health nurse has a major role to play in health education and promotion regarding the use of psychoactive substances and in meeting the health and safety needs of the employees. Aspects of intervention include screening, health promotion, harm reduction and controlled drinking, smoking cessation clinic and referral to another agency.

PRISON HEALTHCARE NURSES

Prison healthcare services deal with the health needs of the prison population. This includes provision of general medical service and psychiatric treatment. The prison populations have a high concentration of people with a history of drug misuse. Over one-third of the people received into British prisons each year are treated for opiate dependence (Home Office 2003a). Opiate dependence and injecting are more common still among women entering prison. Crack was the drug most frequently used by the sample of men from ethnic minority groups (80% of whom were Black and 20% Asian or mixed race). The use of this drug was often combined with harmful levels of alcohol consumption, and associated with psychotic or manic experiences (Home Office 2003b).

The priority issues for the prison healthcare staff are the assessment of alcohol and drug misuse, assessment of high-risk behaviour, random drug screening, the management of alcohol and drug withdrawal, harm reduction, secondary prevention and liaising with general health services, substance-misuse services and self-help groups.

PRIMARY CARE MENTAL HEALTH WORKERS

The primary care mental health workers provide additional, specialist services in primary care settings for people with mental health needs. This new role, created by the government in 2004, was a response to research showing that as many as one in four GP consultations concern mental health. One of the key functions was to help facilitate the transition towards primary care becoming the major arena of community mental health care rather than providing a limited 'gatekeeper' function, guarding access to specialist mental health services available within secondary care (Strain et al. 2006). In addition, the role of the primary care mental health workers was intended to facilitate the supply of basic therapeutic interventions such as cognitive behaviour therapies.

They have a role in providing counselling, health information and harm reduction and brief interventions.

DOCTORS

In recent years, there has been a large increase in the number of doctors from a range of professional backgrounds working with substance misusers. Doctors' competencies encompass the following domains: advice, identification, assessment, patient management, training, supervision and teaching, research and audit, and management and service development (Royal College of Psychiatrists & Royal College of General Practitioners 2005). The updated *Models of Care* for the treatment of adult drug misusers (NTA 2006) describe the functions required within a system and the doctors who work within it. See Chapter 6. Most doctors will provide some Tier 1 interventions, even though they may mainly be providing interventions at other tiers. GPs providing enhanced services may run Tier 2 interventions within primary care, but, in some areas, there will also be a consultant in addiction psychiatry or another specialist involved. Addiction psychiatrists or GPs may provide Tier 3 interventions, but substance-misuse specialists (normally addiction psychiatrists) will have the competencies to manage clients who have more complex needs. Consultants in addiction psychiatry usually supervise specialist prescribing services, though, in some cases, suitably competent specialists from other professions manage them. Services headed by consultant psychiatrists usually provide specialist inpatient addiction (Tier 4) provision (NTA 2005).

ALCOHOL AND DRUG WORKERS

Alcohol and drug workers or substance-misuse workers come from a variety of professional backgrounds, including nursing, social work and the criminal justice system, and are found in statutory services, statutory and voluntary agencies and the private sectors. They are regarded as drug and alcohol specialists. Their work covers broad categories of substance misuse: alcohol, drugs (illicit drugs, prescribed drugs and over-the-counter drugs), tobacco (for smoking cessation) and volatile substances. They may be involved in residential services, social work, outreach services, arrest referral scheme, general practitioner surgery, needle exchange services, day services, street agencies, prison healthcare services and other criminal justice system and community services.

Alcohol and drug workers provide a range of physical and psychosocial interventions in the management and comprehensive treatment of substance misusers. The interventions include support, advice and basic counselling, harm reduction, family therapy and cognitive behavioural therapies such as relapse prevention. They also have a key worker role in the shared care approach, perform risk assessment and act as advocates. Some drug workers practise in a 'social work model' and can address family and personal relationships, childcare, housing, income support and criminal justice issues (Department of Health 1999).

CLINICAL PSYCHOLOGISTS

Clinical psychologists can play a major role in the treatment of alcohol and drug misuse. They contribute to the specialist substance-misuse services by the provision of assessments and psychological treatments (counselling, relapse prevention, motivational intervention, solution-based therapy and participating in multidisciplinary and or multi-agency care planning.

SOCIAL WORKERS

Social workers in local authority social service departments bring general social work skills into many community and residential settings where there are alcohol and drug misusers. Alcohol and drug misuse are associated with child abuse and neglect, sexual abuse, domestic violence, homelessness, poverty, social exclusion, criminal behaviours, juvenile delinquency and mental health. Social workers trained in addictions can be found in specialist inpatient and outpatient treatment settings and residential rehabilitation centres. Aspects of interventions with alcohol and drug misusers include community care assessment, case management, group and individual therapy, family counselling, advocacy for jobs and housing needs, community development of resources and liaising with other health and social care professionals.

PROBATION OFFICERS

Probation officers protect the public by helping offenders not to re-offend, and by making offenders aware of the effect of their crimes on their victims and the public. A report published by HM Inspectorate of Probation (Home Office 2006) suggests that over recent years there has been a significant shift in the treatment of drug misusing offenders from a system that focused on the health perspective to one that recognises involvement in the criminal justice system as a legitimate catalyst for treatment. The widespread use of drug treatment as a condition of a court order for offenders has increased (Home Office 2006). However, the document shows that there has been a substantial improvement in the availability of treatment for drug misusing offenders, but a continuing scarcity of treatment for alcohol misusers. Probation officers work with offenders before, during and after sentencing and liaise with alcohol and drug services. They are responsible for enforcing Community Orders and for making sure offenders go to regular supervision appointments and take part in group programmes.

HOSPITAL AND COMMUNITY PHARMACISTS

Hospital pharmacists have an important role in advising general hospital clinicians when a patient, maintained on substitute medication, is admitted whether to accident and emergency or as a planned medical or surgical admission (Department of Health

1999). Part of the role of the hospital pharmacist is to advise clinicians on the use and interactions of psychoactive substances in the pharmacological treatment and overall treatment regime of substance misusers. Their duties are also liaising with hospital, community and primary care professionals.

Community pharmacists provide a significant point of contact as part of primary healthcare services and have regular (often daily) contact with the patient (Department of Health 1999). The services to substance misusers include the dispensing of controlled drugs prescriptions; monitoring prescriptions for drug interactions and adverse drug reactions; supplying clean injecting equipment, whether by sale or through needle exchange; referring clients to drug treatment agencies; and providing oral and written information and advice. The community pharmacist can play an important role in identifying inappropriate prescribing of controlled drugs and monitoring the misuse potential of 'over-the-counter' medications.

ADDICTION NURSES

Historically, occupational labels such as alcohol nurse, drug dependency nurse, chemical substance nurse, specialist nurse in addiction and community psychiatric nurse (addiction) have been ascribed to those working with substance misusers (Rassool 1997). It was not until the mid-1980s that addiction nursing as a clinical speciality, within the broader framework of mental health nursing, began to put down its clinical and academic roots. The concept of addiction nursing was introduced in the literature in the UK by Rassool (1996). It is defined as a specialist branch of mental health nursing concerned with the care and treatment interventions aimed at those individuals whose health problems are directly related to the use and misuse of psychoactive substances and to other addictive behaviours such as eating disorders and gambling (Rassool 1997).

Thus, the scope of professional practice in addiction nursing incorporates the activities of clinical practice (nursing, a range of psychosocial interventions strategies including complementary therapies), education, policy-making, research and all other pursuits through which nurse practitioners contribute to the care and in the interests of the clients. An expanded role is the prescribing of drugs (Rassool 2004). Addiction nurses practise in both residential and community settings and have an excellent track record in developing innovative healthcare initiatives and community-oriented programmes for substance misusers, and many of the key developments in recent years have been nurse-led. These include smoking cessation clinics, mobile methadone clinics, outreach work with drug-using commercial sex workers, satellite clinics for homeless drinkers and development of multi-professional postgraduate educational programmes in addictive behaviour (Rassool and Gafoor 1997, Rassool 2000).

KEY POINTS

* Health and social care professionals in both primary healthcare and residential settings are usually the first point of contact for clients who have potential or early alcohol and drug problems.

- The extent and nature of the substantial health and social problems associated with substance misuse highlight the pressing need for members of the primary healthcare team, nurses, social workers and those working in the criminal justice system to respond to the needs of substance misusers.
- A wide variety of roles exist in the substance-misuse field and include not only specialist workers but also professionals whose work brings them into contact with drug and alcohol misuse.
- Roles in the substance misuse field are characterised by the level and frequency of contact with substance misuse and substance misusers.

REFERENCES

Advisory Council on the Misuse of Drugs (ACMD) (1982) *Treatment and Rehabilitation*. London: HMSO.

Alcohol Concern (2006) *Toolkit for School Nurses*. London: Alcohol Concern. http://www.alcoholandfamilies.org.uk/documents/SN/sn-tools_index.htm.

Bolton, J. (2006) Accident and emergency psychiatry. *Psychological Medicine*, 5, 3: 73–6.

Brooker, C. and White, E. (1998) *The Fourth Quinnenial Survey of CPNs*. Manchester: Department of Nursing, University of Manchester.

Deehan, A., Templeton, L., Taylor, C., Drummond, C. and Strang, J. (1998) Are practice nurses an unexplored resource in the identification and management of alcohol misuse? Results from a study of practice nurses in England and Wales in 1995. *Journal of Advanced Nursing*, 28: 592–97.

Department of Health (1992) *The Health of the Nation*. London: HMSO.

Department of Health (1998) *Why Mothers Die. Report on Confidential Enquiries into Maternal Deaths in the United Kingdom 1994–1996*. London: The Stationery Office.

Department of Health (1999) *Drug Misuse and Dependence: Guidelines on Clinical Management*. London: UK Department of Health.

Department of Health (2002) *Mental Health Policy Implementation Guide: Dual Diagnosis Good Practice Guide*. London: Department of Health. www.dh.gov.uk/PublicationsAnd Statistics/Publications/PublicationsPolicyAndGuidance/PublicationsPolicyAndGuidanceArticle/ fs/en?CONTENT_ID=4009058&chk=sCQrQr.

Department of Health (2004) *Choosing Health: Making Healthy Choices Easier*, London: Department of Health.

Department of Health (2006) *From Values to Action: The Chief Nursing Officer's Review of Mental Health Nursing*. London: Department of Health.

Gafoor, M. and Rassool, G. Hussein (1998) The co-existence of psychiatric disorders and substance misuse: working with dual diagnosis patients. *Journal of Advanced Nursing*, 27: 497–502.

Gossop, M., Marsden, J., Edwards, C., Wilson, A., Segar, G., Stewart, D. and Lehmann, P. (1995) *The October Report: The National Treatment Outcome Research Study: A Report Prepared for the Task Force*. London: Department of Health.

Hepburn, M. (2004) Substance abuse in pregnancy. *Current Obstetrics and Gynaecology*, 14: 419–25.

Hillman, A., McCann, B. and Walker N.P. (2001) Specialist alcohol liaison services in general hospitals improve engagement in alcohol rehabilitation and treatment outcome. *Health Bulletin*, 59: 420–3.

Home Office (2002) Tackling Drugs to Build a Better Britain Updated Strategy. London: HMSO. www.homeoffice.gov.uk.

Home Office (2003a) *An Analysis of CARAT Research Data as at 3 December 2002*, Research, Development and Statistics Directorate. London: Home Office.

Home Office (2003b) *The Substance Misuse Treatment Needs of Minority Prisoner Groups: Women, Young Offenders and Ethnic Minorities*. London: Home Office Development and Practice Report. www.homeoffice.gov.uk/rds.

Home Office (2005) *Work Force Briefing. Tackling Drug Changing Lives. Recruitment Guidance for Employers*. London: Home Office. www. homeoffice.gov.uk/publication-search/drug strategy/WorkforceBriefing-Jobs?view=Binary.

Home Office (2006) *Probation Inspectorate Report on Substance Misuse Work with Offenders – 'Half Full and Half Empty'*. London: Probation Inspectorates.

Kennedy, J. and Faugier, J. (1989) *Drug and Alcohol Dependency Nursing*. London: Heinemann.

Lock, C.A. and Kaner, E.F.S. (2004) Implementation of brief alcohol interventions by nurses in primary care: do non-clinical factors influence practice? *Family Practice*, 21, 3: 270–5.

McEwen, J. (1991) Interventions in the workplace. In I. Glass (ed.) *The International Handbook of Addiction Behaviour*. London: Routledge.

McMenamin, J.P. (1997) Detecting young adults with alcohol use disorder in a general practice. *New Zealand Medical Journal*, 110: 127–8.

Maxwell, D. (1990) Medical complications of substance abuse. In A.H. Ghodse and D. Maxwell (eds) *Substance Abuse and Dependence*. London: The Macmillan Press.

Newton, A., Sarker, S.J., Pahal, G.S., van den Bergh, E. and Young, C. (2007) Impact of the new UK licensing law on emergency hospital attendances: a cohort study. *Emergency Medicine Journal*, 24: 532–4.

NTA (2002) *Models of Care for Treatment of Adult Drug Misusers*. London: National Treatment Agency.

NTA (2004) *Dealing with Drugs. Reducing Deaths: A Resource for A&E Staff*. London: National Treatment Agency.

NTA (2005) *Roles and Responsibilities of Doctors in the Provision of Treatment for Drug and Alcohol Misusers*. Briefing. London: National Treatment Agency.

NTA (2006) *Models of Care for the Treatment of Adult Drug Misusers. Update 2006*. London: National Treatment Agency. http://www.nta.nhs.uk/publications/Models_of_care.pdf.

Ockene, J.K., Adams, A., Hurley, T.G., Wheeler, E.V. and Hebert J.R. (1999) Brief physician and nurse practitioner-delivered counseling for high-risk drinkers: does it work? *Archives of Internal Medicine*, 159: 2198–205.

Owen, L., Gilmore, I.T. and Pirmohamed, M. (2000) General practice nurses' knowledge of alcohol use and misuse: a questionnaire survey. *Alcohol and Alcoholism*, 35, 3: 259–62.

Owen, L., Gilmore, I.T., and Pirmohamed, M. (2005) How do the NHS general hospitals in England deal with patients with alcohol-related problems? A questionnaire survey. *Alcohol & Alcoholism*, 40, 5: 409–12.

Patton, R., Strang, J., Birtles, C. and Crawford, M.J. (2006) Alcohol: a missed opportunity. A survey of all accident and emergency departments in England. *Emergency Medicine Journal*, 24: 529–31.

Peckover, S. and Chidlaw, R.G. (2007) Too frightened to care? Accounts by district nurses working with clients who misuse substances. *Health & Social Care in the Community*, 15, 3: 238–45.

Prime Minister's Strategy Unit (2004) *Alcohol Harm Reduction Strategy for England*. London: Cabinet Office. http://www.cabinetoffice.gov.uk/strategy/work_areas/alcohol_misuse.aspx.

Ramirez, A. and House, A. (1997) ABC of mental health: common mental health problems in the general hospital. *British Medical Journal*, 314: 1679–81.

Rassool, G. Hussein (1993) Nursing and substances misuse: responding to the challenge. *Journal of Advanced Nursing*, 18, 9: 1401–7.

Rassool, G. Hussein (1996) Addiction nursing and substance misuse: a slow response to partial accommodation. *Journal of Advanced Nursing*, 24, 2: 425–7.

Rassool, G. Hussein (1997) Addiction nursing towards a new paradigm: the UK experience. In G. Hussein Rassool and M. Gafoor (eds) *Addiction Nursing Perspectives on Professional and Clinical Practice*. Cheltenham: Nelson Thornes.

Rassool, G. Hussein. (1998) Health care professionals and substance misuse. In G. Hussein Rassool (ed.) *Substance Use and Misuse: Nature, Context and Clinical Interventions*. Oxford: Blackwell Publications.

Rassool, G. Hussein (2000) Addiction: global problem and global response complacency or commitment? *Journal of Advanced Nursing*, 32, 3: 505–8.

Rassool, G., Hussein and Gafoor, M. (1997) *Perspectives in Professional and Clinical Practice*. Cheltenham: Stanley Thornes.

Rassool, G. Hussein (2004) Prescription for change: perspectives on prescribing authority for addiction nurses in the United Kingdom. *Journal of Addictions Nursing*, 15, 4: 193–7.

Rassool, G. Hussein and Marshall, F. (2001) Substance use and misuse: a public health perspective. *Nursing Research*, 6, 6: 906–18.

Royal College of Physicians (2001) *Alcohol – Can the NHS Afford It, Recommendations for a Coherent Alcohol Strategy for Hospitals*. London: Royal College of Physicians.

Royal College of Psychiatrists (1997) *Community Psychiatric Nursing*, Occasional paper OP40. London: Royal College of Psychiatrists.

Royal College of Psychiatrists and the British Association of Accident and Emergency Medicine (2004) *Psychiatric Services to Accident & Emergency Departments*, Council Report CR118. London: Royal College of Psychiatrists.

Royal College of Psychiatrists and Royal College of General Practitioners (2005) *Roles and Responsibilities of Doctors in the Provision of Treatment for Drug and Alcohol Misusers*. London: Royal College of Psychiatrists. http://www.rcgp.org.uk/drug/docs/toolkit.pdf.

Strain, J. Hutnik, N., Gregory, J. and Bowers, G. (2006) *Graduate Primary Care Mental Health Workers: The Process of Introducing the Role Into Primary Care Trusts*. Health Sciences and Practice Subject Centre, Guildford, University of Surrey.

UK Alcohol Forum (1997) *Guidelines for the Management of Alcohol Problems in Primary Care and General Psychiatry*. London: Tangent Medical Education.

WHO (2001) *Role of the Occupational Health Nurse in the Workplace*. Copenhagen: World Health Organization Regional Office for Europe, EUR/01/5025463.

WHO/ICN (1991) *Roles of the Nurse in Relation to Substance Misuse*. Geneva: ICN.

CHAPTER 21

PREVENTION AND HEALTH EDUCATION APPROACHES TO SUBSTANCE MISUSE

OBJECTIVES

■ Have an awareness of the relevant literature on the key concepts, theories and current debates that inform prevention, health education and promotion practices.

■ Describe the types of prevention strategies.

■ Discuss the various health education approaches to alcohol and drug misuse.

■ Critically reflect on your own role and experiences as a health educator.

■ Discuss your role in the rational use of psychoactive substances.

■ Have an understanding of health promoting institutions in relation to substance misuse.

In the current climate of the pattern of alcohol drinking and drug-taking behaviours, health education, prevention and harm reduction increasingly form part of the role of the health and social care professionals. Every encounter with a patient affords an opportunity for health and social care professionals to transmit knowledge about healthcare and harm reduction in relation to tobacco smoking, alcohol, psychoactive drugs and sexual health. The prevention of alcohol and drug misuse is the promotion of constructive lifestyles to delay or avoid the onset of alcohol and drug misuse in the general population and is achieved through the application of multiple strategies. Health promotion has emerged as an integral part of public health policy and now forms an important part of the health and education services. Harm reduction approaches involve reducing the harm caused by substance misuse, especially in the area of injecting behaviour and sexual health. The WHO/UNODC (2007) Global Initiative project on the primary prevention of substance abuse was implemented in several countries to prevent and reduce the use of psychoactive substances and related problems among young people (7 to 24 years). In a global initiative on primary prevention of substance misuse in several countries (WHO/UNDOC 2007), the study findings showed that the overall evaluation achieved positive outcomes. Where psychoactive substance use among young people did not (markedly) decrease, the age of onset of psychoactive substance use rose. In certain demographic or age groups, youth psychoactive substance use remained stable and/or decreased.

The updated government alcohol strategy (Department of Health 2007) sets out clear goals and actions to promote sensible drinking and reduce the harm that alcohol can cause. It specifically focuses on the minority of drinkers who cause the most harm to themselves, their communities and their families. The government will target information and advice at people who drink at harmful levels, their families and their friends, achieving this through government media campaigns, the NHS and local communities. There is evidence to suggest that brief interventions consisting of simple advice are effective in reducing heavy alcohol consumption to more sensible levels (Babor and Grant 1992). It is estimated that, if the government's updated strategy is consistently implemented across the UK, simple alcohol advice would result in 250,000 men and 67,500 women reducing their drinking levels from hazardous and harmful to low risk each year.

The Department of Health and the National Treatment Agency for Substance Misusers (2007) approach has wider goals of preventing drug misuse and of encouraging stabilisation in treatment and support for abstinence. In relation to harm reduction, the aim is to reduce the number of drug-related deaths and blood-borne virus infections. Providing effective substitution treatments and effective support for abstinence are complementary aims of such a balanced response. The health education and promotion campaigns, including work on hepatitis B immunisation, targeted high-risk groups such as service user groups and carers; homeless drug users; heroin and crack injectors ('speedballers'); potential or new injectors; and people in contact with the criminal justice system, including those in prison. Additional strategies include new campaign materials, reflecting current patterns of drug use; hosting of regional road shows that focus on local implementation and highlight key messages to local stakeholders; and 'engagement projects' for regional service users and carers to support local campaigns and provide peer education and training.

The aims of this chapter are to examine the relationships of health education and and concepts of prevention in the context of substance misuse.

HEALTH EDUCATION AND PREVENTION

Health education and health promotion can be identified in all professional practice from giving advice to more structured interventions. Health promotion includes the provision of information on healthier lifestyles for patients, and how to make the best use of health services, with the intention of enabling people to make rational health choices and of ensuring awareness of the factors determining the health of the community (Department of Health 2008). According to Tones (1990) health education is 'any planned activity which promotes health or illness related learning, that is, some relatively permanent change in an individual's competence or disposition'. This is an acceptable definition but it is too vague to be operationalised in the context of prevention of alcohol and drug misuse. Some writers have incorporated the concept of health education within the aegis of health promotion.

Maben and Macleod Clarke (1995) propose a definition of health promotion which incorporates the concept of health education. Health promotion is seen as

> an attempt to improve the health status of an individual or community, and is also concerned with the prevention of disease . . . At its broadest level it is concerned with the wider influences on health and therefore with the policy and legislative implications of these. Health education through information-giving, advice, support and skills training is part of, and necessary prerequisite to, health promotion.

That is, health education is a component of health promotion activities where the goal is to enhance and promote health through the implementation of effective educational and training programmes taking into account the socio-political influences. Health promotion has been defined by the World Health Organization (WHO 1986a) as 'the process of enabling people to increase control over, and to improve, their health . . . to reach a state of complete physical, mental and social well-being, an individual or group must be able to identify and to realize aspirations, to satisfy needs, and to change or cope with the environment'.

It is not within the scope of this chapter to provide a fuller exposition of health promotion and health education. For a more comprehensive examination of concepts of health promotion and health education the reader is referred to Ewles and Simnett (2003). In the context of substance misuse, the goal of health education is to promote the health of the general population and to enable people to make informed choices about tobacco smoking, alcohol and drug-taking.

In public health, health education activities have been viewed as existing on three levels: primary, secondary and tertiary prevention. This three-stage model has been modified by the Advisory Council on the Misuse of Drugs (ACMD 1984) on the grounds that it was not sufficiently comprehensive to cover all the element of prevention policies. The ACMD's approach to prevention is based on meeting two basic criteria: reducing the risk of an individual engaging in substance misuse and reducing the harm associated with substance misuse.

PRIMARY PREVENTION

Primary prevention is a process that includes efforts to reduce the demand and stop the occurrence of illegal drug use, any drinking behaviour or tobacco smoking. For example, primary prevention campaigns would seek to discourage any alcohol drinking behaviour among young people and those who are in high-risk groups. Prevention has been defined as 'a process to inhibit or reduce physical, mental, emotional or social impairment which results in or from the abuse of chemical substances' (NIDA 1989). Thus, primary prevention involves the provision of health information or teaching, media campaigns and the mobilisation the community. The focus of primary prevention should be targeted not only to the non-using population but also to experimental, recreational and dependent users. Certain groups are more vulnerable as regards to high-risk behaviour: these include binge drinkers, pregnant women, youth offenders, injecting drug users, prisoners, sex workers and the homeless.

SECONDARY PREVENTION

Secondary prevention is the prevention of the sequelae of the misuse of the psychoactive substances and limiting of disability or dysfunction. It seeks to reduce and limit further health and social harms done by the use and misuse of psychoactive substances through early recognition, intervention or rehabilitation. Examples include the rational use of prescribed medication (see below), health information on safer alcohol and drug use and safer sexual practices. The harm reduction approach, as part of secondary preventive strategies, has been widely implemented in the drug and alcohol field as a response to the threat presented by blood-borne viruses such as HIV and hepatitis infections.

TERTIARY PREVENTION

The tertiary level of prevention seeks to limit and reduce further complications or dysfunctions through effective care, treatment and rehabilitation services. The aim is to restore the individual to an optimal level of functioning and to prevent relapse. In particular, tertiary prevention includes the engagement of residential and community facilities for those who are seeking help for their alcohol or drug-related problems. Unlike primary and secondary prevention, tertiary prevention involves actual treatment for the disease and is conducted primarily by specialist substance-misuse services.

The focus of preventive interventions for generic health and social care professionals is based on primary and secondary interventions in an approach combining assessment, intervention and evaluation. It is worth pointing out that the notion of completely 'stopping' the whole population using a variety of mind-altering psychoactive substances is extremely idealistic and of course is unachievable in reality. Professionals in healthcare and allied medicine need to acknowledge this limitation and address the areas where health education can reduce the harm caused as a result of continuing use and misuse.

FRAMEWORK FOR CLASSIFYING PREVENTION

An increasingly popular way of classifying prevention initiatives is the universal, selective and indicated prevention programmes (Mrazek and Haggerty 1994). The focus of universal programmes is the promotion of health and healthy lifestyles and behaviour and preventing the onset of alcohol and drug use of individual, communities or schools. Universal prevention activities may include schools-based prevention programmes or mass media campaigns, or they may target whole communities, or parents and families but focusing on children and young people. Selective prevention programmes target groups or subsets of the population who may have already started to use drugs or are at an increased risk of developing substance-use problems compared to the general population, or both (Edmonds *et al.* 2005). The prevention programmes are aimed at reducing the influence of the 'risk factors', developing resilience (the protective factors) and preventing substance-use initiation. Indicated prevention programmes (harm reduction) target those exhibiting problematic drug or alcohol use which requires specialist interventions. However, this group of people has not yet met DSM-IV criteria for substance dependence (McGrath *et al.* 2005)

HEALTH EDUCATION APPROACHES AND INTERVENTIONS

Part of the goal of health education includes the process of enabling an individual to change his or her lifestyle and behaviour. In the context of substance misuse, helping people to make informed choices about tobacco smoking, alcohol and drug-taking is part of that process. Health education materials may be used to assist in reducing demand for substances through promotion of healthy lifestyles and suitable alternatives. However, there is also a need to shift substance-use education and prevention from its narrow focus of simply providing health information or leaflets to those at risks of alcohol and drug-related problems to the provision of advice and brief interventions. There is ground for optimism that if information, advice and health teaching about sexual health and the dangers in the misuse of drugs, alcohol and tobacco smoking are provided by healthcare professionals, that this may reduce the casualties of health-related harms. Early recognition and minimal interventions are also part of the process of preventive health education (WHO 1986b, Babor and Grant 1992). There is evidence that patients both in hospital and in primary healthcare are critical of the information and advice they receive and would welcome clearer guidance concerning a healthier lifestyle including information about sensible drinking practices and smoking (Hartz *et al.* 1991). Early recognition and minimal interventions can be simultaneously achieved during a brief assessment which includes taking a drug, alcohol and tobacco history, risk assessment and counselling (see Chapters 24 and 26).

The most appropriate means of generic and specific interventions to support attitude and behaviour change at population and community levels has peen published by the National Institute of Clinical Excellence (NICE 2007). The guidance is for National Health Service staff and other professionals for helping people to change their health-related knowledge, attitudes and behaviour. At community level, primary healthcare teams are more likely to be involved with preventative health behaviour. Helping people to change their lifestyle and behaviour is not only about targeting individuals but also about helping the community to change. An element of this approach is mobilising the community, and suggestions on mobilising the community for the nurse as a primary healthcare worker have been documented elsewhere (WHO 1986). But the strategy of preventative health education cannot be operated by nurses in isolation. However, a workable strategy for nudging the community towards healthier lifestyles and behaviour requires positive partnerships with key agents of change within the community. This community partnership includes community leaders, members of the public, social services, education services, non-statutory and voluntary agencies, police services and the media. It has been suggested that the effectiveness of any drug campaign and safer sex strategies need 'ground roots' prevention campaigns using credible trained peers (Kelly and Murphy 1991). Within the framework of this approach, the focus is also directed towards the promotion of general health and raising the consciousness of the individual to maintain a healthier lifestyle by developing alternative activities such as physical and recreational activities, techniques of stress reduction and other coping skills. Helping people to make informed choices about the rational use of licit psychoactive substances is part of that process.

A variety of approaches have been used in an attempt to prevent and reduce substance misuse demand (Gossop and Grant 1990). Table 21.1 summarises the models, goals and interventions of health education in relaion to alcohol and drugs.

RATIONAL USE OF PSYCHOACTIVE SUBSTANCES

In the context of this book the term 'rational use' means that the right drug is taken by the right patient, in the right dose and for the right duration of therapy, and that the risks of therapy are acceptable (WHO 1989). The consequences of the use of licit (prescribed and over-the-counter) and illicit psychoactive substances are of significant public health concerns. Almost half of all medicines globally are used irrationally and can have severe consequences: adverse drug reactions, drug resistance, protracted illness, mortality and financial cost, particularly in developing countries where patients often pay for medicines out of their own pockets (WHO 2004a). In 2000, the UK was 19th among the 20 countries with the highest levels of consumption of psychoactive substances for the treatment of moderate to severe pain (INCB 2003). Opioid analgesics such as fentanyl, morphine and pethidine are most commonly used worldwide.

In recent years, the appropriate use and distribution of psychoactive drugs has been of particular concern because of increasing consumption reported from a number of countries as a result of over-prescribing, irrational use and increases in adverse effects resulting in both psychological and physical dependence. Many of the prescribed psychoactive drugs such as hypnotics, sedatives and tranquillisers are frequently the subject of widespread misuse and can result in health-related problems and dependence. With the advent of self-care approach, consumerism and popular demands for increased self-control have led to the use and misuse of over-the-counter drugs (Rassool 2005). Many medications contain alcohol, hallucinogenic compounds and narcotics such as codeine which can be addictive. The availability and accessibility of medications over the internet has highlighted the need to be vigilant in public health education about the use of psychoactive substances and other drugs (Rassool 2005). Some of the compounds sold over the internet may have addictive potential and be life-threatening. There seems to be a parallel development in the therapeutic uses of psychoactive substances and the non-medical or recreational use of these drugs (Rassool 2000). Irrational use is the use of psychoactive substances that does not conform to good clinical practice. Irrational prescribing may be regarded as 'pathological' prescribing, where the criteria in the

Table 21.1 Health education approaches to substance misuse

Approach	Goals	Health education intervention	Examples
Public health or medical problems	Reduction of morbidity and mortality	Prevention of ill health	Early recognition, care, treatment and rehabilitation. Clinical interventions
Behaviour change	Change of lifestyle and behaviour	Media campaign. Health information: Controlled drinking, safer drug use and safer sex. Alcohol and driving	Prevent non-smokers from starting smoking. Persuade smokers to stop. Counselling. Harm reduction: reducing or minimising ill effect or harm from alcohol and drugs
Educational	Changing attitude. Increasing knowledge and awareness. Developing skills in decision-making and resilience	Health information on smoking, drinking and drug taking. Learning coping skills and stress management	Information about effects of substance misuse and health-related problems. Provision of resources. Referral to specialist services
Consumer empowerment	Enabling individuals to identify their health concerns	Advocacy. Meeting specific health and socio-economic needs	Clients identify health needs, types and access to services. Community anti-drug campaign
Social change	Enabling changes to health and social policies. Bringing changes to the social environment. Improvement in health and social equality in access to services and treatment interventions	Lobbying. Political and social actions	Alcohol and drug policy in workplace. Limit of marketing and advertising of alcohol and tobacco. Decriminalisation of drugs. Labelling on alcoholic beverages.

Source: Adapted from Rassool and Gafoor (1997)

process of prescribing are not fulfilled (WHO 2004c) – for example, extravagant prescribing, over-prescribing, incorrect prescribing, multiple prescribing, indiscriminate uses of injections and under-prescribing of medication of sedative-hypnotics drug and antibiotics.

Prescribing and medication management have expanded the role and authority of healthcare professionals within the multidisciplinary teams. The nursing, midwifery, medical and pharmaceutical professions are all participants in medication management and other intervention strategies, and this would enhance the provision of a more comprehensive and streamlined service and an improvement in the quality of care. The process of rational prescribing and the rational use of drugs includes assessing the healthcare needs of the patient (making a diagnosis); planning and setting goals for care; administering and monitoring the effects of medications; providing patient education and discharge planning; interdisciplinary collaboration; evaluating desired and adverse effects of medications and documenting the process (Manias and Street 2000, Rassool 2005).

Healthcare professionals have professional responsibility to ensure the rational use of psychoactive drugs. The importance of promoting the rational use of psychoactive drugs and the need to educate healthcare professionals in this area has been recognised (Ghodse and Khan 1988, Rassool and Winnington 1993). Their knowledge and clinical skills in relation to a wide range of medications and to the sequelae of their misuse can form a basis for effective nursing interventions (Rassool and Winnington 1993). Non-pharmacological therapies such as counselling, relaxation and other therapies may be an alternative to medication of psychoactive substances. It is asserted that, while focusing on the misuse of psychoactive drugs, consideration must also be given to the proper use of therapeutic medications (Rassool and Winnington 1993).

HEALTH PROMOTING HOSPITALS

During the past two decades, the idea of 'health promoting hospitals' has been slowly emerging in Europe with its emphasis on health gain through health promotion and disease prevention. The Budapest Declaration on Health Promoting Hospital (WHO 1991) states that 'Beyond the assurance of good quality medical services and health care, the health promoting hospital encourages and supports health promoting perspectives and activities among staff, patients, relatives and the wider community'. In England the report on *The Health of the Nation* (Department of Health 1992) reinforced the same theme and stated that 'hospitals exist to provide treatment and care but they also offer unique opportunities for more general health promotion for staff, patients and all who come into contact with them'. The principle behind this movement is to use hospitals to promote positive health within their own environs and the wider community.

The shifting focus from illness to health-oriented approaches within the hospital environments would enable organisations to implement health education and health promotion activities for both staff and patients. A number of initiatives in the creation of health promoting hospitals are under way, and the key principles are derived from the Ottawa Charter for Health Promoting Hospitals (HPHs) (World Health Organization 1992) as a strategic basis. Hospitals are in a strong position within the healthcare system to be advocates for health promotion as they represent the main concentration of health service resources, professional skills and medical technology (Johnson and Baum 2001). Using the hospital as a setting for the promotion of health means that a hospital can incorporate into its culture, and daily work activity, actions that are designed to ensure that an individual's health is promoted and protected at the same time as treating ill-health (Whitehead 2004). Hospitals joining the International Network of Health Promoting Hospitals aim to provide high-quality comprehensive medical and nursing services by introducing health promotion activities for patients, staff and the community into their corporate identity and routine practice (WHO 1998). The World Health Organization (WHO 2003) has set five standards that describe the principles and actions that should be part of care in every hospital. The five standards address management policy; patient assessment; information and intervention; promoting a healthy workplace and continuity and co-operation. The standards include:

- the health improvement or promotion policies or initiatives which are an integral part of an organisation's quality management system (for example, alcohol & drug policy)
- initiatives to support patient treatment, to improve prognosis and promote patients' health and well-being
- initiatives that ensure that patients are informed about planned activities that enable them to participate actively in such activities, and that facilitate integration of health improvement or promotion initiatives in all patient care
- policies or initiatives that support a healthy and safe environment for staff, or promote staff health and well-being
- initiatives involving other health service facilities, voluntary organisations or multi-professional groups within an organisation (Health Promotion Agency 2005).

Alcohol and drug policy is now part of hospital and institutional policies.

HEALTH PROMOTION: SUBSTANCE MISUSE AND THE WORKPLACE

The workplace is an ideal environment for the capture of sizeable numbers of adults in the prevention and health promotion towards the use and misuse of tobacco smoking, alcohol and drugs. In a review of current approaches to health promotion in the workplace at preventing and controlling alcohol- and drug-related problems, the World Health Organization (1993) draws attention on the emphasis of workers' participation in programme development and implementation, and on information dissemination and education that take account of the needs of specific occupational groups and the diversity of cultural settings. According to the World Health Organization (2004c), a comprehensive workplace health promotion scheme empowers social partners from both inside and outside workplace enterprises for the health maintenance of workers and their families and creates healthy working environments for the same. It adds that those who implement such schemes must have a good working knowledge of health factors as they relate to lifestyle, structural, occupational, environmental, ecological and social determinants of health within and outside of organizations.

However, the implementation of health-promoting programmes in the workplace has benefited the organisations from the reduction of stress, absenteeism and sickness among staff, has reduced staff turnover and increased organisational efficiency. In addition, investing in workplace health schemes provides organizations with motivated workforces, higher morale, reduced absenteeism, reduced personnel and welfare problems, reduced industrial relationship disputes, increased overall efficiency and improved organisational performance, competitiveness and public image (Chu *et al.* 2000, Kramer and Cole 2003). It has been suggested that workplace occupational health initiatives are now at the very forefront of nursing-related healthcare and are more prevalent than at any other time (Dawes 2001). Gossop and Grant (1990) identified three focuses of employee-drug-education activities:

- 'impersonal' information
- employee participation
- health promotion activities.

It is anticipated that organisations will encourage the participation of all staff, management, trade unions or professional organisations in decision-making related to healthcare policy. Healthcare professionals have an important contribution to make in the development of occupational health services and policy regarding health in the workplace, including substance-misuse educational programmes.

HEALTH PROMOTING SCHOOLS

Young people constitute one of the high-risk groups who experiment with legal and illicit psychoactive substances. Within this age group, primary prevention initiatives are the most appropriate in motivating young people to avoid drug experimentation. Health promoting schools are part of the World Health Organization Global Schools Health Initiative which was launched in 1995. A health promoting school is one in which all members of the school community work together to provide pupils with integrated and positive experiences and structures, which promote and protect their health (WHO 1995). This includes both the formal and the informal curriculum in health, the creation of a safe and healthy school environment, the provision of appropriate health services and the involvement of the family and wider community in efforts to promote health.

The WHO model of a health promoting school is one that is characterised by constantly strengthening its capacity as a healthy setting for living, learning and working. Health promoting schools focus on:

- caring for oneself and others, creating conditions conducive to health
- making healthy decisions and taking control of life circumstances
- preventing leading causes of death, disease and disability
- influencing health-related behaviours through knowledge, skills and attitudes
- building the capacity for peace, education, social justice, sustainable development and more.

The report on *Updated Strategy* (Home Office 2002) sets out a range of policies and interventions which concentrate on the most dangerous drugs, the most damaged communities and the individuals whose addiction and chaotic lifestyles are most harmful, both to themselves and to others. The most effective way of reducing the harm drugs cause is to persuade all potential users, but particularly the young, not to use drugs. The report adds that success will be achieved only if we stop young people from developing drug problems, reduce the prevalence of drugs on our streets and reduce the numbers of those with existing drug problems by getting them into effective treatment. A key aim under the *Every Child Matters* 'Be Healthy' (Home Office 2005) programme for children and young people is to encourage young people to choose not to take illegal drugs. To be effective in helping young people avoid drug problems, several governmental departments are focusing on the following objectives: reforming delivery and strengthening accountability; ensuring that provision is built around the needs of vulnerable children and young people; and building service and workforce capacity.

The primary goal of school health education is to help individuals adopt behaviours and create conditions that are conducive to health. Skills-based drug education is a key component of the school's overall drug prevention programme (including drug-related school policies, the creation of a safe, healthy and drug-free environment and efforts to provide appropriate health services) because it focuses on developing the knowledge, attitudes and skills that young people need to choose not to use drugs and to stick to their decision (Parsons *et al.* 2002).

The plan of action in relation to young people and substance misuse includes the training of teachers and support innovative projects in drug education and prevention; the development of school policies on managing drug-related incidents; and drug education. Other initiatives are focusing on new interdepartmental publicity campaigns with advertising and media expertise, and on role models aimed at helping young people to resist drugs and treatment services. At school level, it is important to adopt a school policy that recognises a variety of responses to tackle substance misuse. Prevention of substance use and misuse is the primary target for schools, but for those few who have been entangled with psychoactive substances beyond experimentation, treatment and rehabilitation (if appropriate) should be made available rather than adopting a punitive sanction.

CONCLUSIONS

The role of nurses and other healthcare professionals in relation to substance misuse is to support, educate, prevent and provide care, all of which are covered by the general term of 'health intervention'. Both primary and secondary health prevention initiatives in substance use and misuse are within the realm of most healthcare professionals. Prevention, health education and health promotion in the use and misuse of psychoactive substances should be part of the agenda for health and educational policies' development. A review of models of health education and health promotion suggests that the best form of alcohol and drug education makes no reference to alcohol or drugs per se, and is not substance-focused. A better approach is to 'focus on the general personal and social development of people within the context of general health promotion strategies which seek to make healthy choices, easy choices by removing the social concomitants of drug misuse – poverty and deprivation, disadvantage and lack of self fulfilment' (Tones 1987). The success of any health-promoting activities depends upon a co-ordinated approach in utilising existing prevention strategies. Healthcare professionals, schools, families and other interested parties should combine their efforts in preventing and reducing the casualties from substance misuse. Above all, we should not forget the health education of caring practitioners.

KEY POINTS

- Health education, prevention and harm reduction increasingly form part of the role of the health and social care professionals.
- Every encounter with a patient affords an opportunity to transmit knowledge about healthcare and harm reduction in relation to tobacco smoking, alcohol, psychoactive drugs and sexual health.
- Health promotion has emerged as an integral part of public health policy and now forms an important part of the health and education services.
- Health promotion includes the provision of information on healthier lifestyles for patients, and how to make the best use of health services, with the intention of enabling people to make rational health choices and of ensuring awareness of the factors determining the health of the community.
- Health education activities have been viewed as existing on three levels: primary, secondary and tertiary prevention.
- Alcohol and drug policy is now part of hospital policies.
- Health promoting schools are part of the World Health Organization Global Schools Health.
- The primary goal of school health education is to help individuals adopt behaviours and create conditions that are conducive to health.
- The importance of promoting the rational use of psychoactive drugs and the need to educate health care professionals in this area has been recognised.
- A comprehensive workplace health promotion scheme empowers social partners from both inside and outside workplace enterprises for the health maintenance of workers and their families and creates healthy working environments for the same.

ACTIVITY 21.1

There is only one answer to the following multiple choice questions

All of the following are types of prevention except
a.   Primary prevention
b.   Secondary prevention
c.   Social behaviour prevention
d.   Tertiary prevention

The prevention of alcohol and drug misuse is
a.   The promotion of constructive lifestyles
b.   To delay or avoid the onset of substance misuse
c.   Part of public health policy
d.   All of the above

Which of these is not part of the government alcohol strategy?
a.   Promoting sensible drinking
b.   Reducing the harm that alcohol can cause
c.   Helping families with alcohol problems
d.   Focusing on the minority of harmful drinkers

High-risk groups are
a.   Homeless drug users
b.   Heroin and crack injectors
c.   Potential or new injectors
d.   All of the above

Which of these is not part of primary prevention?
a.   Reducing the demand for substance misuse
b.   Reducing the supply for substance misuse
c.   Encouraging good drinking behaviour
d.   Provision of health information

Primary prevention programmes are those aimed mainly at
a.   Individuals who have not yet tried psychoactive substances
b.   Individuals who have tried psychoactive substances
c.   Individuals who have been treated for substance misuse
d.   Individuals who are currently being treated for substance misuse

The aim of secondary prevention is to
a.   Reduce and limit health and social harms
b.   Promote healthy lifestyles
c.   Reduce the demand for substance misuse
d.   Prevent the onset of substance misuse

Secondary prevention programmes are those aimed mainly at
a.   Individuals who have not yet tried psychoactive substances
b.   Individuals who have tried psychoactive substances
c.   Individuals who have been treated for substance misuse
d.   Individuals who are currently being treated for substance misuse

Tertiary level of prevention seeks
a.   To limit and reduce further complications
b.   To promote treatment
c.   To limit dysfunctions
d.   All of the above

Tertiary prevention programmes are those aimed mainly at
a. Individuals who have not yet tried psychoactive substances
b. Individuals who have tried psychoactive substances
c. Individuals who have been treated for substance misuse
d. Individuals who are currently being treated for substance misuse

Universal prevention activities may include
a. Schools-based prevention programmes
b. Mass media campaigns
c. Selective prevention programmes
d. All of the above

Selective prevention programmes
a. Target groups or subsets of the population
b. Target those using psychoactive substances
c. Reduce the influence of the risk factors
d. All of the above

Indicated prevention programmes
a. Target groups or subsets of the population
b. Target those using psychoactive substances
c. Reduce the influence of the risk factors
d. Target those requiring specialist interventions

Rational use of psychoactive substance means that
a. The right drug is taken by the right patient
b. The right dose is taken by the right patient
c. The right dose is taken for the right duration
d. All of the above

Irrational prescribing may be
a. Extravagant prescribing
b. Over-prescribing
c. Incorrect prescribing
d. All of the above

An alternative to medication of psychoactive substances is
a. Counselling and relaxation therapies
b. Pharmacological therapies
c. Reduction in medications
d. None of the above

The goal of health education programmes is to
a. Impart substance misuse knowledge
b. Modify alcohol or drug-using behaviour
c. Identify alcohol and drug users
d. Meet alcohol and drug education requirements

ACTIVITY 21.2

- What is meant by the terms health education, health promotion and prevention?
- What is meant by the terms rational use and irrational use?
- Describe two systems for classifying prevention programmes
- Reflect on the terms rational prescribing and rational use of drug. What do they mean to you now?
- List some examples of effective prevention programmes that have been adopted at your place of work (if appropriate) or at community level
- Describe the features of workplace prevention programmes
- Examine your local or institutional alcohol and drug policy

REFERENCES

Advisory Council on the Misuse of Drugs (1984) *Prevention*. London: HMSO.

Audit Commission (1993) *What Seems to Be the Matter: Communication between Hospitals and Patients*. London: HMSO.

Babor, T.F. and Grant, M. (eds) (1992) *Project Identification and Management of Alcohol-related Problems. Report on Phase II: A Randomized Clinical Trial of Brief Interventions in Primary Health Care*. Geneva: World Health Organization.

Chu, C., Breucker, G., Harris, N., Stizel, A., Xingfa, G. and Dwyer, S. (2000) Health promoting workplaces – international settings development. *Health Promotion International*, 15: 155–67.

Dawes, B.S.G. (2001) Focusing on the safe, healthy workplace. *AORN Journal*, 73: 16–18.

Department of Health (1992) *The Health of the Nation – A Strategy for Health in England*. London: HMSO.

Department of Health (2007) *Safe. Sensible. Social. The Next Steps in the National Alcohol Strategy*. London: Department of Health.

Department of Health (2008) *Glossary*. Appendix 2, London: Department of Health. www.dh.gov.uk/en/Publicationsandstatistics/Publications/PublicationsPolicyAndGuidance/Browsable/DH_4894623.

Department of Health and National Treatment Agency for Substance Misuse (2007) *Reducing Drug-related Harm: An Action Plan*. London: Department of Health.

Edmonds, K., Sumnall, H., McVeigh, J. and Bellis, M.A. (2005) *Drug Prevention among Vulnerable Young People*, Liverpool: The National Collaborating Centre for Drug Prevention [NCCDP]. www.cph.org.uk/cph_pubs/reports/SM/Q3factsheets.pdf.

Ewles, L. and Simnett, I. (2003) *Promoting Health, A Practical Guide*, 5th edition. London: Baillière Tindall.

Ghodse, A.H. and Khan, I. (1988) *Psychoactive Drugs: Improving Prescribing Practices*. Geneva: World Health Organization.

Gossop, M. and Grant, M. (1990). *Preventing and Controlling Drug Abuse*, 76–7. Geneva: World Health Organization.

Hartz, C., Plant, M. and Watts M. (1991). *Alcohol and Health*. London: Medical Council on Alcoholism.

Health Promotion Agency for Northern Ireland (2005) *Health Promoting Hospitals: Part of a Wider Programme of Support and Action towards a Healthier Health Service*. www.healthpromotionagency.org.uk/work/hphospitals/menu.htm (accessed 20 September 2007).

Home Office (2002) *Updated Drug Strategy 2002*. London: Home Office.

Home Office (2005) *Every Child Matters: Change for Children, Young People and Drugs*. London: Home Office.

INCB (2003) *Annual Report 2003*. Vienna: International Narcotic Control Board. www.incb.org.

Johnson, A. and Baum, F. (2001) Health promoting hospitals: a typology of different organizational approaches to health promotion. *Health Promotion International*, 16, 3: 281–7.

Kelly, J.A. and Murphy, D.A. (1991) Some lesson learned about risk reduction after ten years of the HIV/Aids epidemic. *Aids Care*, 3, 3: 8.

Kramer, D.M. and Cole, D.C. (2003) Sustained, intensive engagement to promote health and safety knowledge transfer to and utilisation by workplaces. *Science Communication*, 25, 1: 56–82.

McGrath, Y., Sumnall, H., Edmonds, K., McVeigh, J. and Bellis M. (2005) *Review of Grey Literature on Drug Prevention among Young People*. Liverpool: The National Collaborating Centre for Drug Prevention [NCCDP].

Maben, J. and Macleod Clarke, J. (1995) Health promotion: a conceptual analysis. *Journal of Advanced Nursing*, 22: 1158–65.

Manias, E. and Street, A. (2000) Legitimation of nurses' knowledge through policies and protocols in clinical practice. *Journal of Advanced Nursing*, 32: 1467–75.

Mrazek, P.J. and Haggerty, R.J. (eds) (1994) *Reducing Risks for Mental Disorders: Frontiers for Preventive Intervention Research*. Washington DC: National Academy Press.

NICE (2007), *Behaviour Change*. London: National Institute of Clinical Excellence. www.nice.org.uk/PH006.

NIDA (1989) Prevention NIDA, Rockville, MD: National Institute of Drug Abuse.

Parsons, C., Stears, D. and Thomas, C. (2002) *Models of Health Promoting Schools in Europe. United Kingdom – The Eco-Holistic Model of The Health Promoting School*. Copenhagen: WHO Regional Office for Europe.

Rassool, G. Hussein (2000) Addiction: global problem and global response complacency or commitment? *Journal of Advanced Nursing*, 32, 3: 505–8.

Rassool, G. Hussein (2005) Nursing prescription: the rational use of psychoactive substances. *Nursing Standard*, 19, 21: 45–51.

Rassool, G. Hussein. and Winnington, J. (1993) Using psychoactive substances. *Nursing Times*, 89, 47: 38–40.

Rassool, G. Hussein and Gafoor, M. (1997) *Addiction Nursing: Perspectives on Professional and Clinical Practice*. Cheltenham: Nelson-Thornes.

Whitehead, D. (2004) The European Health Promoting Hospitals (HPH) project: how far on? *Health Promotion International*, 19, 2: 259–67.

WHO (1986a) 'Ottawa charter for health promotion'. *Journal of Health Promotion*, 1: 1–4.

WHO (1986b) *Drug Dependence and Alcohol Related Problems – A Manual for Community Health Workers with Guidelines for Trainers*. Geneva: World Health Organization.

WHO (1989) *Report of the WHO Meeting on Nursing/Midwifery Education in the Rational Use of Psychoactive Drugs*. DMP/PND/89.5. Geneva: World Health Organization.

WHO (1991) *Europe. Budapest Declaration on Health Promoting Hospitals. HPH Networking Documents*. Geneva: World Health Organization Regional Office for Europe.

WHO (1992) *Europe. Health Promoting Hospitals. Networking Documents*. Geneva: World Health Organization Regional Office for Europe.

WHO Expert Committee (1993) *Health Promotion in the Workplace: Alcohol and Drug Abuse*. Technical Report Series, No. 883 iii–33. Geneva: World Health Organization.

WHO (1995) *WHO's Expert Committee Recommendation on Comprehensive School Health Education and Promotion*. Geneva: World Health Organization.

WHO (1998) *Health Promotion Glossary*. Geneva: World Health Organization. www.who.int/hpr/nph/docs.

WHO (2003) *Developing Standards for Health Promotion in Hospitals*. Copenhagen: World Health Organization Regional Office for Europe. www.euro.who.int/Document/IHB/hph standardsfinrpt.pdf

WHO (2004a) *Promoting Rational Use of Medicines Saves Lives and Money*. The International Conference on Improving Use of Medicines, Thailand, from 30 March to 2 April. Geneva: World Health Organization.

WHO (2004b) *Promoting Rational Drug Use*. A CD-Rom Training Programme in collaboration with Boston University School of Public and International Health. Geneva: World Health Organization.

WHO (2004c) *Healthy Workplaces*. Copenhagen: World Health Organization Regional Office for Europe. www.euro.who.int/healthyworkplaces.

WHO/UNDOC (2007) *Outcome Evaluation Summary Report: WHO/UNODC Global Initiative on Primary Prevention of Substance Abuse*. Geneva: World Health Organization.

CHAPTER 22

STRATEGIES IN HELPING PEOPLE TO CHANGE

OBJECTIVES

- Discuss the nature of motivation and readiness to change.

- Identify the reasons why people change.

- Describe the models of helping people to change.

Healthcare professionals need to accept the challenge to become agents of change, nudging, motivating, educating, coaching and supporting individuals throughout the process of change. To do this, providers of healthcare need to understand the nature of change, assess the readiness of individuals to change and communicate in ways that facilitate behavioural change. The practice of health education and promotion on strategies in helping people change is based on a number of theories and models. The theories or models include the health action model, the health belief model, the theory of reasoned action, the trans-theoretical stages of change model, social learning theory, social cognitive theory, the theory of planned behaviour, community development and models of organisational change. When planning work on behaviour change with individuals, NICE (2007) suggested that a number of concepts drawn from the psychological literature are helpful. These concepts include:

- outcome expectancies (helping people to develop accurate knowledge about the health consequences of their behaviours)
- personal relevance (emphasising the personal salience of health behaviours)
- positive attitude (promoting positive feelings towards the outcomes of behaviour change)

- self-efficacy (enhancing people's belief in their ability to change)
- descriptive norms (promoting the visibility of positive health behaviours in people's reference groups – that is, the groups they compare themselves to, or aspire to)
- subjective norms (enhancing social approval for positive health behaviours in significant others and reference groups)
- personal and moral norms (promoting personal and moral commitments to behaviour change)
- intention formation and concrete plans (helping people to form plans and goals for changing behaviours, over time and in specific contexts)
- behavioural contracts (asking people to share their plans and goals with others)
- relapse prevention (helping people develop skills to cope with difficult situations and conflicting goals).

This chapter will focus on two models: the health action model and the trans-theoretical stages of change model. Both models are relevant in the prevention of alcohol and drug misuse and helping people change their health behaviour.

MOTIVATION AND READINESS TO CHANGE

Individuals are resistant to change, even when a simple behavioural change is vital such as taking medications. In fact, a study showed that more than a third of patients fail to take one or both medications as prescribed for reducing high blood pressure and cholesterol within six months (Chapman *et al.* 2005). Some individuals with alcohol and drug problems are not only resistant to change but are not even thinking about changing their drinking or drug-taking behaviours. Their lack of readiness to change may be due to personality factors, psychosocial circumstances and environmental and cultural contexts.

In the trans-theoretical model of change (Prochaska and DiClemente 1983, 1986), among precomtemplators (individuals who have been thinking about change or have no insight into the consequences of their alcohol or drug misuse), 'four Rs' – reluctance, rebellion, resignation and rationalisation – have been identified. Reluctant precontemplators are those who, through lack of knowledge or inertia, do not want to consider change. The impact of the problem has not become fully conscious. Rebellious precontemplators have a heavy investment in drug-taking or drinking and in making their own decisions. They are resistant to being told what to do. Resigned precontemplators have given up hope about the possibility of change and seem overwhelmed by the problem. Many individuals have made many attempts to quit or control their drinking or drug-taking. Rationalising precontemplators have all the answers; they have plenty of reasons why drinking or drug-taking is not a problem, or why drinking or drug-taking is a problem for others but not for them. In fact, individuals may not change because they believe they cannot change.

In a study (Matzger *et al.* 2005) of why people change in a sample of 659 problem drinkers, the findings suggest that, among individuals who identified as 'hitting rock bottom', having traumatic events, and spiritual or religious experiences were given as reasons for cutting down on alcohol. In addition, an interventions performed by family members (receiving a spouse's warning) or medical doctors are negatively related to positive outcomes. There is evidence to suggest that a community reinforcement and family training (CRAFT) approach, teaching behaviour change skills to use at home, was the most effective method for engaging unmotivated drinkers in treatment (Miller *et al.* 1999). From a psychoanalytic perspective, a central reason that individuals are resistant to change is their fear of the threats that they believe change entails. These threats or dangers include relinquishment of infantile wishes and fantasies, anxiety, guilt, fantasies that change would threaten a vital relationship, defences, unconscious pathogenic beliefs, devotion and loyalty to early figures and stable internal working models of self (Eagle 1999).

There is a consensus of opinion that incremental changes are recommended for alcohol and drug users to change their behaviour. However, there is evidence to suggest that radical, sweeping, comprehensive changes are often easier for people than small, incremental ones (Ornish 2002). For example, Ornish (2002) stated that individuals who make moderate changes in their diets get the worst of both worlds: the individuals feel deprived and hungry because they are not eating everything they want, but they are not making big enough changes to see quickly an improvement in how they feel, or in measurements such as weight, blood pressure, and cholesterol. In the context of alcohol and drug misuse, some individuals may require incremental changes and others may require radical changes. Whether the paradox holds that big changes are easier than small ones in the addiction field remains inconclusive. Some of the reasons why people change are presented in Table 22.1.

The motivation to change and adopt new lifestyle and behaviour are both internally and externally construed. Alcohol and drug misusers who have the desire to change need to have the readiness to adopt new behaviours which require some form of action. Motivation and readiness to change require both conviction and confidence (Rollnick *et al.* 1999). 'Confidence' relates to the person's belief that they have the ability to adopt a new behavior. 'Conviction' is a belief that a new behaviour, or why change is needed, is important and worth the effort to achieve it. Without these two core beliefs, individuals are not motivated to take action and make necessary changes. Motivated individuals actively seeking to make changes in their behaviour require a different approach from those who are unmotivated (NICE 2007). The latter may need more information about the benefits of change, as well as a realistic plan of action.

Table 22.1 Why do people change?

- Possess competencies, knowledge and skills
- Participate in decision to change
- Find that rewards of change exceed the pain of change
- Change as a result of others changing
- Prefer an environment free from threat and judgement
- Trust the motives of the persons trying to induce change
- Can influence reciprocally the person or persons attempting to influence them
- See the change has been successful
- Change either in a series of small steps or as a total change in their way of life
- Maintain change as the change is supported by their environment
- Maintain change if there is public commitment to the change
- Resist change to the degree that they feel it is being imposed upon them

Source: Adapted from research done at the National Training Laboratories, Bethel, Maine. USA

Equally, it is important to note that an intervention aimed at changing one behaviour may inadvertently lead to another undesirable behaviour. For example, someone who gives up heroin use may start drinking more alcohol. Matching intervention strategies to behavioural changes may be required to meet individual need.

THE HEALTH ACTION MODEL

The health action model (Tones 1987, Tones *et al.* 1990) incorporates the health belief model, the theory of reasoned action and other health-related theories, and takes account of the need for an ecological and multi-factorial approach in the prevention of alcohol and drug misuse. The health action model describes the interaction of knowledge, beliefs, values, attitudes, drives and normative pressures and seeks to show how these relate to individual intentions to act. It also indicates how environmental circumstances, information and personal skills may facilitate the translation of intentions into health actions (Tones 1987). According to Tones *et al.* (1990), the significance of this model is its recognition of three major factors that influence individual's decision-making: environmental factors, interpersonal factors and intrapersonal factors and the supply of post-decisional support. The health action model shows the stages a person goes through during the process of behaviour change and can act as a framework for a range of possible interventions by health educators. The health action model is divided into two main sections: behavioural intention and socio-cultural and environment factors.

Behavioural intention or an individual's intention to act comprises a set of interacting systems involving knowledge and beliefs (cognitive system), values, attitudes and drives (motivating system) and pressure from social norms including significant others (normative system). The second facet is concerned with the physical, cultural and socio-economic environment, and the acquisition of relevant knowledge and skills which may act as either facilitating or inhibiting factors in the translation of behavioural intention or action. The process of feedback is a crucial element in this model because the experience of performing a particular health action, a break in a routine or other related event can either consolidate action or, as it were, 'switch it off' (Tones, Tilford and Keeley-Robinson 1990). In the context of this model, it is important to provide the necessary environmental and social support once an individual has made that decision to change their behaviour. However, the model recognises the gap between attitude and practice by drawing attention to the potential barriers such as environmental factors, lack of knowledge and skills deficit. Alcohol and drug prevention strategy must take into account factors relating to the individual, educational, environmental, political and socio-cultural factors with an integrated community-based approach to be effective.

THE TRANS-THEORETICAL STAGES OF CHANGE MODEL

The trans-theoretical model (Prochaska *et al.* 1992, Prochaska and Velicer 1997) is an integrative model of behaviour change. Its most popular construct has been the stages of change, which reflect the temporal dimension of health behaviour change (Prochaska and Velicer 1997): the model involves emotions, cognitions and behaviour. The stages of change model evolved from research in smoking cessation but has now been applied to a wide variety of problem behaviours such as alcohol and drug interventions, exercise, weight control and condom use for HIV protection.

In this model, behavioural change is viewed as a process with individuals at various levels of motivation or stages for 'readiness' to change. Individuals will be at different stages in this process of change, and intervention strategies should match their particular stage. The trans-theoretical model construes change as a process involving progress through a series of six stages: pre-contemplation, contemplation, preparation, action, maintenance, termination or relapse.

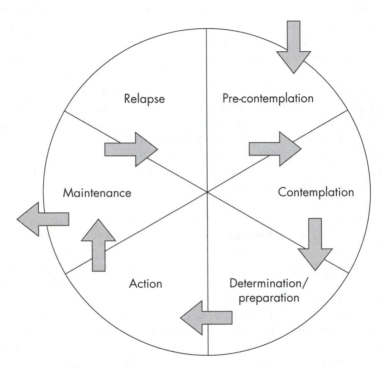

FIGURE 22.1 A model of the process of change

Source: Prochaska and DiClemente (1986)

Pre-contemplation

In this stage, the individuals have no insight of the problem or are unaware of the problem. Individuals may lack the awareness that life can be improved by a change in behaviour despite their high risk behaviour. Pre-contemplators are often characterised as resistant or unmotivated and tend to avoid information, discussion, or thought with regard to the targeted health behaviour (Prochaska *et al.* 1992).

Contemplation

The individuals are seriously comtemplating a change in behaviour. They are aware of the pros and the cons of behavioural change. Ambivalence develops as a result of the balance between the costs and benefits of changing. The individuals may be trapped in this stage for long periods of time and this characteristic is termed chronic contemplation or behavioural procrastination.

Preparation

At the preparation stage, individuals are planning and making final adjustments before changing behaviour; they plan to take action in the immediate future, usually measured as the next month. The preparation stage is viewed as a transition rather than a stable stage, with individuals intending progress to action in the next 30 days.

Action

Action is the stage in which people have made specific overt changes in their lifestyles and behaviour. In this stage, individuals must attain adequate changes in reducing their high-risk behaviours. This is a critical stage where there is the possibility of relapse.

Maintenance

At this stage, the individuals continue with desirable and acceptable actions and these are working to prevent relapse and consolidate gains secured during the action phase. Maintainers are distinguishable from those in the action stage in that they report the highest levels of self-efficacy and are less frequently tempted to relapse (Prochaska and DiClemente 1984).

Termination or relapse

In the termination phase, the individuals have gained adequate self-efficacy to eliminate the risk lapse or relapse. Their former lifestyles and behaviours are no longer perceived as desirable. Most substance misusers experience relapse on the journey to permanent cessation or stable reduction of high-risk behaviours. In relapse, the individual reverts to old behaviour: this can occur during either action or maintenance and the individual will experience an immediate sense of failure that can seriously undermine their self-confidence.

This model of change is a circular rather than a linear model (see Table 21.1). The individual may go through several cycles of contemplation, action and relapse before either reaching maintenance or termination or exiting the system without remaining free from substance misuse. The 'revolving-door schema' explains the sequence that individuals pass through in their efforts to become free from alcohol or drugs. An individual enters and exits at any point and often recycles several times. The stages of change model considers relapse to be normal. Relapsed individuals may need to learn to anticipate high-risk situations more effectively, control environmental cues and learn how to handle unexpected episodes of stress to reach the stage of termination. An important aspect of this model is the belief that the counselling outcome can be improved when there is a match between the client's stage of change and the type of counselling interventions offered (Prochaska and DiClemente 1982).

MATCHING INTERVENTIONS

The stage of model of change is of practical value when selecting appropriate interventions. See Chapter 26 for the different methods of intervention strategies. By identifying an individual position in the change process, intervention strategies can be tailored in matching individual readiness to change. A summary of the stages model of change and intervention strategies is presented in Table 22.2.

Table 22.2 Summary of stages model of change and intervention strategies

Stages of model	Individual stage	Intervention models
Pre-contemplation	Denial Rationalisation Feeling of no control Not thinking about change Lack of awareness of severity of consequences Resistant to change	Support Locus of control Health belief model Motivational interviewing
Contemplation	Weighing benefits and costs of proposed change	Counselling Motivational interviewing
Preparation	Decided on action Making the steps necessary to prepare for action	Counselling Cognitive-behavioural therapy Motivational interviewing
Action	Taking a definitive action to change	Cognitive-behavioural therapy 12-Step programme
Maintenance	Maintaining new behaviour over time	Counselling Support Cognitive-behavioural therapy (relapse prevention) 12-Step programme
Termination	Self-efficacy	Support Self-help groups
Relapse	Recycling – learning from relapse	Motivational interviewing

KEY POINTS

- Health care professionals need to accept the challenge to become agents of change, nudging, motivating, educating and supporting individuals throughout the process of change.
- There are a number of theories or models that are aimed at the prevention of alcohol and drug misuse and helping people change their health behaviour.
- Individuals are resistant to change even when a simple behavioural change is vital such as taking medications.
- Individuals may not change because they believe they cannot change.
- The health action model shows the stages a person goes through during the process of behaviour change and can do so as a framework for a range of possible interventions by health educators.
- The health action model is divided into two main sections: behavioural intention and socio-cultural and environment factors.
- Motivation and readiness to change require both conviction and confidence.
- The trans-theoretical model is an integrative model of behaviour change.
- Its most popular construct has been the stages of change, which reflect the temporal dimension of health behaviour change and involve emotions, cognitions and behaviour.
- The trans-theoretical model involves the process of six stages: pre-contemplation, contemplation, preparation, action, maintenance, termination or relapse.
- Individuals will be at different stages in this process of change, and intervention strategies should match their particular stage.

ACTIVITY 22.1

State whether the following statements are true or false by ticking where appropriate

	True	False
In the trans-theoretical model of change pre-comtemplators are individuals who have been thinking about change		
Reluctant pre-contemplators are those who through lack of knowledge or inertia do not want to consider change		
Rebellious pre-contemplators do not have a heavy investment in drug taking or drinking		
Resigned pre-contemplators have given up hope about the possibility of change		
Rationalising pre-contemplators have plenty of reasons why drinking or drug taking is a problem		
Many individuals have made many attempts to quit or control their drinking or drug taking		
Having traumatic events, and spiritual or religious experiences are given as		

reasons for cutting down on alcohol

There is no evidence to suggest that radical, sweeping, comprehensive changes are often easier for people than small, incremental ones

Confidence relates to the person's belief that they have the ability to adopt a new behaviour

Conviction is a belief that a new behaviour is important and worth the effort to achieve it or why change is needed

In the health belief model, there is omission of environmental circumstances, information and personal skills that may facilitate the translation of intentions into health actions

In the stage of change model, behavioural change is viewed as a process with individuals at various levels of motivation or stages for 'readiness' to change

The stage model of change is a linear model

Most substance misusers experience relapse on the journey to permanent cessation or stable reduction

---

ACTIVITY 22.2

There is only one correct answer to the following multiple-choice questions

The stage of change in which ambivalence develops as a result of the balance between the costs and benefits of changing is
a.   Stage 1, pre-contemplation
b.   Stage 2, contemplation
c.   Stage 3, preparation
d.   Stage 4, action

The stage of change in which people decide to take action in the immediate future is
a.   Stage 1, pre-contemplation
b.   Stage 2, contemplation
c.   Stage 3, preparation
d.   Stage 4, action

The stage of change in which people are not thinking of changing is
a.   Stage 1, pre-contemplation
b.   Stage 2, contemplation
c.   Stage 3, preparation
d.   Stage 4, action

The stage of change in which people are planning and making final adjustments before changing behaviour is
a.   Stage 1, pre-contemplation
b.   Stage 2, contemplation
c.   Stage 3, preparation
d.   Stage 4, action

Confidence is shown when an individual
a.   Discounts the importance of contemplation
b.   Is aware of their feelings
c.   Understands the value of motivation
d.   Believes they can achieve an objective

Julie would like to stop smoking, but when she comes home from work she just wants to sit down and have a cigarette. She is exhibiting
a.   Ambivalence
b.   Lack of ambition
c.   Limited conviction
d.   Confidence

ACTIVITY 22.3

Questions
• Discuss the nature of motivation and readiness to change
• List the reasons why people change
• Can you apply the models of helping people to change in your work or speciality? Reflect on how you would apply this model of change to your patient or client

REFERENCES

Chapman, R.H., Benner, J.S., Petrilla, A.A., Tierce, J.C., Collins, S.R., Battleman, D.S. and Schwartz, J.S. (2005) Predictors of adherence with antihypertensive and lipid-lowering therapy. *Archives of Internal Medicine*, 165: 1147–52.

Eagle, M. (1999) Why Don't People Change? A Psychoanalytic Perspective. *Journal of Psychotherapy Integration*, 9, 1: 30–2.

Matzger, H., Kaskutas, L.A. and Weisner, C. (2005) Reasons for drinking less and their relationship to sustained remission from problem drinking. *Addiction*, 100: 1637–46.

Miller, W.R., Meyers, R.J. and Tonigan, J. (1999) Engaging the unmotivated in treatment for alcohol problems: a comparison of three strategies for intervention through family members. *Journal of Consulting and Clinical Psychology*, 67: 688–97.

NICE (2007) *Behaviour Change*. London: National Institute of Clinical Excellence, www.nice.org.uk/PH006.

Ornish, D. (2002) *Intensive Lifestyle Changes in Management of Coronary Heart Disease.* Harrison's Advances in Cardiology. New York: McGraw-Hill.

Prochaska, J.O. and DiClemente, C.C. (1982) Transtheoretical therapy: toward a more integrative model of change. *Psychotherapy: Theory, Research and Practice* 19, 3: 276–88.

Prochaska, J.O. and DiClemente, C.C. (1983) Stages and processes of self change of smoking: toward an integrative model of change. *Journal of Consulting and Clinical Psychology*, 51: 390–5.

Prochaska, J.O. and DiClemente, C.C. (1984) Self-change processes, self-efficacy and decisional balance across five stages of smoking cessation. In *Advances in Cancer Control – 1983*. New York: Alan R. Liss, Inc.

Prochaska, J.O. and DiClemente, C.C. (1986) Towards a comprehensive model of change. In W.R. Miller and N. Heather (eds) *Treating Addictive Behaviors: Processes of Change*. New York: Plenum.

Prochaska, J.O., DiClemente, C.C. and Norcross, J.C. (1992) In search of how people change. *American Psychologist*, 47: 1102–14.

Prochaska, J.O. and Velicer, W.K. (1997) The trans-theoretical model of health behaviour change. *American Journal of Health Promotion*, 12, 1: 38–48.

Rollnick, S., Mason, P. and Butler, C. (1999) *Health Behaviour Change: A Guide for Practitioners*. Edinburgh: Churchill Livingstone.

Tones, K. (1987) Devising strategies for preventing drug misuse: the role of the Health Action Model. *Health Education Research*, 2, 4: 305–17.

Tones, K., Tilford, S. and Keeley-Robinson, Y. (1990) *Health Education: Effectiveness, Efficiency and Equity*. London: Chapman and Hall.

WORKING WITH DIVERSITY: CULTURAL COMPETENCE

OBJECTIVES

■ Define culture and cultural competence.

■ Identify the goals of cultural competence services.

■ Discuss how an understanding of culture allows us to provide cultural competence care.

■ Describe culturally competent attitudes, knowledge and skills.

■ Describe the challenges and problems in the provision and delivery of cultural competent care.

There is a growing recognition that culture is an important component and determinant of health (Department of Health 1999a). The National Service Framework for Mental Health (Department of Health 1999b) states that mental health services need to develop and demonstrate cultural competence, with staff having the knowledge and skills to work effectively with diverse communities. The provision of culturally competent approach in working with Black and ethnic minority substance misusers has also been advocated by Black and ethnic minority drug treatment professionals (Sangster *et al*. 2002). For nurses, the provision of culturally competent care is both a legal and a moral requirement for nurses in the Nursing and Midwifery Council's Code of conduct (NMC 2004).

The National Treatment Agency for Adult Substance Misusers (NTA) recognises the significant discrimination faced by Black and ethnic minority groups within the drug treatment field. In response to this, the NTA produced a race equality scheme in

(NTA 2002), which is reviewed on an annual basis. The NTA is committed to action to ensure:

- equal access to relevant and appropriate drug treatment services for the whole population
- the eradication of unlawful discrimination and the promotion of equal opportunities with respect to ethnicity, age, culture, gender, sexuality, mental ability, mental health, geographical location, offending background, physical ability, political beliefs, religion, health or status or any other specific factors which result in discrimination.

Given the growing diversity within the UK population, health, social care and criminal justice agencies and agencies will need to evolve culturally competent systems if they are to meet the needs of Black and ethnic minority communities in an integrated service delivery systems. The chapter aims to discuss how and why cultural differences affect health and social care and provides a framework for a culturally competent system of care.

CULTURE

In order to understand cultural competence, it is important to define what culture is. Culture has many definitions. One of the definitions is that culture is the shared beliefs, values and practices that are learned and transmitted throughout a society, and influence the way that a group of people live and make decisions and interact (Leininger 1991). Another definition of culture is 'the integrated pattern of human behaviour that includes thoughts, communications, actions, customs, beliefs, values and institutions of a racial, ethnic, religious or social group' (Cross *et al.* 1989). What is clear is that we need to understand culture so that we become aware of how others interpret their 'world view' and respond to it. Understanding culture allows us to be more aware of cultural differences and stereotypes.

Culture is also related to health and healthcare provision and delivery. The 'world view' of health and illness and their causes is determined by cultural factors. So how people seek and respond to health and social care and how we care for patients are fundamentally influenced by cultural factors. Understanding cultural health behaviour can reduce barriers and promote equity in the delivery of health and social care. Thus, there is a need for substance-misuse services to develop practices and procedures to deliver culturally competent care.

CULTURAL COMPETENCE

The area of cultural competence in general suffers from a lack of an agreed-upon definition and is not universally accepted. It is often interrelated with terms like cultural awareness, cultural sensitivity, cultural appropriateness, cultural specificity and others (Rassool 2006). Cultural competence is most appropriately viewed as an umbrella term which describes an ability to meet the needs of diverse communities; cultural appropriateness provides the mechanism through which cultural competence is achieved; and cultural sensitivity and cultural specificity form the building blocks for culturally appropriate ways of working (Sangster *et al.* 2002). Cultural competence is a process of change that is developed over time in order to increase understanding and knowledge of cultural differences that affect the healthcare experience (Cross *et al.* 1989)

Papadopoulos *et al.* (1998) describe cultural competence as the capacity to provide effective healthcare, taking into consideration people's cultural beliefs, behaviours and needs. A more comprehensive and operational definition is that cultural competence is the integration and transformation of knowledge about individuals and groups of people into specific standards, policies, practices and attitudes used in appropriate cultural settings to increase the quality of services, thereby producing better outcomes (Davis 1997). In the context of substance misuse, cultural competence is the willingness and ability of the workforce, the services and the system to value the importance of cultural diversity and be culturally responsive in the provision and delivery of services of quality services to Black and ethnic minority groups (Rassool 2006). In a study on delivering drug services to Black and ethnic minority communities (Sangster *et al.* 2002) cultural competence is described as an ability to meet the different needs of a community.

CHALLENGES FOR PROVIDERS OF CULTURAL COMPETENCE CARE

There are major challenges facing health and social care providers in the provision and delivery of service provision for alcohol and drug users from Black and ethnic minority groups. These difficulties are accentuated in the recognition and assessment of substance misuse because of cultural variations in presentation symptoms and where a 'dual diagnosis' – substance misuse and psychiatric disorders – is ascribed (Rassool 2006). Black and ethnic minority communities are a heterogeneous group with varying values, attitudes, religious beliefs and customs that affect the patterns of substance misuse. Cultural and religious beliefs should not be applied equally in a stereotypical fashion to members of a particular Black and ethnic minority group. There are often differences among Black and ethnic minority communities and differences between members of the same ethnic group. This cultural diversity, with a wide variation in lifestyles, health behaviours, religion and language, has profound effects on the use of alcohol and drug. Owing to cultural and religious diversity, there is the recognition of differences in the nature and extent of substance misuse among Black and ethnic minority communities. For example, cocaine is reported as a main drug of use by Black Caribbean, African and 'other' groups than by either South Asian or white drug users. Amongst Black and ethnic minority communities, those exceeding the daily recommended alcohol limit were Irish.

A study by Fernandez (2004) shows that many clients from the Bengali community requested a community or outpatient detoxification regime rather than an inpatient detoxification. From the user's point of view this was a quick and easy way of getting 'clean' and, from a clinician's point of view, uncomplicated drug profiles and small drug histories seemingly make Asian clients suitable for an outpatient detoxification programme (Fernandez 2004). This kind of diversity has strong implications for the provision and kind of substance-misuse services which are based on the local needs of those communities.

The notion of cultural competence is applied to service provision, service delivery and system of care. This is a significant development as it provides the basis for moving beyond individually focused anti-racism training and brings into play the culture of organisations, their aims and core competencies, their management structures and their use of monitoring (Chandra 1996). Services with 'cultural competence', according to Chandra (1996), are those 'perceived by black and minority ethnic users being in harmony with their cultural and religious beliefs' – and offer a range of ways for health purchasers to work towards this with providers. Cross *et al.* (1989) list five essential elements that contribute to an institution's or agency's ability to become more culturally competent:

- valuing diversity
- having the capacity for cultural self-assessment
- being conscious of the dynamics inherent when cultures interact
- having institutionalised cultural knowledge
- having developed adaptations of service delivery reflecting an understanding of cultural diversity.

These five elements should be manifested at every level of an organisation, including policy-making, administration and practice. Further, these elements should be reflected in the attitudes, structures, policies, and services of the organisation. A summary of the core elements needed in the development and provision of cultural competence drug services for Black and ethnic minority communities (Sangster *et al.* 2002) is provided in Table 23.1.

Table 23.1 Cultural competence and service delivery in substance-misuse services

- Cultural ownership and leadership (the extent to which race and ethnicity are considered important by a service)
- Symbols of accessibility (something that shows Black and ethnic minority people that they are welcomed by a service, for example posters, leaflets, culturally specific newspapers and magazines)
- Familiarity with, and ability to meet, the distinct needs of communities
- Holistic, therapeutic and social help
- A range of services
- Black and ethnic minority workers
- Community attachment and ownership and capacity building (the process through which the skills and structures needed to provide drug services are developed)

Source: Sangster *et al.* (2002)

GOALS OF CULTURALLY COMPETENT CARE

The goals of cultural competent care are cultural awareness, cultural knowlege, cultural skill and cultural encounters (Campinha-Bacote *et al.* 1996, Kavanagh and Kennedy 1992, Tervalon and Murray-Garcia 1998).

- *cultural awareness*: appreciating and accepting cultural differences
- *cultural knowledge*: deliberately seeking out various world views and explanatory models of disease. Knowledge can help promote understanding between cultures.

- *cultural skill*: learning how to assess a patient culturally to avoid relying only on written 'facts'; explaining an issue from another's perspective; reducing resistance and defensiveness; and acknowledging interactive mistakes that may hinder the desire to communicate.
- *cultural encounters*: meeting and working with people of a different culture will help dispel stereotypes and may contradict academic knowledge. Although it is crucial to gather cultural knowledge, it is an equally important, but sometimes neglected, culturally competent skill to be humble enough to let go of the security of stereotypes and remain open to the individuality of each patient.

MODEL OF CULTURAL COMPETENCE

A model to promote the inclusion of cultural competence in nursing and healthcare sciences education has been developed by Papadopoulos *et al.* (1998). A model of cultural competence is shown in Figure 23.1.

The model consists of four stages. The first stage in the model is *cultural awareness* and is the basis for a critical examination of our personal values and beliefs. The nature of construction of cultural identity as well as its influence on people's health beliefs and practices is viewed as a learning foundation. *Cultural knowledge* (the second stage) can

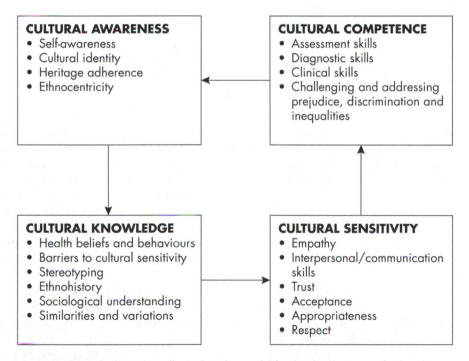

CULTURAL AWARENESS
- Self-awareness
- Cultural identity
- Heritage adherence
- Ethnocentricity

CULTURAL COMPETENCE
- Assessment skills
- Diagnostic skills
- Clinical skills
- Challenging and addressing prejudice, discrimination and inequalities

CULTURAL KNOWLEDGE
- Health beliefs and behaviours
- Barriers to cultural sensitivity
- Stereotyping
- Ethnohistory
- Sociological understanding
- Similarities and variations

CULTURAL SENSITIVITY
- Empathy
- Interpersonal/communication skills
- Trust
- Acceptance
- Appropriateness
- Respect

FIGURE 23.1 The Papadopoulos, Tilki and Taylor model for the development of cultural competence in nursing

Source: Papadopoulos *et al.* 1998

be gained in a number of ways. Meaningful contact with people from different Black and ethnic minority groups can enhance knowledge around their health beliefs and behaviours as well as raise understanding around the problems they face. An important element in achieving *cultural sensitivity* (the third stage), is how professionals view people in their care: clients should be seen as equal partners. This includes trust, acceptance and respect as well as facilitation and negotiation. The achievement of the fourth stage (*cultural competence*) requires the synthesis and application of previously gained awareness, knowledge and sensitivity. Cultural competence activities include the development of skills in the assessment of need, clinical diagnosis and clinical skills; practices are responsive to the culture and diversity within the populations served. A most important component of this stage of development is the ability to recognise and challenge racism and other forms of discrimination and oppressive practice. It is argued that this model combines both the multiculturalist and the anti-racist perspectives and facilitates the development of a broader understanding around inequalities and human and citizenship rights, whilst promoting the development of skills needed to bring about change at the patient/client level (Papdopoulos *et al.* 1998).

It is worth pointing out that it is not practical for health and social care professionals to have knowledge of all Black and ethnic minority groups but they can learn to appreciate diversity and provide culturally sensitive care to heterogeneous populations. However, health and social care professionals should have the cultural knowledge and traditions of the population they serve. The goal of interventions is the provision of culturally competent care that diminishes the barriers and improves health outcomes.

HEALTHCARE APPROACHES: CLINICAL AND EDUCATIONAL

The Nursing and Midwifery Council in England *Code of Professional Conduct: Standards for Conduct, Performance and Ethics* (NMC 2004) points out that nurses and midwives 'are personally accountable for ensuring that you promote and protect the interests and dignity of patients and clients, irrespective of gender, age, race, ability, sexuality, economic status, lifestyle, culture and religious or political beliefs'. The General Social Care Council is committed to the strategy for delivering equality and diversity both in terms of the services provided for its customers and stakeholders and in the GSCC's employment policies. The General Medical Council sets out the principles and values on which good medical practice is founded. Other clinicians, including psychologists, pharmacists and occupational therapists, have their guidance regarding equality and diversity.

In addition to the client's cultural beliefs, health and social care professionals must be aware of their own beliefs, practices and perceptions as these may have an impact on the care they provide to clients from diverse cultural backgrounds. Awareness of one's own values and those of the healthcare system is the foundation of culturally competent nursing (Leonard and Plotnikoff 2000). Burr (2002) identified some stereotypical views of South Asian patients held by qualified and experienced healthcare professionals and warned against the dangers of imposing one's own values systems wittingly or otherwise on to others. The imposition of our own values implicitly suggests that underlying these sentiments is the belief that one's own value system is superior to that of others and the expectation that once in England one should think and conduct oneself in keeping with the ways of the majority (Burr 2002). Some ethnic and racial groups may feel powerless when faced with institutionalised racism and other forms of privilege enjoyed by the dominant group (Singer and Clair 2003). Respect for the belief systems of others and the effects of those beliefs on health behaviour are critically important to culturally competent care. The main source of problems in caring for patients from diverse cultural backgrounds is the lack of understanding and tolerance and the inability to ask questions sensitively.

Health and social care professionals must be aware of their own cultural expectations and not impose these upon communities from different cultures. They need to challenge and confront their own prejudice and negative perceptions of Black and ethnic minority groups and to consider the different composition of ethnic and cultural backgrounds of their patients in order to deliver safe and effective care.

Culturally competent approaches are necessary to ensure the best possible access to substance-misuse services and for better healthcare outcomes. Healthcare professionals who are culturally knowledgeable and competent can provide care that ensures that Black and ethnic minority groups receive the best and most appropriate health care interventions. Gerrish (2000) has put forward a philosophy of individualised care that incorporates notions of equity and fairness, holism, respect for individuality, establishing partnerships between patients and professionals and promoting independence. In this framework individualised care entails a holistic assessment of physical, psychological, social and spiritual needs, an assessment approach that can be used across Black and ethnic minority groups.

Some ethnocentric health interventions are clearly biased towards the dominant culture, and mainstream counselling may be inappropriate for some Black and ethnic minority groups. Ethnocentrism is a belief that one's way of life and view of the world are inherently superior to others and more desirable (Leininger and McFarland 2002). Studies have shown the predominance of Eurocentric counselling and support by treatment staff, and staff ignorance of cultural factors that impact on drug use and drug treatment (Abdulrahim et al. 1994, NTA 2003). The literature has also shown how ethnocentrism among professionals shapes the experience of mental health services by Black and ethnic minority users (Littlewood and Lipsedge 1989). Unaddressed ethnocentrism can compromise nurse–patient relationships and lead to misdiagnosis, mistreatment, and insufficient treatment (Greipp 1995). This is applicable also to professionals in the substance-misuse services.

Many ethnic minorities have very little knowledge or real experience of counselling and counselling process (Rassool 2006). A client-centred approach, as advocated by the literature, may not be the type of approach that the client is looking for. A transcultural approach may be more appropriate as part of the therapeutic intervention strategies in the management of dual diagnosis in Black and ethnic minority groups. The use of transcultural therapy or counselling has been advocated for dealing with mental health and substance-use problems. Intercultural therapy and counselling recognise the importance of internal realities of culture (beliefs, values, attitudes, religion and language) for both therapist and patient and are sensitive to the external realities of the patient's life (e.g. poverty, refugee status, racism, sexism). Recognising and working with the unconscious aspects of culture, the similarities and differences, in the therapy are considered vital for successful outcome of the therapy (Kareem and Littlewood 2000).

D'Ardenne and Mahtani (1989) stated that 'transcultural counselling is not about being an expert on any given culture but a way of thinking about clients where culture is acknowledged and valued'.

However, there is ample evidence to indicate that nurses frequently fall short of providing sensitive and appropriate care to ethnic minority patients. Gerrish *et al.* (1996) demonstrated how, in the earlier 1990s, nurses in England were inadequately prepared through their education to address the challenge of delivering multi-ethnic nursing care. Whereas the idea of culturally competent nursing has become a recognised theoretical strategy, the elements involved in its application and practices are sometimes vaguely utilised or understood (Kirkland 1998). If cultural competence policy objectives are to be met, it is essential to examine policies and procedures regarding cultural sensitivity and competence to improve the experiences of Black and ethnic minority services users (Loudon *et al.* 1999).

Professional development is essential to develop a workforce in the provision of competence care. In a recent review of cultural competence in mental health care, Bhui *et al.*'s (2007) study shows that there is limited evidence on the effectiveness of cultural competency training and service delivery. The educational curriculum of nurses and allied health and social care professionals should include cultural awareness, cultural knowledge and cultural sensitivity. The curriculum must also address issues of stereo-typing, discrimination and racism that are prevalent in society, and an examination of societal and institutional issues that affect minority cultures should be included (Bhui *et al.* 2007). Classroom discussions that challenge biases, generalisations, and language used, such as the terms 'us' and 'them', are beneficial for student cultural knowledge building (Browne *et al.* 2002). It is stated that, when a person has an inherent caring, appreciation and respect for others, they can display warmth, empathy and genuine-ness and this enables them to have culturally congruent behaviours and attitudes (Administration on Ageing 2001). However, when these three essentials intersect, practitioners can exemplify cultural competence in a manner that recognises values and affirms cultural differences among their clients (Administration on Ageing 2001). Whether this could be achieved through the process of educational and training development remains to be seen.

CONCLUSION

A population-based assessment of local needs would enable us to deliver an acces-sible and effective service provision and delivery based on cultural competence. Understanding cultural variations can help us develop knowledge of how to interact with others and avoid prejudice, stereotypes, biases and clinical uncertainty. In mental health, progress and change are dependent on an inclusive process, involving politicians, policy-makers, service providers from both statutory and voluntary sectors, service users and carers and, most importantly, Black and ethnic minority communities themselves (Sashidaran 2002). Substance misuse in Black and ethnic minority groups in the UK needs to be considered in the context of socio-political perspectives and the permeation of racism. The issues related to working with Black and ethnic minority groups with alcohol and drug problems include language, culture, patriarchy, gender issues, religious beliefs, family pride, health beliefs, stigma, confidentiality, oppression and racism (Rassool 1997).

To work effectively with these client groups requires one not to become an expert in all ethno-cultural groups but to have cultural flexibility, acceptance and understanding; and to perceive the patient or client as an individual (Rassool 1995). What is considered essential is to develop openness to cultural diversity to the relativity of our own beliefs, values and culture. There is an urgent need to prepare nurses and other healthcare professionals in the substance-misuse field on cultural competence and race issues to enable them to work in a culturally sensitive manner. In addition, professional and regulatory bodies and educational institutions should establish standards of care and core competencies to promote standards encouraging culturally competent care and to integrate issues of diversity and culture into curricula.

KEY POINTS

- The provision of culturally competent approach in working with Black and ethnic minority substance misusers has also been advocated by Black and ethnic minority drug-treatment professionals.
- Culture is related to health and healthcare provision and delivery.
- Understanding cultural health behaviour can reduce barriers and promote equity in the delivery of health and social care.
- Cultural competence describes an ability to meet the needs of diverse communities.
- Cultural appropriateness provides the mechanism through which cultural competence is achieved.
- Cultural sensitivity and cultural specificity form the building blocks for culturally appropriate ways of working.
- There are major challenges facing health and social care providers in the provision and delivery of service provision for alcohol and drug users from Black and ethnic minority groups.
- Health and social care professionals must be aware of their own beliefs, practices and perceptions as these may have an impact on the care they provide to clients from diverse cultural backgrounds.
- If cultural competence policy objectives are to be met, it is essential to examine policies and procedures regarding cultural sensitivity and competence to improve the experiences of Black and ethnic minority service users.
- The educational curriculum of nurses and allied health and social care professionals should include cultural awareness, cultural knowledge and cultural sensitivity.

ACTIVITY 23.1

Please state whether the following statements are true or false by ticking where appropriate

	True	False

Culture is an important component and determinant of health

The provision of culturally competent care is not a legal or moral requirement for nurses

Understanding culture allows us to be more aware of cultural differences and stereotypes

The 'world view' of health and illness and their causes is not determined by cultural factors

There are no differences among Black and ethnic minority communities or between members of the same ethnic group

Cultural and religious beliefs should be applied equally to members of a particular Black and ethnic minority group

The goals of cultural competent care are cultural awareness, cultural knowledge, cultural skill and cultural encounters

Awareness of own beliefs, practices and perceptions are important in delivering cultural competence care

Ethnocentrism among professionals shapes the experience of substance-misuse services by Black and ethnic minority users

Unaddressed ethnocentrism can lead to misdiagnosis, mistreatment and insufficient treatment

Transcultural counselling is being an expert on any given culture

ACTIVITY 23.2

There is only one correct answer to the following multiple-choice questions

Cultural competence is
a.   An ability to meet the needs of diverse communities
b.   Understanding and knowledge of cultural differences
c.   The capacity to provide effective healthcare
d.   All of the above

Black and ethnic minority communities are
a.   A heterogeneous group with varying values, attitudes and religious beliefs
b.   A homogeneous group with varying values, attitudes and religious beliefs
c.   A special group with varying values, attitudes and religious beliefs
d.   A group with high prevalence of substance misuse

Essential elements that contribute to become more culturally competent are

a. Valuing diversity and understanding of cultural diversity
b. Awareness of socio-political factors
c. Having limited institutionalised cultural knowledge
d. Provision of existing services

Ethnocentric health interventions are

a. A belief that one's way of life is superior to others
b. A belief that one's view of the world is more desirable
c. A belief that shapes the experiences of professionals
d. All of the above

Intercultural therapy and counselling recognises

a. The importance of internal realities of culture
b. The importance of internal realities of beliefs
c. The importance of external realities of beliefs of the patient's life
d. All of the above

ACTIVITY 23.3

- Define culture
- Define cultural competence
- Discuss the four-stage model of cultural competence
- List the barriers in the provision of cultural competence care
- Identify the core elements needed in the development and provision of cultural competence drug services for Black and ethnic minority communities

REFERENCES

Abdulrahim, D., White, D., Phillips. K., Boyd. G., Nicholson, J. and Elliot, J. (1994) *Ethnicity and Drug Use: Towards the Design of Community Interventions*. Volume 1, London: University of East London, AIDS Research Unit.

Administration on Ageing (2001) *Achieving Cultural Competence: A Guidebook for Providers of Services to Older Americans and Their Families*. www.aoa.gov/prof/adddiv/cultural/addiv cult.asp (accessed 18 September 2007).

Bhui, K., Warfa, N., Edonya, P., McKenzie, K. and Bhugra, D. (2007) Cultural competence in mental health care: a review of model evaluations. *BMC Health Services Research*, 7: 15doi:10.1186/1472-6963-7-15 (accessed 20 September 2007).

Browne, A.J., Johnson, J.L., Bottorff, J.L., Grewal, S. and Hilton, B.A. (2002) Recognizing discrimination in nursing practice. *Canadian Nurse*, 98, 5: 24–7.

Burr, J. (2002) Cultural stereotypes of women from South Asian communities: mental health care professionals' explanations for patterns of suicide and depression. *Social Science and Medicine*, 55, 200: 835–45.

Campinha-Bacote J., Yahle, T. and Langenkamp, M. (1996) The challenge of cultural diversity for nurse educators. *Journal of Continuing Nursing Education*, 27, 2: 59–64.

Chandra, J. (1996) *Facing up to Difference: A Toolkit for Creating Culturally Competent Health Services for Black and Minority Ethnic Communities*. London: The King's Fund.

Cross, T.L., Bazron, B.J., Dennis, K.W. and Isaacs, M.R. (1989) *Towards a Culturally Competent System of Care*. Volume I. CASSP Technical Assistance Center. Washington, DC: Georgetown University Child Development Center.

D'Ardenne, P. and Mahtani, A. (1989) *Transcultural Counselling in Action*. London: Sage.

Davis, K. (1997) *Exploring the Intersection between Cultural Competency and Managed Behavioral Health Care Policy: Implications for State and County Mental Health Agencies*. Alexandria, VA: National Technical Assistance Center for State Mental Health Planning.

Department of Health (1999a) *Reducing Health Inequalities: An Action Report*. London: The Stationery Office.

Department of Health (1999b) *National Service Framework for Mental Health Modern Standards and Service*. London: Department of Health.

Fernandez, J. (2004) Cultural considerations: improving community involvement. *Substance Misuse Management in General Practice, Net Work* (September), 9, 8.

Gerrish, K. (2000) Individualised care: its conceptualisation and practice within a multiethnic society. *Journal of Advanced Nursing*, 32: 91–9.

Greipp, M.E. (1995) Culture and ethics: a tool for analysing the effects of biases on the nurse-patient relationship. *Nursing Ethics*, 2: 211–21.

Kareem, J. and Littlewood, R. (2000) *Intercultural Therapy*. Oxford: Blackwell.

Kavanagh, K.H. and Kennedy, P.H. (1992) *Promoting Cultural Diversity: Strategies for Health Care Professionals*, Newbury Park, CA: Sage Publications, Inc.

Kirkland, S. (1998) Nurses' description of caring for culturally diverse clients. *Clinical Nursing Research*, 7: 125–46.

Leininger, M.M. (ed.) (1991) *Culture Care Diversity and Universality: A Theory of Nursing*. New York: National League of Nursing.

Leininger, M. and McFarland, M. (2002) *Transcultural Nursing: Concepts, Theories, Research, and Practice*, 3rd edition. New York: McGraw-Hill.

Leonard, B.J. and Plotnikoff, G.A. (2000) Awareness: the heart of cultural competence. *Advanced Practice in Acute and Critical Care*, 11, 1: 51–9.

Littlewood, R. and Lipsedge, M. (1989) *Aliens and Alienists: Ethnic Minorities and Psychiatry*. London: Unwin Hyman.

Loudon, R., Anderson, M., Gill, P. and Greenfield, S. (1999) Educating medical students for work in culturally diverse societies. *JAMA*, 282, 9: 875–80.

NTA (2002) *Race Equality Scheme and Workplan*. London: National Treatment Agency.

NTA (2003) *Black and Ethnic Minority Communities: A Review of the Literature on Drug Use and Related Service Provision*. London: National Treatment Agency. www.nta.nhs.uk.

Nursing and Midwifery Council (2004) *The NMC Code of Professional Conduct: Standards for Conduct, Performance and Ethics*. www.nmc-uk.org (accessed 28 September 2007).

Papadopoulos, I., Tilki, M. and Taylor, G. (1998): *Transcultural Care: A Guide for Health Care Professionals*. Wiltshire: Quay Books.

Rassool, G. Hussein (1995) The health status and health care of ethno-cultural minorities in the United Kingdom: an agenda for action. *Journal of Advanced Nursing*, 21: 199–201.

Rassool, G. Hussein (1997) Ethnic minorities and substance misuse. In G. Hussein Rassool and M. Gafoor (eds) *Addiction Nursing: Perspectives on Professional and Clinical Practice*. Cheltenham: Stanley Nelson.

Rassool, G. Hussein (2006) Black and ethnic minority communities: substance misuse and mental health: whose problems anyway. In G. Hussein Rassool (ed.) *Dual Diagnosis Nursing*. Oxford: Blackwell Publications.

Sangster, D., Shiner, M., Sheikh, N. and Patel, K. (2002): *Delivering Drug Services to Black and Ethnic Minority Communities*, DPAS/P16. London: Home Office Drug Prevention and Advisory Service (DPAS). Also available on http://www.drugs.gov.uk.

Sashidaran, S.P. (2002) *Inside Outside: Improving Mental Health Services for Black and Minority Ethnic Communities in England*. London: Department of Health.

Singer, M. and Clair, S. (2003) Syndemics and public health: reconceptualizing disease in bio-social context *Medical Anthropology Quarterly*, 17: 423–41.

Tervalon, M. and Murray-Garcia, J. (1998) Cultural humility versus cultural competence: a critical distinction in defining physician training outcomes in multicultural education. *Journal of Health Care Poor Underserved*, 9, 2: 117–25.

PART 5

CARE PLANNING AND INTERVENTION STRATEGIES

CHAPTER 24

FRAMEWORK FOR ASSESSMENT, RISK ASSESSMENT AND SCREENING

OBJECTIVES

- Describe briefly the client's journey.

- Identify the types of assessment.

- Describe the aims and purpose of screening or initial assessment.

- Describe the aims and purpose of triage screening.

- Describe the aims and purpose of comprehensive assessment.

- Have an awareness of the barriers in assessing those with dual diagnosis.

- Identify and assess possible risk behaviours.

- Assess possible risks and the individual's understanding of services available.

- Carry out assessment to identify and prioritise needs.

- Carry out comprehensive substance-misuse assessment.

- Discuss issues related to confidentiality and records keeping.

TREATMENT JOURNEY

Assessment and care planning are a continuing process and a foundation for good clinical practice. They are a fundamental component within the framework of the systematic approach to the provision of care and interventions. *Models of Care* (NTA 2002) place emphasis on assessment, care planning and co-ordination of care. For a systematic approach to health and social care interventions, evaluation of care should be an important component of the process of care. It is stated that all those who enter into structured drug and alcohol treatment services should receive a written care plan, agreed with the client (NTA 2002). The progression through the drug treatment system has been described as the client journey (Audit Commission 2004) and covers all stages of a person's involvement with services, from referral discharge and continuing care.

The National Treatment Agency's *Treatment Effectiveness Strategy* (NTA 2005) divides the treatment journey into four overlapping components:

- engagement
- treatment delivery (including maintenance)
- community integration (which underpins both delivery and treatment maintenance or completion)
- treatment completion (for all those who choose to be drug-free and who can benefit).

This framework guides assessment and care planning, which should be specifically targeted and focused on setting goals and objectives, and monitoring outcome in relation to these four stages in the client journey (NTA 2006a). The phases of the treatment journey are presented in Figure 24.1.

The treatment journey is considered to be a cyclical process from engagement, retention, follow-up, re-engagement of drop-out clients to completion of treatment. However, in clinical practice, clients may not go through the process of engagement, treatment delivery and exit from treatment in sequential phase. They are more likely to enter or exit at different phases at different times during their alcohol or drug-using careers.

The provision of care and treatment should be needs-led across different care settings and reflected in the capacity to assess needs, diagnose, formulate care plan and implement and evaluate care. The emphasis is on collaborative working or shared care with other members of the team. The empowerment of individuals and their carers to actively participate in the planning, delivery and evaluation of care is also part of the strategy of good practice.

ASSESSMENT

Assessment is only one of the stages in the systematic approach to care and interventions. Assessment is a dynamic and interpersonal process in which patients are given the opportunity to understand their 'addiction' and health-related needs and provides information on what interventions are required. It is a comprehensive analysis of an individual's needs and related problems which is based on the collection of data of the

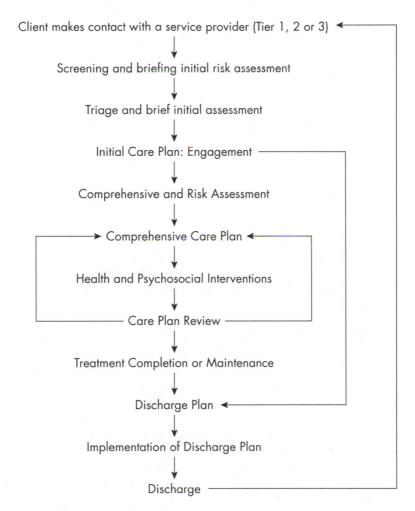

Client makes contact with a service provider (Tier 1, 2 or 3)

Screening and briefing initial risk assessment

Triage and brief initial assessment

Initial Care Plan: Engagement

Comprehensive and Risk Assessment

Comprehensive Care Plan

Health and Psychosocial Interventions

Care Plan Review

Treatment Completion or Maintenance

Discharge Plan

Implementation of Discharge Plan

Discharge

FIGURE 24.1 Service user's treatment journey

Source: Adapted from NTA (2006)

physical or medical, psychosocial and spiritual needs of the individual. Assessment takes the form of interviewing in the taking and recording of a medical or nursing and psychosocial history.

The purposes of assessment are to gather information for the planning of care and health or social care interventions, to intervene in urgent medical and psychological problems, to provide feedback for clients on their level of substance misuse and to build a rapport with the client. The maintenance of rapport, empathy, genuineness and being non-judgemental are critical in the process of assessment. Evidence suggests that the initial clinical encounter has a significant influence in changing the drinker's attitudes, enhance commitment and clarify goals (Edwards *et al.* 2003). The assessment process should result in a written document that can be referred to and used as a basis for discussing care planning, goals and objectives with the client, and implementation and evaluation of the care plan.

LEVELS OF ASSESSMENT

The *Models of Care* (NTA 2002) identified three levels of assessment: screening, triage and comprehensive assessment.

Screening or initial assessment

Screening or initial assessment is a brief process that aims to determine whether an individual has a drug and alcohol problem, health-related problems and risk behaviours. It is likely that this type of assessment is carried out in generic settings (hospital or primary health care). Substance misusers may be present in A&E departments with overdose, self-harm, lost prescriptions, withdrawal seizures, delirium tremens and withdrawal syndrome. The outcome of screening will determine the level of interventions and the urgency of the referral to alcohol or drug treatment services. Screening assessment may be an enabling process that can motivate the substance misusers to move from a pre-contemplation to a contemplation stage of change through brief opportunistic intervention. Through the assessment process, there is a window of opportunity to promote heath education and harm reduction strategies.

The CAGE questionnaire is the simplest, and its four questions could easily be incorporated in the routine assessment process. Two or more positive responses are said to identify the problem drinker. This short questionnaire concentrates on the consequences rather than on the quantity or frequency of alcohol use. It includes the following questions.

1   Have you ever felt that you should *cut* down your drinking?
2   Have people *annoyed* you by criticising your drinking?
3   Have you ever felt bad or *guilty* about your drinking?
4   Have you ever had a drink first thing in the morning to steady your nerves, or get rid of a hangover (*eye-opener*)?

A number of screening instruments have been introduced to assess alcohol and drug problems and comorbidity. Table 24.1 (opposite) presents a summary of screening instruments for alcohol and drug problems. Table 24.2 on page 330 presents the FAST Alcohol Screening Test.

Triage assessment

Triage assessment usually takes place when substance misusers first contact the substance-misuse services. The aim of triage assessment is to determine the severity and urgency of the client's problems and the most appropriate type of treatment for the client (NTA 2006b). Triage assessment involves a complete assessment including a client's readiness to engage in treatment, risk behaviours and the urgency to access treatment. Subsequently, a client might be offered services or referred to another specialist service.

Table 24.1 Screening tools for alcohol and drug problems

Screening tool	Description	Reference
CAGE	This easy-to-use patient questionnaire is a screening test for problem drinking and potential alcohol problems	Ewing 1984
AUDIT: The Alcohol Use Disorders Identification Test	Brief self-report questionnaire (World Health Organization) to identify people whose alcohol consumption has become hazardous or harmful to their health	Babor *et al.* 1992
CUAD: The Chemical Use, Abuse and Dependence scale	Brief (20 minutes to administer), reliable and validated tool for the identification of substance-use disorders in severely mentally ill inpatients	Appleby *et al.* 1996
FAST: The FAST Alcohol Screening Test	Brief 4-item questionnaire, potentially the shortest screening tool	Hodgson *et al.* 2002
DAST-10: The Drug Abuse Screening Test	Self-report questionnaire for measuring the severity of drug (not alcohol) dependence	Skinner 1982
DALI: The Dartmouth Assessment of Lifestyle Instrument	An 18-item interviewer-administered tool (on average 6 minutes to complete). It was developed primarily to detect alcohol, cannabis and cocaine use disorders	Rosenberg *et al.* 1998
MMSE: Mini-Mental State Examination	Brief, quantitative measure to screen for cognitive impairment, to estimate its severity, to follow cognitive changes over time and to document response to treatment	Folstein *et al.* 1975
PRISM: The Psychiatric Research Interview for Substance and Mental Disorders	Diagnostic interview based on DSM-IV. More reliable for assessing psychiatric disorders in those who have co-morbid substance-use disorders	Hasin *et al.* 1996
SATS: The Substance Abuse Treatment Scale	To evaluate treatment progress or as an outcome measure. The scale is intended for assessing a person's stage of substance-misuse treatment	McHugo *et al.* 1995

Source: Adapted from Crawford and Crome, 2001

Comprehensive assessment

Alcohol and drug misusers with complex needs require assessment that is comprehensive and multi-professional to plan effective care and treatment. Comprehensive assessment is carried out when a client may (NTA 2006b):

- require structured and/or intensive intervention
- have significant psychiatric and/or physical co-morbidity
- have significant level of risk of harm to self or others
- be in contact with multiple service providers
- have a history of disengagement from drug treatment services
- be pregnant or have children 'at risk'.

Table 24.2 The FAST alcohol screening test

1. **How often do you have eight or more drinks on one occasion?**

   __ Never   __Less Than Monthly · __ Monthly   __ Weekly   __ Daily or Almost Daily

2. **How often during the last year have you been unable to remember what happened the night before because you had been drinking?**

   __ Never   __Less Than Monthly   __ Monthly   __ Weekly   __ Daily or Almost Daily

3. **How often during the last year have you failed to do what was normally expected of you because of your drinking?**

   __ Never   __Less Than Monthly   __ Monthly   __ Weekly   __ Daily or Almost Daily

4. **Has a relative or friend, a doctor or other health worker been concerned about your drinking or suggested you cut down?**

   __ No   __ Yes, but not in the last year.   __ Yes in the last year.

Source: Hodgson *et al.* (2001)

Scoring the FAST test
Score questions 1, 2 and 3 as follows:

- Never – 0 points
- Less than monthly – 1 point
- Monthly – 2 points
- Weekly – 3 points
- Daily or almost daily – 4 points
- Score question 4 as follows:
- No – 0 points
- Yes, but not in the last year – 2 points
- Yes, in the last year – 4 points

The maximum score is 16. A total score of 3 indicates hazardous drinking.

If a person answer 'never' on the first question, he or she is not a hazardous drinker and the remaining questions are not necessary.

If a person answers 'weekly' or 'daily or almost daily' on the first question, he or she is considered a hazardous drinker and the rest of the questions are skipped.

If a person answers 'monthly' or 'less than monthly' to the first question, the other three questions are needed to complete the screening for hazardous drinking.

Taking a drug and alcohol history is a detailed assessment of the current presentation of an individual's drug- and alcohol-taking pattern of use. One of the initial tasks of the assessment is to discern the individual's views of their drug and/or alcohol consumption. The assessment should then focus on the current pattern of substance misuse, the type of drug used, quantities of substances used, level of dependence, risk behaviours, associated problems, source of help, source of access to psychoactive substance(s) and periods of abstinence and relapse. In order to ascertain the level of dependency, it is important to ask about experiences of withdrawal symptoms or any medical complications. An outline of the assessment is shown in Table 24.3.

Table 24.3 Assessment of substance use

• Statement of the need or problem	Consider the individual's concerns, issues, needs or problems
• Current drug and alcohol use	Type, quantity, frequency and route of administration (drug)
• Pattern of drug or alcohol use	Details of drug or alcohol taking for past week or month
• Current use of other substances	Prescribed, illicit or over-the counter drugs
• Level of dependence	Any withdrawal symptoms. Evidence of increasing tolerance
• Associated problems	Any medical, psychiatric, social or legal problems
• Risk behaviours	Source of injecting equipment. Sharing of equipment. Knowledge about sterilisation and needle-exchange services. Sexual behaviour when intoxicated
• Periods of abstinence or relapse	Duration, periods of abstinence – voluntary or enforced. Reasons for lapse or relapse
• Sources of help	Social support systems. Statutory agencies. Local authorities. Voluntary agencies. Self-help groups
• Coping strategies and strengths	Previous strategies in coping with use of alcohol and drug use. Achievements, strengths and positive aspects of the individual

Source: Rassool and Winnington (2006)

Assessment all too often focuses only on the individual's negative aspects of substance misuse such as an individual's weakness, risks and problems. The inclusion of an assessment of positive aspects of the individual regarding substance misuse may highlight and enhance the self-efficacy and self-esteem of the individual. This positive approach may enable the individual to engage with the service with less resistance and also influence the individual's coping strategies and treatment outcomes (Rassool and Winnington 2006). The position of strengths should focus on strategies that the individual has 'successfully' used in previous attempt to manage substance misuse and psychiatric symptoms – for example, previously using coping strategies that were drug- or alcohol-free.

A comprehensive assessment is an ongoing process and may take place over a few weeks and involve assembling information from a variety of sources including partners, significant others, key workers, doctors and nurses. However, the accountability for completion of the comprehensive assessment must be clear, and services often have a named key or allocated worker leading for each case. The usefulness of self-report or check list in the assessment of the levels of substance misuse is limited. Additional and independent collateral data and laboratory investigations would provide confirmation of the presence or absence of substance use.

ASSESSMENT OF SUBSTANCE MISUSE AND PSYCHIATRIC DISORDERS

Individuals with dual diagnosis have complex or multiple needs which are often difficult to assess comprehensively. Prior to undertaking a full and comprehensive assessment, there are some observations that may indicate substance misuse and/or mental health problem(s). This may warrant further investigations in the process of assessment and diagnosis. Table 24.4 presents the indicators for further assessment.

Table 24.4 Indicators for further assessment

- Use of psychoactive substances to control thoughts and feelings
- Self-medication of psychoactive substances for alleviating mental health problems
- Use of psychoactive substances to balance or reduce side effects of prescribed medications
- Misuse of prescription and over-the-counter drugs
- Unable to reduce alcohol and/or drug use
- Previous detoxification and/or rehabilitation
- Symptoms of withdrawal
- High tolerance of psychoactive substances
- Drug-seeking behaviour
- Self-harm
- Frequency of mood swings and sadness
- Anger and impulsiveness
- Over-suspiciousness

Source: Adapted from Rassool and Winnington (2006)

Clinical assessment for those with substance-misuse and psychiatric disorders is difficult because substance misuse can mask psychiatric symptoms or distort diagnosis. The inability to distinguish the effects of psychoactive substances on the individual's mental state from symptoms of mental health problems add to the complexities of assessing an individual with dual diagnosis (Rassool and Winnington 2006). Since many psychiatric symptoms are a temporary result of substance-misuse withdrawal or drug or alcohol intoxication rather than 'dual diagnosis', it would be reasonable for workers to manage the immediate symptoms until the individual has had time to recover from drug intoxication or drug withdrawal state. That is why it is unlikely that a comprehensive assessment can be completed at first contact with individuals.

The lack of knowledge and skills in assessing mental health or taking a drug and alcohol history and the attitudes towards substance misusers or individuals with drug and alcohol problems may influence the assessment process and subsequent interventions (Rassool and Winnington 2006). Many individuals with dual diagnosis remain unnoticed in both drug and alcohol services and mental health services. The lack of integration or segregation of mental health and drug and alcohol services perpetuates this problem, as staff from different service domains often focus on observation and assessment that are part of their repertoire of knowledge and skills. That is, mental health workers may identify mental health problems but overlook drug and alcohol problems, whereas workers in drug and alcohol services focus on substance misuse and fail to recognise mental health problems. Assessment may therefore become focused on the need to establish primacy rather than the pursuit of meeting the individual's needs (Banerjee *et al.* 2002). It is argued that individuals with dual diagnosis can become system misfits when they do not conform to the expectations established with drug and alcohol and mental healthcare systems (Bachrach 1986).

A central aspect of working in dual diagnosis is the ability to provide a comprehensive assessment of mental health history and current symptoms, current and historical substance use and misuse, current physical health, assessment of social needs and the awareness of diversity amongst those individuals with dual diagnosis and how these major aspects impact on the current presentation or baseline behaviour. One feature of a dual diagnosis assessment is the use of 'time lines', by recording the sequence of events for both substance misuse and mental health problems over a given time period. Time lines can provide invaluable information, particularly in relation to which event occurs first, substance misuse or mental health problems; additionally they can be used to help indicate priority for treatment actions (Moore and Rassool 2001).

The art of completing a substance-misuse assessment relies on incorporating the following elements (Rassool and Winnington 2006):

- assessment of history and current nature of the type and frequency of psychoactive substances used
- assessment of mental health history and current symptoms
- assessment of current physical health
- assessment of level and nature of risks in evidence
- assessment of social needs (housing, employment, social networks)
- assessment with self-awareness of diversity issues and cultural competence.

A number of screening instruments have been introduced to assess dual diagnosis (Rassool and Winnington 2006). A good practice suggestion for assessment of clients with dual diagnosis (Rethink & Turning Point 2004) includes the following:

- Consider the client's concerns.
- Consider a range of needs.
- Avoid assumptions and keep an open mind.
- Remember that timelines can be a useful tool (Moore and Rassool 2001).
- Monitor regularly.
- Recognise positive achievements.

RISK ASSESSMENT

Risk assessment and management are a core element of good practice in substance-misuse services. The need for risk assessment and management appears to be in response to perceived failings in the policy of community care; to criticisms of current practice following inquiries into tragedies involving people with serious mental illness; to government initiatives to reduce self-harm and improve community management of people with mental illness; and to the need for mental health providers to reduce the increasing costs associated with litigation and complaints (Doyle 2004). It is good practice to carry out risk assessment as part of screening, triage and comprehensive assessment (NTA 2006a).

The aim of risk assessment is to identify risk factors which can be used to determine the likelihood of 'harm' to self and others. This information is subsequently used to provide appropriate health interventions as part of a comprehensive care plan. The severity of alcohol and substance misuse, including the use of combined psychoactive substances, is related to the risk of overdose and/or suicide. The exploration of the possible association between substance misuse and increased risk of aggressive or antisocial behaviour forms an integral part of the risk assessment, and should be explicitly documented if present (Department of Health 2002).

Risk assessment should fully involve the individual being assessed, relevant professionals and any informal carer or significant other. Individuals may fail to disclose 'risky behaviours' or self-harm: that is why it is important to seek information from a variety of sources. Risk assessment is an ongoing process and there are several critical points when practitioners need to conduct further assessment of 'risky behaviours' – for example, before individuals are discharged from hospital or are referred to any agency or service provision or return to be looked after by their informal carers.

The principal elements of risk assessment and management are:

- risk of suicide or self-harm – ideas, plans and intentions
- risk of overdose, polydrug use and unsafe injecting practices
- risk of harm or violence to others
- risk of harm or abuse or exploitation by others
- risk of severe self-neglect
- risk related to physical condition.

There is no specific method of predicting 'risky behaviour' but there are several factors that have been reported in the literature to be associated with an increasing probability of risk behaviours. There may be patterns of past and current factors of psychosocial and physical problems that may be indicative of risk behaviours. A summary of the predisposing and precipitating risk factors is presented in Table 24.5.

Assessment of a risk of violence to others should be notified to informal carers and all agencies and key people involved in their care and support. Where there is such a risk, it is crucial that adequate personal care, supervision and treatment are provided. A special consideration regarding the assessment harm or violence to others is the potential victim(s) of the perpetrator. It is worth exploring the issues of the likely victims and whether the victims are aware of the risks posed to them and to others. Another element of risk assessment that requires attention from practitioners includes the

Table 24.5 Predictors of risk

Precipitating factors	Predisposing risk factors
• Specific plan	• Previous history of harm to self or others
• Neurological (Organic disorders)	• Family history of harm or mental illness
• Continuing high suicidal and behavioural intent	• Borderline or impulsive personality
• Hopelessness	• Social exclusion
• Hallucinations and persecutory delusions	• Lack of support network
• Social isolation	• Past sexual or physical abuse
• Recent loss or separation	• Depression
• Recent psychiatric hospitalisation	• Schizophrenia
• Relationship breakdown	• Substance misuse
• Unemployment	
• Imprisonment or threat of imprisonment	
• Homelessness	
• Cultural and diversity issues (e.g. shame)	
• Intoxication with alcohol or drugs	
• Poor compliance with medication or treatment programmes	
• Poor communications between professionals	

Source: Adapted from Evans and Sullivan (2001)

individuals' vulnerability to dangers or exploitations such as sexual, financial, occupational and familial, particularly when their judgement or cognitive functioning is seriously impaired (Rassool and Winnington 2006).

It is critical to assess the risk of self-harm and attempted suicide of individuals with dual diagnosis as they are more likely to pose risk to themselves than to others. An examination should cover previous incidents of self-harm and their frequency and seriousness, whether the previous attempt(s) was accidental or intended, previous coping or intervention strategies and current intensions, plan, access and means to carry out the plan (Rassool and Winnington 2006). This assessment should be conducted with a sensitive approach and in a non-judgemental manner despite the difficulties that the practitioners may face in asking about such 'risky behaviours'. It is a myth that raising the subject of 'risky behaviours' or self-harm is likely to encourage the individual to engage in them. By acknowledging the thoughts and feelings relating to the 'risk' behaviour, practitioners can work through with them using techniques such as anger management, individual therapy and group work (Rethink & Turning Point 2004).

An examination of the' risky behaviours' should include the following questions:

- Does the individual have a suicide plan or serious intentions?
- How specific is the plan?
- What method will be used?
- Does the individual have the means to carry out the plan?
- When will the 'risky behaviour' happen?

Finally, it is stated that effective risk management should not disempower people but should minimise risk through open discussion, standardised assessment and the use of up-to-date, jointly owned care plans: the key to all these is greater collaboration and communication (O'Rourke and Bird 2001). Equally, it is important that risk assessment is based on an appropriate evidence base and the management of risk is planned in a systematic way by the multidisciplinary team to enable more effective interventions. Consultations and communications about risk assessment and management of the individual between members of the multidisciplinary team and appropriate personnel from other agencies or services are good clinical practice. The importance of documentations or records and information-sharing is fundamental when assessing the future potential risk of an individual.

TESTING FOR CURRENT DRUG AND ALCOHOL USE

If self-reported assessment indicates current use of drugs and/or alcohol, laboratory investigations may be undertaken to aid early identification and diagnosis. The investigations are also helpful in contributing objective information to the overall assessment. Drugs and alcohol can be measured directly in serum, urine, exhaled air and hair. Urine analysis is widely undertaken to measure or assess for drug use.

There are two main methods for testing a urine sample. Special immunological procedures called immunoassay tests are based on detecting antibodies to ingested drugs but gas chromatography is more accurate. Hair testing can be used to detect drugs laid down within the growing hair follicle but is more expensive than urine testing. However, hair analysis carries a major advantage over urine testing in that it covers much longer periods than a single urine test (McPhillips *et al.* 1997). Serum saliva tests are currently under evaluation. These tests only estimate whether drugs are present or absent and do not measure the amount of drugs in the body. The detection periods for urine drug screening are presented in Table 24.6.

A number of blood tests can be undertaken to assess the presence of drugs or alcohol. Essential investigations include liver function tests (LFT), gamma-glutamyl transferase (GGT), asparate transaminase (AST) and mean corpuscles volume (MCV). A summary of those special blood tests for drug and alcohol is given in Table 24.7. When injecting drug users share needles, syringes or other paraphernalia, cross infections are likely to occur. Blood tests can also be carried out to determine HIV and hepatitis B and C. These tests must always be accompanied by pre-test and post-test counselling. Guidance on hepatitis C (Department of Health 2001) is available for those working with drug users.

Table 24.6 Detection periods for urine drug screening

Substance	Maximum range (hours and days)
Amphetamine	48 hours
Methamphetamine	48 hours
Barbiturates	
• Short-acting	24 hours
• Intermediate-acting	48–72 hours
• Long-acting	7 days or more
Benzodiazepines (therapeutic dose)	3 days
• Ultra-short-acting (e.g. Midazolam)	12 hours
• Short-acting (e.g. Triazolam)	24 hours
• Intermediate-acting (e.g. Temazepam or Chlordiazepoxide)	40–80 hours
• Long-acting (e.g. Diazepam or Nitrazepam)	7 days
Cannabinoids (Marijuana)	
• Single use	3 days
• Moderate use (4 times per week)	4 days
• Heavy use (daily)	10 days
• Chronic heavy use	21–7 days
Cocaine metabolites	2–3 days
Codeine/Morphine/Propoxyphene (Heroin is detected in urine as the 48 hours metabolite morphine)	48 hours
Methaqualone	7 days or more
Methadone (maintenance dosing)	7–9 days (approximate)
Norpropoxyphene Phencyclidine (PCP)	6–48 hours 8 days (approximate)

Source: Department of Health (1999a)

Table 24.7 Special laboratory alcohol and drug tests

Tests	Detected substance(s)	Observations
Gamma glutamyl transferase (GGT)	Alcohol	Elevated before liver damage. More likely to have liver damage at higher readings
Liver functions tests (LFT)	Alcohol and drug	Liver damage due to alcohol
Full blood count	Alcohol	Mean red blood cells raised in heavy chronic drinkers
Asparate transaminase (AST)	Alcohol	Suggest alcohol-related liver damage
Uric acid	Alcohol	Increase of urates and possibly gout
Haemoglobin	Drug and alcohol	Anaemia due to poor nutrition or vitamin deficiencies
Tests for HIV, hepatitis B and C	Drug	History of injecting

Source: Rassool, G. Hussein and Winnington, J. (2006) Framework for multidimensional assessment, in G. Hussein Rassool (ed.), *Dual Diagnosis Nursing*. Oxford: Blackwell Publications

CONFIDENTIALITY

A guide to *Consent and Confidentiality Guidance for Staff in Drug Treatment Services* is published by the Eastern Region Public Health Observatory (ERPHO). The Department of Health has produced a code of practice for NHS staff that addresses confidentiality issues, and is part of the contractual obligation of NHS staff (www.doh.gov.uk). Patient information is generally held under legal and ethical obligations of confidentiality. Information provided in confidence should not be used or disclosed in a form that might identify a patient without his or her consent (Department of Health 2007). For more comprehensive information see *Patient Confidentiality* (Department of Health 2007) and *Guidance for Access to Health Records* (Department of Health 2003).

The exchange and sharing of information is part of good practice and is vital to the health and social care process. This has to be done in observing the code of practice regarding confidentiality and underpinned by clear policies and procedures. It is important as part of the assessment to inform clients how information relating to them may be shared and what happens if information has to be shared. Information contained in the care plan can be divulged to all named participants including the user. In exceptional circumstances some or all of the information contained in the care plan can be withheld from the user if divulging the information would compromise safety to the user, the user's children, the professionals or the wider public (NTA 2006b).

Informed consent is an ongoing agreement by a person to receive treatment, undergo procedures (or participate in research), after risks, benefits and alternatives have been adequately explained to them (Royal College of Nursing 2005). The consent should be documented, accessible in the client's notes and subject to regular review. A decision by the user to provide informed consent to disclosure of information should also be subject to regular review and the disclosure should take place within the professional codes of conduct of the service (NTA 2006b).

RECORD KEEPING (CASE NOTES)

Record keeping is a basic health and social care practice and is applicable to all services. A record is 'anything that contains information (in any media) which has been created or gathered as a result of any aspect of the work of NHS employees' (Department of Health 1999b). This definition can be applied to all addiction specialists in contact with patients. All record systems, whether written or computerised, must have processes in place that follow the Caldicott guidelines (Caldicott Report 1987) and are compatible with the Data Protection and Freedom of Information Acts. Within the Data Protection Act 1998 a health record is defined as a record consisting of information about the physical or mental health or condition of an identifiable individual made by or on behalf of a health professional in connection with the care of that individual. The Data Protection Act 1998 gives every living person or their authorised representative the right to apply for access to their health records irrespective of when they were compiled.

The record may be a compilation of every episode of care for that individual or may contain information about the current episode of care only. Record keeping should be simple, accurate, legible and up-to-date. Clinical records must be kept confidential at all times and stored in a secure place. The process of keeping records involves consideration by third parties, including courts of law and other health or social care professionals.

NHS ELECTRONIC CARE RECORDS

Under the system, everyone will have a computer-based care file with basic information to provide healthcare staff with quicker access to reliable information. The NHS Care Records Service aims to make caring across organisational boundaries safer and more efficient. This will mean that instead of having separate records in all the different services key workers will have access to the information they need. The electronic patient records are available to staff whenever a client visits hospital or community-based services. Access to the electronic record is strictly password-controlled to maintain patient confidentiality at all times.

KEY POINTS

- The progression through the drug treatment system has been described as the client journey and covers all stages of a person's involvement with services, from referral to discharge and continuing care.
- Assessment and care planning are a continuing process and a foundation for good clinical practice.

- *Models of Care* place emphasis on assessment, care planning and co-ordination of care.
- Three are three levels of assessment: screening, triage and comprehensive assessment.
- Screening or initial assessment is a brief process that aims to determine whether an individual has a drug and alcohol problem, health-related problems and risk behaviours.
- Triage assessment usually takes place when substance misusers first contact substance-misuse services.
- Triage assessment involves a complete assessment including a client's readiness to engage in treatment, risk behaviours and the urgency to access treatment.
- Alcohol and drug misusers with complex needs require assessment that is comprehensive and multi-professional to plan effective care and treatment.
- Taking a drug and alcohol history is a detailed assessment of the current presentation of an individual's drug- and alcohol-taking pattern of use.
- Assessment all too often focuses only on the individual's negative aspects of substance misuse such as an individual's weakness, risks and problems.
- Clinical assessment for those with substance misuse and psychiatric disorders is difficult because substance misuse can mask psychiatric symptoms or distort diagnosis.
- Many individuals with dual diagnosis remains unnoticed in both drug and alcohol services and mental health services.
- Risk assessment is an ongoing process, and there are several critical points when practitioners need to conduct further assessment of 'risky behaviours'.
- The exchange and sharing of information has to be done in observing the code of practice regarding confidentiality and underpinned by clear policies and procedures.
- Record keeping is a basic health and social care practice and is applicable to all services.

ACTIVITY 24.1

There is only one correct answer to the following multiple-choice questions

The progression through the drug treatment system has been described as
a.   Referral discharge
b.   The client journey
c.   Continuing care
d.   Engagement

Assessment is
a.   A continuing process
b.   A foundation for good clinical practice
c.   A component of the systematic approach
d.   All of the above

The purposes of assessment are

a.   To gather information for the planning of care
b.   To intervene in urgent medical and psychological problems
c.   To provide feedback for clients
d.   All of the above

The initial clinical encounter in the process of assessment is critical because

a.   It saves time and effort
b.   It enables building of rapport
c.   It is routine procedure
d.   It is part of the referral process

Recording of the assessment is important because it can used as a basis for

a.   Discussing care planning with the client
b.   Discussing goals and objectives with the client
c.   Evaluation of care plan
d.   All of the above

Screening or initial assessment is a brief process that

a.   Aims to determine whether an individual has a drug and alcohol problem
b.   Aims to determine whether an individual has health-related problems
c.   Aims to determine whether an individual has risk behaviours
d.   All of the above

Screening or initial assessment is carried out in

a.   Specialist substance-misuse services
b.   Generic or primary healthcare services
c.   Alcohol specialist services
d.   Drug specialist services

The outcome of screening will determine

a.   The level of interventions
b.   The urgency of the referral to other services
c.   The urgency to meet healthcare needs
d.   All of the above

Triage assessment usually takes place when substance misusers first contact health services except

a.   Alcohol services
b.   Generic services
c.   Drug services
d.   Substance-misuse services

The aim of triage assessment is to determine

a.   The severity of the client's problems
b.   The urgency of the client's problems
c.   The most appropriate type of treatment
d.   All of the above

Alcohol and drug misusers with complex needs require

a.   Screening assessment
b.   Triage assessment
c.   Initial assessment
d.   Comprehensive assessment

Comprehensive assessment is carried out when a client may

a.   Require structured and/or intensive intervention
b.   Have significant psychiatric co-morbidity
c.   Be pregnant or have children 'at risk'
d.   All of the above

Assessment focusing on the client's positive aspects

a.   May enhance the self-efficacy of the client
b.   May enable less resistance from the client
c.   May influence the client's coping strategies
d.   All of the above

A comprehensive assessment is

a.   An ongoing process
b.   May take place over a few weeks
c.   Involve assembling information from a variety of sources
d.   All of the above

Assessment for those with dual diagnosis is difficult because

a.   Substance misuse can mask psychiatric symptoms
b.   Psychiatric problems can distort diagnosis
c.   It may be difficult to distinguish the effects of psychoactive substances
d.   All of the above

'Time lines' are

a.   The recording of the sequence of events for substance misuse
b.   The recording of the sequence of events for mental health
c.   Used to help indicate priority for treatment actions
d.   All of the above

The aim of risk assessment is to

a.   Identify risk factors
b.   Provide appropriate health interventions
c.   Be part of a comprehensive care plan
d.   All of the above

Critical points of 'risky behaviours' include being

a.   Discharged from hospital
b.   Discharged from prison
c.   Looked after by informal carers
d.   All of the above

Confidentiality refers to
a.   Information held under legal and ethical obligations
b.   Exchange and sharing of information
c.   Information disclosure
d.   Information withheld

Informed consent refers to
a.   An ongoing agreement by a person to receive treatment
b.   An agreement to undergo procedures
c.   Explanation of risks, benefits and alternatives given to patient
d.   All of the above

REFERENCES

Audit Commission (2002) *Changing Habits: The Commissioning and Management of Community Drug Treatment Services for Adults.* London: Audit Commission.

Bachrach, L. (1986) The context of care for the chronic mental patient with substance abuse. *Psychiatric Quarterly*, 87, 58: 3–14.

Banerjee, S., Clancy, C. and Crome, I. (2002) *Co-existing Problems of Mental Disorder and Substance Misuse (Dual Diagnosis): An Information Manual.* London: The Royal College of Psychiatrists' Research Unit.

Caldicott Report (1997) *Confidentiality Guidelines.* Oxford: Oxford Radcliffe Hospitals NHS Trust.

Department of Health (1999a) *Drug Misuse and Dependence – Guidelines on Clinical Management.* Norwich: Her Majesty's Stationery Office.

Department of Health (1999b) *For The Record: Managing records in NHS Trusts and Health Authorities*, HSC 1999/053. www.doh.gov.uk/nhsexec/manrec.htm (accessed 30 November 2007)

Department of Health (2001). *Hepatitis C: Guidance for Those Working with Drug Users.* London: Department of Health. www.drugs.gov.uk.

Department of Health (2002) *Mental Health Policy Implementation Guide: Dual Diagnosis Good Practice Guide.* London: Department of Health. www.doh.gov.uk.

Department of Health (2003) *Guidance for Access to Health Records.* London: Department of Health. www.doh.gov.uk.

Department of Health (2007) *Patient Confidentiality.* London: Department of Health. www.doh.gov.uk.

Doyle, M. (2004) Organisational responses to crisis and risk: issues and implications for mental health nurses. In T. Ryan (ed.) *Managing Crisis and Risk in Mental Health Nursing*, 2nd edition, pp. 40–56, Cheltenham: Nelson Thornes.

Eastern Region Public Health Observatory (ERPHO) (2007) *Consent and Confidentiality Guidance for Staff in Drug Treatment Services.* Regional Drugs Health Information Unit, Cambridge: Institute of Public Health. http://www.erpho.org.uk/Download/Public/16123/1/Consent.pdf. (accessed on 22 January 2008).

Edwards, G., Marshall, E.J. and Christopher, C.H. (2003) *The Treatment of Drinking Problems: A Guide for the Helping Professions.* Cambridge: Cambridge University Press.

Hodgson, R., Alwyn ,T., John, B., Thom, B. and Smith, A. (2002) The fast alcohol screening test. *Alcohol and Alcoholism*, 37, 1: 61–6.

McPhillips, M.A., Kelly, F.J., Barnes, T.R.E., Duke, P.J., Gene-Cos, N. and Clark, K. (1997) Detecting comorbid substance misuse among people with schizophrenia in the community: a study comparing the results of questionnaires with analysis of hair and urine. *Schizophrenia Research*, 25: 141–8.

Moore, K. and Rassool, G. Hussein. (2001) Synthesis of addiction & mental health nursing: an approach to community interventions. In G. Hussein Rassool (ed.) *Dual Diagnosis: Substance Misuse and Psychiatric Disorders*. Oxford: Blackwell Publishing.

NTA (2002) *Models of Care for Treatment of Adult Drug Misusers*. London: National Treatment Agency.

NTA (2005) *Treatment Effectiveness Strategy*. London: National Treatment Agency.

NTA (2006a) *Care Planning Practice Guide*. London: National Treatment Agency.

NTA (2006b) *Models of Care updated 2006*. London: National Treatment Agency.

O'Rourke, M. and Bird, L. (2001) *Risk Management in Mental Health: A Practical Guide to Individual Care and Community Safety*. London: Mental Health Foundation Publications.

Rassool, G. Hussein and Winnington. J. (2006) Framework for multidimensional assessment. In G. Hussein Rassool (ed.) *Dual Diagnosis Nursing*. Oxford: Blackwell Publications.

Rethink & Turning Point (2004) *Dual Diagnosis Toolkit: Mental Health and Substance Misuse. A Practical Guide for Professionals and Practitioners*. London: Rethink & Turning Point.

Royal College of Nursing (2005) *Informed Consent in Health and Social Care Research*. London: Royal College of Nursing.

CHAPTER 25

CARE PLANNING: PRINCIPLES AND PRACTICE

OBJECTIVES

- Define what is a care plan.

- Identify the key principles in care planning.

- Differentiate between initial and comprehensive care plan.

- Describe the stages of a client's treatment journey.

- Develop an initial care plan based on the identified needs of clients.

- Understand and discuss the need for client involvement in the care planning process.

- Contribute to care planning and review.

- Identify skills in developing a therapeutic relationship to help engage clients in the assessment and care planning processes.

- Understand and discuss the importance of multi-agency working, information sharing and communication throughout the assessment and care planning processes.

CARE PLANNING AND TREATMENT JOURNEY

The planning phase of the client's treatment journey involves the development of a care plan for the client based on their needs. Care planning provides a 'road map' of the client's treatment journey and a is a key component of structured alcohol and drug treatment interventions. The role of care planning and care co-ordination as key components of an integrated system of treatment for drug and alcohol misusers was identified in *Models of Care for Treatment of Adult Drug Misusers* (NTA 2002). *Models of Care: Update 2006* (NTA 2006a) also identifies the need for service provision to increase their focus on improving the client journey, through a structured care planning approach.

A review of substance-misuse services by a joint working party of the Health Care Commission and NTA (2006) outlines the positive benefits of involving service users at all levels: in their own treatment, in planning specific services and in planning the treatment system at a strategic level. One of the areas that the report draws attention to is that not enough service users had a care plan. The report recommends that all service users should have a comprehensive assessment of their needs and a personal care plan outlining the best course of treatment. The satisfaction of service users is strongly linked to having an up-to-date care plan, which they understand and feel involved in, which meets their individual needs and which is reviewed regularly and as needed (Health Care Commission and NTA 2006)

The client journey may start with primary healthcare services or generic services (A&E departments, maternity services) which may provide interventions across the Tiers 1 to 3 of the *Model of Care* (NTA 2002, 2006a). These services should provide screening and risk assessment to identify the nature and extent of drug and alcohol problems. Interventions at this stage may be the provision of health information, harm reduction strategies and information about specialist services. Depending on the complexities of the health needs of the client, referral to a more specialist service should occur if appropriate. The progression of the client journey (if appropriate) is presented in Figure 25.1.

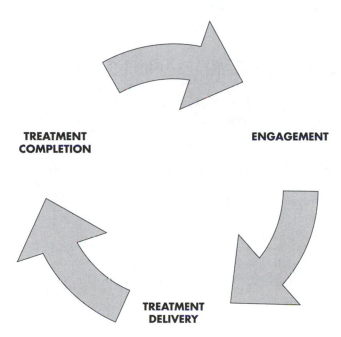

FIGURE 25.1 Treatment journey

WHAT IS A CARE PLAN?

The care planning process, an essential component of the client treatment journey, is a method for setting goals based on the needs identified by an assessment and planning intervention to meet those goals with the client (NTA 2006a). A care plan is a structured and task-oriented plan of action between the client and the health or social care professional. The care plan, a written document, is based on the identification of needs or goals, strengths and risks identified by the assessment process and the main focus of intervention strategies. The care plan is also a tool to monitor any changes in the service user's needs and progress and provides valuable information to other relevant multi-professional professionals. The effectiveness of the care plan is based on the engagement of the service user throughout the assessment and care planning process and he or she should be actively involved in the formulation of the care plan. The care plan should be perceived as a contractual agreement between the client and care provider(s) and show accountability. A care plan should be reviewed and evaluated at regular intervals, and at the request of the service user, their carer or a member of the care team.

The NTA has produced a standard national *Care Planning Practice Guide* (NTA 2006b) and e-learning package (see NTA website). The NTA has designed this course to ensure that service providers are up to date with best practice in care planning. The learning package is a self-teaching tool in three parts. The first part focuses on the aspects of developing a care plan, including confidentiality, risk assessment and goal setting. The second part consists of three interactive case studies, where you apply the principles of good care planning to a pregnant heroin user, a long-term heroin and crack user, and a polydrug user who has just been remanded on bail. Finally, there is an online quiz to evaluate the learning.

KEY PRINCIPLES IN CARE PLANNING

The first step in care planning is the accurate and comprehensive assessment that should form the key elements for decisions about healthcare interventions, care and support. The principles of care planning is based on the holistic needs of the individual, the setting of the goals of treatment, targets to be achieved, the interventions or treatment modalities to be provided and the responsibility and accountability of the agency and professional in the delivery of the interventions. A comprehensive care plan should be agreed with the client and cover the client's needs as identified in one or more of four key domains (NTA 2006b):

- drug and alcohol misuse
- physical and psychological health
- offending behaviour
- social functioning.

Table 25.1 shows the four key domains and associated health and social care outcomes.

Table 25.1 Four key domains

Alcohol and drugs
Drug use, including types of drugs, quantity and frequency of use, pattern of use, route of administration, source of drug (including preparation) and prescribed medication

Alcohol use, including quantity and frequency of use, pattern of use, whether in excess of 'safe' levels and alcohol dependence symptoms

Physical and psychological health
Physical problems, including complications of drugs and alcohol use, blood-borne infections and risk behaviours, liver disease, abscesses, overdose and enduring severe physical disabilities. Pregnancy may also be an issue

Psychological problems include personality problems or disorders, self-harm, history of abuse or trauma, depression and anxiety and severe psychiatric co-morbidity. Contact with mental health services will need to be recorded

Criminal involvement and offending
Legal issues including arrests, fines, outstanding charges and warrants, probation, imprisonment, violent offences and criminal activity. Involvement with workers in the criminal justice system, for example probation workers

Social functioning
Social issues, including childcare issues, partners, domestic violence, family, housing, education, employment, benefits and financial problems

---

Source: NTA (2006a)

Every service user should have a documented care plan which is individualised to the client's needs, develops with the client and significant others, reflects evidence-based practice and interventions and provides for continuity of after-care. The Health Care Commissions and NTA (2006) highlighted the need for services to improve the way they explain and agree care plans with service users. The care plan should be client-centred and the contents should be agreed between client and service provider. Considerations need to be taken of the client's cultural and ethnic background so as to provide cultural competence care.

A care plan should have SMART (specific, measurable, achievable and realistic, time-limited) goals or objectives. The goal must be stated in terms of client achievement and each goal must state a target date for evaluation. Each goal must be accompanied by the treatment intervention which is evidence-based. References to the risk behaviours, management of risk and emergency planning should be made explicit in the care plan. The intervention strategies must also be specific, not global, and appropriate. It may be the case that several interventions are needed to achieve any particular goal. The agency and service provider are responsible for carrying out these interventions, which should always be negotiated with those they name.

The planning of care for the individual in an integrated way will depend on good communication and liaison between agencies and service providers. This should help to ensure sharing of information and a smooth transition between services. It is important to be clear what information will be given to other third parties. The care plan should have a contingency plan should the outcomes fail to be realised. A care plan should be monitored, reviewed and evaluated at regular intervals, and at the request of the client, their significant other or a member of the care team. Reviewing a care plan provides a framework within which the key worker and client can decide whether a goal has been achieved. In addition, a review provides information on any unmet needs and the effectiveness of the care plan. It is important to draw conclusions on the interventions used and consider changes in the intervention strategies that might improve goal achievement. The principles of care planning are presented in Table 25.2.

Table 25.2 Key principles in care planning

Client-centred approach
- Client-directed
- Holistic needs of client
- Client involved in decision-making on the components of the care plan and how it will be delivered

Diversity
- Reflect the cultural and ethnic background, gender and sexuality

Goals
- Need to reflect the outcome of the assessment
- Based on philosophy of care
- SMART – specific, measurable, achievable, realistic and time-bound
- Taking account of individual's current state and motivation
- Short-term and long-term goals

Intervention strategies
- Type of interventions. Pharmacological and psychosocial interventions. Harm reduction

Risk management
- Identification of risk factors as per assessment
- Risk management and contingency plan

Communication and liaison
- Sharing of information in line with service policies on confidentiality and the sharing of information

Key worker
- Developing, implementing and evaluating a care plan
- Deliver heath and psychosocial interventions

Promoting and enhancing engagement
- Where an individual has been difficult to engage in treatment and rehabilitation, the plan should identify a plan for promoting and enhancing their engagement

Monitor
- Monitor plan and changes in client's needs

Review
- Identity their review date

KEY ISSUES IN PLANNING AND DELIVERING CARE

A care programme approach (CPA) aims to ensure effective collaboration between agencies so as to provide a seamless service for individuals with severe mental health problems. CPA addresses both health and social care needs through an integrated and co-ordinated approach. The care programme entitles clients to have a systematic assessment of health and social care needs; an agreed care plan; allocation of a care co-ordinator; and a regular review of progress. This holistic approach to management, treatment, care and support of the client enables links to be made across social work or care services, health, education and employment, housing, criminal justice and voluntary agencies to facilitate access for individuals to the range of services required to meet their needs (Scottish Executive Effective Interventions Unit 2002). When implemented well, it enables multidisciplinary staff to provide an agreed plan of care whilst minimising inter-professional conflict and maximising opportunities for joint working (Simpson 2006). For clients with co-existing substance-misuse and psychiatric disorders who meet the national criteria for the 'enhanced' version of the care programme approach, enhanced care plans should include instructions on what to do in a crisis and details of how to contact someone during non-office hours. They should also incorporate contingency plans so that continuous care and support are provided even when key personnel are not available, whether through sickness, holidays or any unforeseen situations (Department of Health 1999). For dual diagnosis clients, a care plan co-ordinator is a stipulation. The care co-ordinator takes a lead in the formulation of the care plan on behalf of the whole team and other service providers who are involved in the care of the client. For young substance misusers, the responsibility for care planning and delivery of treatment interventions may be located with child and adolescent mental health services, social services or young offenders team.

INITIAL CARE PLAN

During the triage assessment, if the client has been found to have urgent health needs, an initial care plan may be developed. In this instance, this is done prior to a comprehensive assessment. The identification of health or social care needs, setting goals and planning interventions should be part of the initial care plan. The initial care planning stage is an opportunity to engage clients in treatment by delivering advice on harm reduction and ensuring fast-track treatment delivery. Any such initial care plan should address a range of immediate needs, such as referral for rapid prescribing and urgent housing concerns (NTA 2006b). A key worker has the responsibility for the client's initial care plan and to ensure that a comprehensive assessment is undertaken or that appropriate referral is made to another service provider. Examples of the contents of care plan are presented in Table 25.3.

Table 25.3 Examples of care plan contents

Background	Goal	Interventions
A client presents to a drug service with a history of amphetamine use. In a triage assessment she is found to be street homeless	Client to make contact with housing services and obtain temporary housing	Referral to specialist vulnerable housing worker. Completion of assessment of substance misuse
A client who is new to treatment presents with a history of self-harm. Under the care of a community psychiatric nurse (CPN)	To co-ordinate mental health interventions with substance-misuse interventions	To reduce the frequency of self-harming behaviour. To stabilise client mood and reduce drug and/or alcohol use
A client who is new to treatment identifies a history of sharing injecting paraphernalia. The client is very anxious about hepatitis C and worried about having a test	To increase the client's knowledge of blood-borne viruses in preparation for taking a HCV antibody test within three months and to stop needle sharing within three months	To attend the HCV education group the service provides and to discuss the issue in keyworking sessions
A client is using crack cocaine weekly although stable on a daily methadone prescription	To reduce crack cocaine use by 50% over the next three months, as evidenced by production of 50% cocaine-free oral fluid tests	Relapse prevention techniques. Drug diaries. Psycho-education. Skills development to manage cravings and high risk situations. Weekly oral fluid tests
A client is now stable on buprenorphine daily and has been for three months. The client has abstinence as an eventual goal	To reduce the dose to over the next three months	Relapse prevention techniques. Monitoring

Source: Adapted from NTA (2006b)

COMPREHENSIVE CARE PLAN

Comprehensive assessment underlies planning and delivery of structured pharmacological or psychosocial interventions. One technique that might assist the development of a care plan is node-link mapping (also referred to as mapping). Node-link mapping is a technique for visually displaying thoughts, feelings and actions as nodes, with the relationships between them represented by named links (Dees *et al.* 1994). Node-link mapping provides a structure for key workers and clients to explore problems (and personal strengths), identify goals, develop plans and undertake specific actions to address goals (NTA 2006b). This process is described in more detail in a separate document on nodal link mapping (NTA 2007). The comprehensive care plan may be formulated by a key worker or in conjunction with other members of the multi-disciplinary team. The plan will include the setting of goals or objectives based on the four key domains, identified through the initial and ongoing comprehensive assessment, and intervention strategies. The comprehensive care plan is based on the key principles of care planning.

PLANNING INTERVENTIONS

The planning of interventions is based upon the needs or goals identified in the care planning process. The process includes the engagement stage, interventions delivery stage, and long-term treatment and continuing care stage. Within the stages exist various intervention strategies such as pharmacological treatment, harm reduction, motivational interviewing, individual cognitive behavioural counselling, lifestyle change, relapse planning and prevention and family education.

STAGE OF ENGAGEMENT

Engagement is concerned with the development and maintenance of a therapeutic alliance between staff and client. Attempts to make a confrontational and judgemental approach may exacerbate the potential for clients to disengage with treatment services. The aim at this stage is to understand the clients and their views, to respond to their behaviour and language, to recognise their often unspoken needs and thereby to develop some trust and genuineness (Price 2002). This can be enhanced by the style of interaction, which should be non-confrontational, empathetic and respectful of the client's subjective experiences of substance misuse. The strength of the therapeutic alliance will depend upon the value a client attributes to the service, the social marketing of the services by the staff and meeting the client's immediate needs (Rassool 2006). Issues of alcohol and drug misuse are not addressed directly until the end of the engagement process when a working alliance has developed. The client's immediate needs such as emergency care, accommodation, financial issues and legal issues are often more important to the client at that time than dealing with their substance misuse. Guidelines that will help promoting engagement (Rethink & Turning Point 2004) with the service provider are presented in Table 25.4.

The engagement stage draws upon the principles of motivational interviewing (see Chapter 26) to effect change and is contingent upon regular contact and a working alliance between staff and client. In this context, its purpose is to empower the client to gain insight into their problems and to strengthen a client's motivation and commitment to change whilst avoiding confrontation and resistance.

Table 25.4 Promoting engagement

- Motivate clients to see the benefits of the treatment process – this requires a clear idea of what they need and value
- Have a non-confrontational, empathetic and committed approach
- Offer help with meeting initial needs such as food, shelter, housing, clothing
- Provide assistance with benefit entitlements
- Provide assistance with legal matters
- Involve family or carers wherever possible
- Meet clients in settings where they feel safe. This may be more constructive than expecting them to come to services

Source: Rethink & Turning Point (2004)

A variety of simple techniques (Department of Health 2002) can be used for this purpose, including:

- education about substances and the problems that may be associated with misuse including the effects on mental health
- presentation of objective assessment data (for example, liver function tests, urinalysis)
- balance sheets on which the client lists the pros and cons of continued use/ abstinence
- exploration of barriers to the attainment of future goals
- reframing of problems or past events emphasising the influence of substance misuse
- reviewing medication and the use of an optimal medication regime.

The engagement often continues through the client's treatment journey, and interventions delivered at this stage include harm reduction interventions, provision of health and social care information relevant to their substance misuse, and treatment and engaging with significant others to support clients in treatment.

INTERVENTIONS DELIVERY STAGE

This stage involves maintaining the therapeutic relationships and the persuasion of the client of the value and benefits of treatment. This may take a few months before a client is ready to receive active treatment interventions for their substance misuse. It is important at the outset of the care planning to agree the anticipated goal of treatment and to intervene on intermediate goals that represent reductions in the harm incurred from drug and alcohol misuse whilst not focusing prematurely on complete cessation. In some cases, clients may wish to reduce their substance misuse altogether, in which case pharmacological intervention will be necessary to enable a safe detoxification. Clients will need high levels of support, and detoxification should not be used without other concurrent interventions. Interventions at this stage will include a range of treatment modalities including pharmacological management, health information, motivational interviewing and other psychosocial interventions, harm reduction approach, interventions to prevent relapse occupational therapy, welfare advice, community prescribing interventions and employment services. In the delivery of drug treatment, a greater emphasis is required on improving service users' physical and mental health, especially those with hepatitis C infections and those misusing alcohol (NTA 2006a).

The client and key worker should discuss a timetable for the first review at the outset and the precise timing of subsequent reviews will be subject to local policies and client needs (NTA 2006b). For many clients, a change in healthcare needs or situation or a crisis provides an opportunity for a review of the care plan. However, a care plan with its goals and associated interventions should be monitored and reviewed when necessary.

LONG-TERM OR CONTINUING CARE STAGE

This stage is the completion phase when clients have achieved changes in one or more of the above domains of functioning: drug and alcohol misuse; physical and psychological health; offending behaviour; and social functioning In this stage, interventions are targeted at assisting clients to maintain the actual changes achieved during the treatment journey. Alcohol and drug misuse are chronic relapsing conditions. Given the relapsing nature of substance misuse, it is important once a client has reduced their misuse, or become abstinent, to offer interventions aimed at the prevention and management of future relapses. It is also crucial that both client and staff accept relapse and do not perceive it as a weakness or failure. If the substance use is a sustained use, a return to the motivation for change stage is necessary and attention is given to the development of new action plans. For the principles and strategies of 'relapse prevention' for substance misuse see Chapter 26. This approach aims to identify high-risk situations for substance misuse and rehearse coping strategies proactively.

Clients should continue to receive the community integration interventions that they began to receive in the intervention delivery phase to address specific social needs that will enable them to successfully integrate back into the wider community (NTA 2006b). It is important at this stage to encourage the client to establish or maintain contact with self-help groups such as Narcotics Anonymous (NA), Alcoholics Anonymous (AA) or non-12-Step equivalents; to target social needs such as housing, relationships and childcare; and to support training, education, employment and life opportunities (NTA 2006b).

This is the completion stage and may be the last stage of the road map in the client's treatment journey. However, in clinical practice owing to the relapse rate among substance misusers, the client journey may include a return to an earlier stage of the treatment journey.

KEY POINTS

- The planning phase of the client's treatment journey involves the development of a care plan for the client based on their needs.
- Care planning provides a 'road map' of the client's treatment journey and is a key component of structured alcohol and drug treatment interventions.
- The role of care planning and care co-ordination as key components of an integrated system of treatment for drug and alcohol misusers was identified in *Models of Care*.
- The client journey may start with primary healthcare services or generic services.
- The care planning process, an essential component of the client treatment journey, is a method for setting goals based on the needs identified by an assessment and planning interventions to meet those goals with the client.
- A care plan is a structured and task-oriented plan of action between the client and the health or social care professional.
- The effectiveness of the care plan is based on the engagement of the service user throughout the assessment and care planning process: the user should be actively involved in the formulation of the care plan.

- The first step in care planning is accurate and comprehensive assessment.
- Every service user should have a documented care plan which is individualised to the client's needs, develops with the client and significant others, reflects evidence-based practice and interventions and provides for continuity of after-care.
- The identification of health or social care needs, setting goals and planning interventions should be part of the initial care plan.
- The comprehensive care plan is based on the key principles of care planning.
- The planning of interventions is based upon the needs or goals identified in the care planning process.
- The process includes the engagement stage, interventions delivery stage, and long-term treatment and continuing care stage.

ACTIVITY 25.1

There is only one correct answer to the following multiple-choice questions

The planning phase of the client's treatment journey involves
a. The development of a care plan
b. The implementation of intervention
c. The evaluation of intervention
d. The part of an integrated system

Care planning provides
a. A 'road map' of the client's treatment journey
b. A key component of treatment interventions
c. Co-ordination of an integrated system of treatment
d. All of the above

The satisfaction of service users is strongly linked to
a. A reviewed care plan
b. A care plan drawn up solely by the service provider
c. Having an up-to-date care plan
d. None of the above

Primary healthcare services or generic services
a. Provide screening and risk assessment
b. Identify the nature and extent of drug and alcohol problems
c. Provide harm reduction strategies
d. All of the above

A care plan is
a. A structured plan
b. A task-oriented plan of action
c. The identification of needs or goals
d. All of the above

The effectiveness of the care plan is based on
a.   The engagement of the client in assessment process
b.   Being actively involved in the formulation of the care plan
c.   Feeling the ownership of the care
d.   All of the above

The principle of care planning is based on
a.   The holistic needs of the individual
b.   The setting of the goals of treatment
c.   The targets to be achieved and the interventions provided
d.   All of the above

A comprehensive care plan should include the following domains
a.   Drug and alcohol misuse and offending behaviour
b.   Physical and psychological health
c.   Offending behaviour and social functioning
d.   All of the above

Consideration of the client's cultural and ethnic background enables
a.   The provision of a comprehensive care plan
b.   The provision of cultural competence care
c.   The provision of measurable goals
d.   The provision of achievable goals

A care plan should include
a.   SMART goals or objectives
b.   Treatment interventions
c.   Risk behaviour and management
d.   All of the above

Reviewing a care plan provides a framework within which
a.   The key worker can decide whether a goal has been achieved
b.   The client can decide whether a goal has been achieved
c.   Information on unmet needs is provided
d.   All of the above

The aims of the care programme approach are to
a.   Ensure effective collaboration between agencies
b.   Provide a seamless service
c.   Address both health and social care needs
d.   All of the above

If the client has been found to have urgent health needs during triage assessment
a.   Engagement of the client is necessary
b.   Engagement of the client in treatment
c.   A comprehensive care plan should be formulated
d.   An initial care plan should be formulated

A comprehensive care plan underlies

a. Planning of structured pharmacological or psychosocial interventions
b. Delivery of structured pharmacological or psychosocial interventions
c. Its development by a key worker or the multidisciplinary team
d. All of the above

Node-link mapping is a technique for

a. Visually displaying thoughts
b. Visually displaying feelings
c. Visually displaying actions
d. All of the above

Engagement is concerned with

a. The development of a therapeutic alliance between staff and client
b. Intervening with client's immediate needs
c. Understanding the client and their view
d. All of the above

The development of therapeutic alliance is based on

a. A judgemental approach
b. A confrontational approach
c. An empathetic approach
d. A sympathetic approach

The interventions delivery stage involves

a. Maintaining therapeutic relationships
b. Persuasion of the client of the value of treatment
c. Persuasion of the client of the benefits of treatment
d. All of the above

Long-term or continuing care stage is reached when changes occur in

a. Drug and alcohol misuse
b. Physical and psychological health
c. Offending behaviour and social functioning
d. One or more of the above domains of functioning

ACTIVITY 25.2

Write an outline of a care plan for the following scenarios

J.D. is a single 25-year-old unemployed man with a two-year history of injecting heroin use. Despite receiving methadone, he still continues to use illicit heroin. Attempts at outpatient detoxification have been unsuccessful. The client has a stable relationship and has, in the past, managed to hold down a number of jobs. He has a promise of full-time employment on becoming drug-free. He appears well motivated towards detoxification but was not prepared to consider any time beyond this.

S.E., aged 28 years of age, was prescribed temazepam and dihydrocodeine as a result of a car accident. She has attended the A&E department on a number of occasions looking intoxicated. There seems to be an increasing incidence of prescriptions which have been lost or mislaid. Increasingly there has been a series of crises where the client has presented looking for additional prescriptions.

REFERENCES

Dees, S.M., Dansereau, D.F. and Simpson, D.D. (1994) A visual representation system for drug abuse counsellors. *Journal of Substance Abuse Treatment*, 11, 6: 517–23.

Department of Health (1999) *Effective Care Co-ordination in Mental Health Services: Modernising the Care Programme Approach*, A Policy Booklet. London: HMSO.

Department of Health (2002) *Mental Health Policy Implementation Guide Dual Diagnosis Good Practice Guide*. London: Department of Health.

Health Care Commission and NTA (2006) *Improving Services for Substance Misuse: A Joint Review*. London: Commission for Healthcare Audit and Inspection.

NTA (2002) *Models of Care for Treatment of Adult Drug Misusers. Part 2*, Full Reference Report. London: National Treatment Agency.

NTA (2006a) *Models of Care for Treatment of Adult Drug Misusers: Update 2006*. London: National Treatment Agency.

NTA (2006b) *Care Planning Practice Guide*. London: National Treatment Agency.

NTA (2007) *The International Treatment Effectiveness Project: Implementing Psychosocial Interventions for Adult Drug Misusers*. London: National Treatment Agency.

Price, P. (2002) Nursing interventions in the care of dually diagnosed clients. In G. Hussein Rassool (ed.) *Substance Misuse and Psychiatric Disorders*. Oxford: Blackwell Publishing.

Rassool, G. Hussein (2006) Understanding dual diagnosis: an overview. In G. Hussein Rassool (ed.) *Dual Diagnosis Nursing*. Oxford: Blackwell Publishing.

Rethink & Turning Point (2004) *Dual Diagnosis Toolkit: Mental Health and Substance Misuse*. London: Rethink & Turning Point.

Scottish Executive Effective Interventions Unit (2002) *Integrated Care for Drug Users: Principles and Practice*. The Scottish Government Publication. www.scotland.gov.uk/library5/health/icdu-00.asp (accessed 20 November 2007).

Simpson, A. (2006) Shared care and inter-professional practice. In G. Hussein Rassool (ed.) *Dual Diagnosis Nursing*. Oxford: Blackwell Publishing.

CHAPTER 26

PSYCHOSOCIAL AND PHARMACOLOGICAL INTERVENTIONS

OBJECTIVES

▨ Discuss the principle of psychosocial interventions.

▨ Describe the range of psychosocial interventions in the treatment of substance misusers.

▨ Describe the range of pharmacological interventions in the treatment of substance misusers.

▨ Have an understanding of the use of complementary therapies.

▨ Discuss the effectiveness of treatment interventions for alcohol and drug misuse.

There are a wide range of psychosocial and pharmacological interventions for the treatment of alcohol and drug misuse which can be delivered across all the four tiers of the *Models of Care*. Psychosocial interventions encompass a wide range treatment strategy such as brief interventions, counselling, cognitive behavioural therapy, family therapy, social skills training, supportive work and complementary therapy. Pharmacological interventions are categorised as detoxification, medications for relapse prevention and nutritional supplements. There is evidence to suggest that drug misuse treatment is effective in terms of reduced substance misuse, improvements in personal and social functioning; reduced public health and safety risks; reduced criminal behaviour (McLellan *et al.* 1997, Prendergast *et al.* 2002, NTA 2006a). There is also evidence of the effectiveness of psychosocial therapies and pharmacotherapies in achieving reductions in drinking and alcohol problem and reduce longer-term health costs of problem drinkers (NTA 2006b).

Alcohol and drug misusers have complex problems relating to medical, psychosocial, social and legal issues, and intervention strategies should be appropriately responsive to the individual needs of the service users. The nature and severity of their complex needs are likely to influence the type and range of interventions. The appropriateness of the intervention and the readiness of the client to accept voluntarily the need to change are vital components. Service providers should have clear and cogent policies, procedures, goals and objectives that are familiar to staff and clients and should be flexible in order to provide individualised treatment planning and implementation. An explicit treatment alliance, such as a contract and review(s), will measure the expected outcome and overall progress. Local policy will dictate whether a review is undertaken informally or carried out on a more formal basis.

PSYCHOSOCIAL INTERVENTIONS

The goals of psychosocial interventions are to improve the psychosocial well-being of alcohol and drug users. The term 'psychosocial' is used to emphasise the close connection between psychological aspects of our experience (our thoughts, emotions and behaviour) and our wider social experience (our relationships, traditions and culture) (The Psychosocial Working Group 2003). Psychosocial interventions include brief interventions, counselling, motivational interviewing, motivational enhancement therapy, solution-focused therapy, community reinforcement approach, social behaviour and network therapy, coping and social skills training, marital therapy, relapse prevention and complementary therapies.

PRINCIPLES OF PSYCHOSOCIAL INTERVENTIONS

One of the principles of good practice is that the framework of psychosocial interventions is based on the notion of assessment of health and social care needs. The assessment of needs or goals will enable decision-making about what type of intervention to initiate. Key working also forms part of the component of good practice, and usually involves regular contact between a service provider and the client. Key working is a basic delivery mechanism for a range of psychosocial components. The delivery of interventions include: regular reviews of care plans and treatment goals with the patient; provision of alcohol- and drug-misuse-related advice and information; interventions to reduce alcohol- or drug-related harm (especially risk of overdose and blood-borne virus infections); psychosocial interventions to increase motivation; psychosocial interventions to prevent relapse; and help to address social problems (for example, family problems, housing and employment) (Department of Health 2007).

The effectiveness of a therapeutic alliance is crucial to the delivery of any treatment intervention and patient outcomes. It is essential to engage a patient appropriately and to demonstrate satisfactory levels of warmth and trust; to adopt a personal style that is consistent with and meshes with that of the patient; to adjust the nature of the intervention according to the potential of the client; to deal with difficult emotions; and to understand and work with a patient's emotional context including patient motivation (Roth and Pilling 2007). A further principle is that goals of treatment should not be imposed on the service user but based on mutual agreement between the key worker and the service user.

BRIEF INTERVENTIONS

Brief interventions aim to motivate those at risk to change their substance-use behaviour (Babor and Higgins-Biddle 2001). The aim of the intervention is to help the patient understand that their alcohol drinking or drug use is putting them at risk and to encourage them to reduce or give up their substance use. Brief interventions comprise a single brief advice or several short (15–30 minutes) brief counselling sessions. Generally, brief interventions are not intended to treat people with alcohol and drug problems but are aimed at those with problematic or risky substance use. Brief interventions can also be used to encourage those with more serious dependence to accept more intensive treatment within the primary care setting, or referral to a specialised alcohol and drug services (WHO 2005). Targets for intervention are usually identified through the application of a screening tool, which indicates that clients are drinking at hazardous levels (Heather and Kaner 2001).

The acronym FRAMES summarises the elements of effective brief interventions (Bien *et al.* 1993): Feedback, Responsibility, Advice, Menu, Empathy and Self-efficacy. Table 26.1 presents the elements of effective brief interventions. Brief interventions can be delivered in a supportive, non-judgemental manner by health or social services

Table 26.1 Elements of effective brief interventions

	Acronym	Elements	Counselling responses
F	Feedback	Feedback of personal risk or impairment	Your difficulty in getting to work on time may be related to your alcohol or drug use. (Sharing of results of assessments such as cognitive testing, liver function tests)
R	Responsibility	Emphasis on personal responsibility for change	It is your responsibility to make a decision about stopping substance misuse for the next two weeks
A	Advice	A clear advice to change	It is recommended that you stop drinking or drug use for the next two weeks, to see if that makes a difference
M	Menu	Menu of alternative change options	If you cannot reduce or stop your substance misuse, consider other options such as AA or NA, or referral to the specialist service
E	Empathy	Therapeutic empathy as a counselling style	I understand that this will be difficult for you because you feel alcohol helps you to unwind after a stressful working day
S	Self-efficacy	Enhancement of patient self-efficacy or optimism	Considering how difficult you find this, I am confident that you have the abilities or strengths to consider changing your behaviour

workers. The positive approaches of brief interventions have been demonstrated to be associated with better outcomes than more traditional confrontational styles.

There is strong evidence for the effectiveness of brief interventions in a variety of settings for alcohol and tobacco, and growing evidence of effectiveness for other substances. Brief interventions delivered in a variety of settings are effective in reducing alcohol consumption among hazardous and harmful drinkers to low-risk levels (NTA 2006b). The NICE (2007) guideline on psychosocial interventions recommends that opportunistic brief interventions focused on motivation should be offered to people in limited contact with drug services (for example, those attending a needle and syringe exchange or primary care settings) if concerns about drug misuse are identified by the service user or staff member. These interventions should:

- normally consist of two sessions each lasting 10–45 minutes
- explore ambivalence about drug use and possible treatment, with the aim of increasing motivation to change behaviour
- provide non-judgemental feedback.

In addition, NICE recommended that service providers should routinely provide people who misuse drugs with information about self-help groups based on 12-Step principles. These include Alcoholics Anonymous, Narcotics Anonymous and Cocaine Anonymous. The WHO Brief Intervention Study Group (1996) studied 1,260 men and 299 women who were drinking at levels considered to put them at risk of alcohol-related problems but who had no prior history of alcohol dependence. They concluded that brief interventions were consistently robust across healthcare settings and socio-cultural groups. However, it is important to note that using a self-help manual is better than minimal advice alone and that the provision of a brief intervention is preferable to no therapeutic intervention (Heather *et al*. 1986, Heather 1998).

COUNSELLING

Counselling ranges from general psychological support, review and monitoring to offering specific behavioural, cognitive-behavioural and therapeutic techniques. Counselling takes place when a alcohol or drug worker sees a client in a private and confidential setting to explore dealing with losses, past trauma, generalised anxieties or specific psychological problems, relationship difficulties and ill-health, both physical and mental. The aim of counselling is to attempt to address some of the underlying problems which have contributed to, aggravated or derived from alcohol or drug problems.

It is usually a client-centred process using techniques including clarifying, exploring, reflecting, paraphrasing, summarising and restructuring in order to allow ventilation of feelings. In its purest sense it is not about giving advice or directing a client to take a particular course of action. For example, individual counselling may be offered to support and retain a patient waiting for admission into a residential or inpatient unit or it may be a part of an ongoing psychological intervention process.

However, the main factor that usually determines how successful the therapy is does not lie with the technique or approach used but with the actual counsellor. How you connect with the counsellor you choose is likely to determine how successful the treatment is. Acceptance and respect for the client are essentials for a counsellor and, as therapeutic alliance develops, so too does trust between the counsellor and client. Velleman (2001) has developed an approach to counselling substance misusers which highlights the processes irrespective of the theoretical persuasion of the counsellor. He describes six stages, namely developing trust, exploring the problem, helping clients to set goals, empowering clients to take action, helping them to maintain changes, and agreeing with them when the time comes to end the counselling relationship. Some counselling skills are presented in Table 26.2.

Table 26.2 Counselling skills

Techniques	Explanations	Examples
Empathy	Incorporates acceptance and understanding. Seeing the world view of the other person	I understand how you are feeling about reducing your alcohol consumption. That must be difficult for you
Active listening	Involves paying attention to a client's verbal and non-verbal messages	Listening in a way that conveys respect, interest and empathy
Open-ended questions	The 'How', 'What' or 'Why' Questions. Open-ended questions encourage clients to express their feelings and share information about their situation	Can you tell me more about that? How do you feel about that? Why do you feel you are at risk from HIV?
Reflective	To encourage a client to express and explore. Repetition of the last few words or a significant word or phrase can be reflected	I feel that a part of me is . . . missing
Focusing	Attempt to redirect the patient in an understanding manner	
Affirming	Reinforcing or complimenting the client on the positive actions they have taken	You have managed to reduce your alcohol consumption. This is a positive step in managing to do safer injecting practice
Correcting misperceptions	Providing correct information to the patient in a sensitive way that does not put the patient on the defensive. Acknowledge misinformation and correct it	
Summarising	Present the main points to the client	

MOTIVATIONAL INTERVIEWING

No single counselling approach is appropriate for all clients. Matching counselling techniques to a client's goals is crucial in determining successful outcomes. Motivational interviewing is employed when clients present showing no or little commitment to change. Rollnick and Miller (1995) defined motivational interviewing as 'directive, client-centred counselling for eliciting behaviour change by helping clients to explore and resolve ambivalence'. They described it as more focused and goal-directed than non-directive counselling, and said that the counsellor takes a directive approach to the examination and resolution of ambivalence, which is its central purpose. Motivational interviewing is based on the premise that the main obstacle to changing drug or alcohol use and associated behaviour patterns is a lack of motivation; it follows that, if motivation to change can be enhanced, then behaviour change will be more likely (Baker and Reicher 1998).

Motivational interviewing has been employed extensively and successfully among people with alcohol and other drug problems in order to enhance involvement and reduce substance use (Miller and Rollnick 2002). It is a technique that does not require an in-depth counselling knowledge but involves a non-judgemental approach, open-ended questioning and reflective listening. It is used in such a way as to raise the patient's self-esteem and self-efficacy and increase awareness of their problems. It elicits self-motivational statements from the patient and highlights their motivated behaviour whilst underlying that responsibility for change lies with the patient. The four principles of motivational interviewing are: expressing empathy, developing discrepancy, rolling with resistance and supporting self-efficacy. Various tools and strategies have been developed to help apply these principles these include pencil and paper exercises, structured questions and focused reflections (Mason 2006).

Motivational interviewing has been found to increase the effectiveness of more extensive psychosocial treatment for alcohol problems and improved outcomes for drug-related problems (NTA 2006a, 2006b).

CONTINGENCY MANAGEMENT

Contingency Management is the process of using positive reinforcers to increase desired behaviours. It operates by providing a variety of incentives in the form of vouchers, privileges, prizes or modest financial incentives to modify a person's drug misuse or to increase health-promoting behaviours (Department of Health 2007). NICE (2007) has recommended that drug services should introduce contingency management programmes to reduce illicit drug use and/or promote engagement with services for people receiving methadone maintenance treatment. The principles of contingency management (NICE 2007) are presented in Table 26.3.

Table 26.3 The principles of contingency management

- Incentives can be offered (usually vouchers to be exchanged for goods or services of the service user's choice, or privileges such as take-home methadone doses) contingent on each presentation of a drug-negative test (for example, free from cocaine or non-prescribed opioids)
- The frequency of screening should be set at three tests per week for the first three weeks, two tests per week for the next three weeks, and one per week thereafter until stability is achieved
- If vouchers are used, they should have monetary values that start in the region of £2 and increase with each additional, continuous period of abstinence
- Urinalysis should be the preferred method of testing but oral fluid tests may be considered as an alternative
- For people at risk of physical health problems (including transmittable diseases) resulting from their drug misuse, material incentives (for example, shopping vouchers of up to £10 in value) should be considered to encourage harm reduction. Incentives should be offered on a one-off basis or over a limited duration, contingent on concordance with or completion of each intervention.

Source: NICE (2007)

Contingency management would normally be provided as part of a structured care or treatment plan in combination with other interventions provided by the key worker (Department of Health 2007). This approach has been identified in the NICE guideline as having the strongest scientific evidence base for the most effective outcomes. Contingency management has been found to be a useful treatment for 'non-responsive' patients and more effective when they were directed towards changing the use of a single illicit drug than towards reducing multiple drug use (NTA 2006a).

CUE EXPOSURE

Cue exposure is aimed at extinguishing conditioned responses such as craving. Childress *et al*. (1988) recognised that repeated pairings of substance use with particular settings, individuals, affect states, paraphernalia and so on could lead to substantial conditioned craving. They demonstrated 'cue reactivity' including both physiological (changes in skin temperature) and subjective (withdrawal-like symptoms, craving) responses in both opiate and cocaine misusers exposed to drug-related stimuli, such as handling drug paraphernalia etc. The general approach is to expose drug or alcohol users to cues for using (for example, exposing a cocaine user to white powder or drug paraphernalia or an alcohol misuser to a beer bottle) while concurrently addressing and attempting to lessen the desire to use. Cue exposure can reduce the desire to use that was caused by the cue; provides the opportunity to practise coping responses (for example, relaxation) realistically; and can increase self-efficacy, which will increase the likelihood that the response will be utilised in future real-life cue exposures (Monti *et al*. 1989).

Cue exposure shows promise as an alcohol treatment method, particularly when combined with coping and communication skills training as part of a broader cognitive behaviour therapy programme. However, there was limited evidence to support the effectiveness of cue exposure for the treatment of drug problems (Conklin and Tiffany 2002).

RELAPSE PREVENTION

Relapse prevention is a cognitive behavioural technique centred on the teaching of coping skills. The techniques used to teach coping skills include identification of specific situations where coping inadequacies occur, and the use of instruction, modelling, role-plays and behavioural rehearsal. Exposure to stressful situations is gradually increased as adaptive mastery occurs. Clients may need support to identify risks associated with their substance misuse, and a relapse prevention plan is based on the identified risk factors. An important part of any plan should include assertiveness work and social inclusion. Relapse prevention skills training is typically offered in the following areas (Addiction-clinics 2007):

- reducing exposure to alcohol or drug
- exploring the pros and cons of continued use
- self-monitoring to identify high risk situations

- development of strategies for coping with craving
- identification of thought processes that can increase risk for relapse
- preparation for emergencies and coping with relapse
- homework assignments.

There is good evidence of the effectiveness of specific relapse prevention in the treatment of drug and alcohol problems and psychosocial functioning (NTA 2006a and 2006b).

MARITAL AND FAMILY THERAPIES

In marital and family therapies, the role of important or significant 'others' in the addictive process is examined. Marital or family therapy interventions focus on drug misuse, discuss with families the sources of stress associated with drug misuse and tries to support and promote the family in developing more effective coping behaviours (Department of Health 2007). Marital behavioural therapy in particular and various other combinations of family approaches have demonstrated effectiveness in reducing dropout and relapse rates (NICE 2007).

SOLUTION-FOCUSED THERAPY

Solution-focused work is based on Ericksonian's model of human behaviour. It argues that most interventions focus on pathological or negative aspects of a person's life, and the aim of this therapy is to enable the focusing of the client's strengths and successes through a series of future-orientated questions. The therapist and client are able to co-construct new solutions to existing problem behaviours. The prominent features of solution-focused therapy have been characterised by Barret-Kruse (1994) as:

- the view that self and others are essentially able
- the acceptance of the patient's definition of the problem
- the formation of the therapeutic alliance
- the crediting of success to the patient
- the therapist learning from the patient
- the avoidance of a power struggle with the patient
- the objectification, rather than the personalisation, of the patient's behaviour.

TRADITIONAL, MINNESOTA MODEL, 12-STEP-ORIENTED MODEL

These approaches are grounded in the concept of substance misuse as a spiritual and medical disease. Their origin is based on the philosophy of self-help groups such as Alcoholics Anonymous, which is that of reaching out to other alcoholics to help everyone stay sober. Alcoholics Anonymous (AA) began in the US in 1933. It has since spread to many countries and has led to the development of Narcotics Anonymous (NA) for drug users and to Al-Anon and Families Anonymous (FA) for the families of drinkers and drug users. AA groups are prominent in most UK towns, making it possible to attend a meeting on every night of the week in the cities. Groups meet in a variety of community and institutional settings such as church halls, hospitals, prisons and clinics. Use of such premises is not seen to compromise the independence or characteristics of these abstinence-based groups, which are group identity, open confession and confidential sharing of personal information with other members. AA is spiritual and not religious; the requirement is a belief in a higher power, rather than a god, and atheists are welcome at groups. The 12-Step model is presented in Table 26.4.

Table 26.4 The 12-Steps model

- Admitted we were powerless over alcohol; that our lives had become unmanageable
- Came to believe that a Power greater than ourselves could restore us to sanity
- Made a decision to turn our will and our lives over to the care of God as we understood Him
- Made a searching and fearless moral inventory of ourselves
- Admitted to God, to ourselves, and to another human being the exact nature of our wrongs
- Were entirely ready to have God remove all these defects of character
- Humbly asked Him to remove our shortcomings
- Made a list of all persons we had harmed, and became willing to make amends to them all
- Made direct amends to such people wherever possible, except where to do so would injure them or others
- Continued to take a personal inventory and, when we were wrong, promptly admitted it
- Sought through prayer and meditation to improve our conscious contact with God as we understood Him, praying only for knowledge of His will for us and the power to carry that out
- Having had a spiritual experience (awakening) as the result of these steps, we tried to carry this message to alcoholics, and to practise these principles in all our affairs

A meta-analysis of the role of AA in treatment outcomes found the more involved one is with the process, the better the drinking outcome (Tonigan *et al.* 1996). However, the review of the effectiveness of treatment for alcohol problems (NTA 2006b) found that the 12-Step treatment confers no added benefit compared with other forms of treatment.

SOCIAL INTERVENTIONS

The social model engages the interaction between the internal experience of the individual and networks and communities in which they live. There has been increased recognition of the key role that families can play in substance misuse treatment, in terms of preventing and/or influencing the course of the substance-misuse problem, improving substance-related outcomes for the user and also helping to reduce the negative effects of substance-misuse problems on other family members (Copello *et al.* 2006). This model of intervention is based on empowering and supporting the individual and the family social networks in developing strategies to cope with specific social problems and difficulties. The role of advocacy in helping an individual dealing with housing, childcare and welfare benefits issues may directly influence the individual's ability to address their alcohol or drug problems. There is an increasingly robust evidence base that supports both family-focused and social-network-focused interventions and that family and social network approaches either match or improve outcomes when compared with individual interventions (Copello *et al.* 2006).

COMPLEMENTARY THERAPIES

Complementary therapies are gaining increased recognition within the allopathic heathcare system in the UK, and there is a significant interest in the development of its use in the addiction field. The general purpose of acupuncture is to unblock the meridians and allow the passage of Chi. Chi is regarded as the vital energy of all beings. Both physical and psychological problems can cause blockage in the pathways. The use of auricular acupuncture in the treatment of substance misuse was pioneered in the Lincoln Hospital in New York in the early 1970s. The best recognised form of acupuncture used in the field of addiction is auricular (ear) acupuncture. It has been used to treat most forms of substance misuse and addictive behaviours: cigarette smoking, alcoholism, methadone detoxification, detoxification of opiate, cocaine, crack cocaine, alcohol and tobacco addiction and preventing relapse.

The reason for the paucity of acupuncture detoxification therapy is not merely a lack of understanding of its physiological basis of action but primarily the scarcity of controlled objective clinical studies and failure to describe acupuncture in quantitative objective western terminology (Katims *et al.* 1992). The evidence supporting acupuncture's effectiveness in detoxification treatment is largely anecdotal, and, despite its use in some clinics and drug court programmes, acupuncture is still considered an alternative therapy (Spray and Jones 1995). Auricular acupuncture is not a magic solution to substance-misuse treatment but can be a complementary tool in the detoxification process.

Aromatherapy involves the use of the organic essence of aromatic plants for healing the body, mind and spirit. The oils are obtained from the plants using distillation and solvent extraction. Each oil has its own properties, and oils are often used in conjunction with each other to offer a comprehensive treatment to the client. As some of the oils are contraindicated in certain conditions, aromatherapy should be administered only by a qualified practitioner. Massage can be of great benefit to the client, promoting relaxation and calmness. The combination of massage and aromatherapy can be of particular benefit in substance misuse, allowing the client 'time out' from stress (McDonald and Rassool 1997). Aromatherapy is welcomed by most clients attending services. Miller and Walker (1997) argue that anything that holds out hope of being helpful ought to be freely available, or in essence that therapies should be practised (and reimbursed) until proved ineffective or harmful. There is no available literature on the use of aromatherapy in the addiction field.

In the United Kingdom, reflexology is the third most popular complementary therapy used by nurses (Trevelyan 1996). The hands, feet or head are massaged to treat physical psychological and emotional ailments. Reflexology is one of the many complementary treatments on offer to clients who present with substance-misuse problems. The practitioner will work on the feet or hands, feeling for imbalance and energy blockage. These areas will be worked on using a technique of compression massage, with the thumbs and fingers used to apply pressure. The practitioner will remain focused throughout the procedure, allowing the passage of Chi. Most clients enjoy the massage element alone, which allows them time out to relax in a quiet and safe environment. On a deeper level reflexology can help to heal physical, psychological and emotional problems.

Complementary therapies can be of great value in substance misuse services by increasing the options of care for this client group. The advantages of using any of the complementary therapies are that they are more economical in comparison with the expense of drugs such as methadone. There is no danger of therapeutic addiction. However, more research is needed to examine the safety and effectiveness of complementary therapies, and adequate professional and legal regulations are of vital importance.

PHARMACOLOGICAL INTERVENTIONS

Effective pharmacological treatment involves the prescribing of a spectrum of medications. The need for pharmacological treatment and the type of treatment depend on the consequences of substance misuse. The aims of pharmacological interventions are: to reduce harms associated with illicit psychoactive substances by prescribing a substitute opiate-based medication (for example, methadone); to reduce withdrawal syndromes; to enable the maintenance of abstinence and the prevention of relapse; to prevent complications of substance misuse (for example, use of vitamins); and in the treatment of co-existing substance-misuse and psychiatric disorders.

Alcohol, opiates and hypno-sedatives produce substantial physical withdrawal syndromes, and pharmacological treatments are often needed to reduce withdrawal symptoms. Whilst opiate withdrawal is rarely life-threatening, alcohol and hypno-sedative withdrawal are associated with a significant mortality and morbidity rate without pharmacological interventions. Methadone maintenance is used as a substitute for opiate users for stabilisation which permits the client to function without experiencing withdrawal symptoms, craving or adverse effects. Naltrexone, a long-acting opiate antagonist to block the effects of opiate use, is used in the prevention of relapse.

METHADONE

Methadone treatments are the most widely used type of treatment for opiate addiction throughout the world (Kreek and Vocci 2002). Methadone, a long-acting opiate, allows for symptoms to be controlled over a period of time. Taken orally once a day, methadone suppresses opiate withdrawal for between 24 and 36 hours. Methadone has many advantages (Department of Health 1999) such as:

- It is licensed for the treatment of opiate dependence.
- It is longer acting (typically 24–48 hours), making stability from daily dosing easier to achieve.
- It is straightforward to titrate in order to achieve the correct dose.
- It is less likely to be diverted than shorter-acting drugs.
- It is less likely to be injected.
- Its clinical effectiveness is supported by research.

However, methadone is not an effective treatment for other psychoactive substances. For clients with a history of relapse and treatment dropout, methadone is the treatment of choice. Methadone maintenance treatment provides the heroin addict with individualised healthcare and medically prescribed methadone to relieve withdrawal symptoms, reduce the opiate craving, and bring about a biochemical balance in the body (Department of Health 1999). Methadone reduces the cravings associated with heroin use by blocking the high and euphoric rush from heroin. As methadone is effective in eliminating withdrawal symptoms, it is used in detoxifying opiate addicts. Many clients on methadone require continuous treatment, sometimes over a period of years without adverse effects. Ultimately, the patient remains physically dependent on methadone but is freed from the chaotic lifestyles observed in heroin users.

The baseline dose of methadone aims to minimise the severity of the withdrawal, to produce a degree of comfort and to lessen the risk of overdose. Dose reduction of methadone can be undertaken depending on the results of the assessment and treatment plan. The most rapid regime can be carried out by incremental cuts in dose over 7–21 days, and slower regimes may take several months to complete. When there are complex social or other needs, slow reductions of methadone are prescribed, the general principle being that at higher dose levels the greater the reduction possible, as it represents a smaller percentage of the total. As the dose falls, reduction should be more gradual (Department of Health 1999). This gradual reduction of methadone can occur at any time interval, for example, daily, alternate days, weekly. In order to decrease the individual's anxiety and increase their sense of control, it may be necessary to hold the reduction steady at a given dose over a few days. Delays in the rate of reduction should be accompanied by psychological support. Progress should be monitored at intervals and the individual's progress should be discussed with the multidisciplinary team.

There is evidence to suggest that methadone maintenance treatment produces better outcomes on average in terms of illicit drug consumption and other criminal behaviour, leads to reduced levels of HIV risk behaviours and lower HIV seroconversion rates, and reduction in sharing injecting equipment and in having unprotected sex (Institute of Medicine 1990, Sorensen and Copeland 2000, Gossop *et al.* 2002)

NALTREXONE

Naltrexone (naltrexone hydrochloride) is a long-acting opioid antagonist used primarily in the management of alcohol and opiate addiction. Naltrexone should not be confused with naloxone, which is used in emergency cases of overdose rather than for longer-term dependence control. Naltrexone pharmacotherapy provides an almost ideal treatment for opiate addiction and has a potentially important role in helping to prevent relapse (Mello *et al.* 1981). It can be administered orally, or as an implant, and has minimal adverse effects. The euphoric effects of opiates such as heroin are blocked when an individual is being treated with naltrexone and prevents a return to physical dependence. Naltrexone may be indicated for those who are in their early stages of their addiction and those who are highly motivated. Naltrexone as a medication for relapse prevention is indicated to help clients who have lapsed but shows minor positive effects (NTA 2006b).

However, naltrexone has been found to have limited impact on the clinical management of heroin addiction, is costly compared to other pharmacological interventions and the majority of drug-dependent patients are reluctant or resistant to taking naltrexone (NTA 2006a). Furthermore, there is also a problem of high dropout rates from naltrexone treatment (Tucker *et al.* 2004). There is a need for caution when naltrexone is used in the treatment of addiction, since many addicts have liver disease associated with viral hepatitis infections (NTA 2006a)

BUPRENORPHINE AND NON-OPIATES

Buprenorphine is licensed in the UK for the treatment of drug dependence. This drug has an effective duration of at least 24 hours and is taken as a sublingual tablet daily. It is reported to have low euphoric effects at higher doses compared to methadone, less euphoria and physical dependence, lower potential for misuse and relatively mild withdrawal symptoms. Unlike the other pharmacological interventions, buprenorphine produces far less respiratory depression and is thought to be safer in overdose. There is interest in its use as an alternative to methadone maintenance and also in the management of opiate withdrawal as its mixed antagonist properties make it a potentially good agent for the management of opiate withdrawal (Department of Health 1999). However, because of its double actions, it can paradoxically aggravate withdrawal symptoms if used in combination with methadone or other opiates. Buprenorphine needs to be administered at least 24 hours after the last dose of methadone and at least four hours after the use of heroin. It is also reported to have lower overdose potential, which makes it more suitable than methadone.

There are now satisfactory non-opiate treatments (such as lofexidine) for opiate withdrawal. These non-opiate drugs are effective in alleviating opiate-withdrawal symptoms, are not liable to, or less open to, misuse by the patient and are less likely to be diverted on to the black market (Department of Health 1999). Lofexidine, a fully licensed drug in the UK for the management of the symptoms of opiate withdrawal, can be used with supervision in inpatient, residential and community settings. There is evidence to suggest that it is equally as efficacious as methadone in withdrawal and has a role in the treatment of opiate-dependent individuals seeking abstinence and whose drug use is already well controlled. Clonidine is not licensed for the treatment of opiate withdrawal symptoms but is useful as a non-opiate treatment for opiate withdrawal. Because of its substantial hypotensive effect there is a need to monitor blood pressure and to modify or withdraw the treatment if symptomatic hypotension occurs.

KEY POINTS

- There are a wide range of psychosocial and pharmacological interventions for the treatment of alcohol and drug misuse.
- There is evidence to suggest that substance-misuse treatment is effective in terms of reduced substance misuse; improvements in personal and social functioning; reduced public health and safety risks; reduced criminal behaviour.
- The delivery of interventions includes regular reviews of care plans and treatment goals, harm reduction approach, promoting readiness to change, preventing relapse and addressing social problems.

- The effectiveness of a therapeutic alliance is crucial to the delivery of any treatment intervention and patient outcomes.
- Brief interventions comprise a single brief advice or several short (15–30 minutes) counselling sessions.
- Motivational interviewing is 'directive, client-centred counselling for eliciting behaviour change by helping clients to explore and resolve ambivalence'.
- Motivational interviewing has been found to increase the effectiveness of more extensive psychosocial treatment for alcohol problems and to give improved outcomes for drug-related problems.
- NICE has recommended that drug services should introduce contingency management programmes to reduce illicit drug use and/or promote engagement with services for people receiving methadone maintenance treatment.
- Clients may need support to identify risks associated with their substance misuse and a relapse prevention plan is based on the identified risk factors.
- Marital behavioural therapy in particular and various other combinations of family approaches have demonstrated effectiveness in reducing dropout and relapse rates.
- Families can play a key role in substance-misuse treatment, in terms of preventing and/or influencing the course of the substance-misuse problem, improving substance-related outcomes for the user and also helping to reduce the negative effects of substance misuse problems on other family members.
- Auricular acupuncture has been used during detoxification.
- Aromatherapy is welcomed by most clients attending services.
- Reflexology is one of the many complementary treatments on offer to clients who present with substance-misuse problems.
- Complementary therapies can be of great value in substance-misuse services.
- Effective pharmacological treatment involves the prescribing a spectrum of medications.
- Methadone treatments are the most widely used type of treatment for opiate addiction throughout the world.

ACTIVITY 26.1

Please state whether the following statements are true or false. Reflect on the statements and give reason(s) for choosing a particular option

	True	False
Psychosocial and pharmacological interventions for the treatment of alcohol and drug misuse can be delivered across all four tiers of the Models of Care		
Pharmacological interventions are categorised as detoxification, medications for relapse prevention and nutritional supplements		
There is no evidence to suggest that drug-misuse treatment is effective in terms of reduced substance misuse		
There is evidence of the effectiveness of psychosocial and pharmacotherapies in achieving reductions in drinking and alcohol problem		

The nature and severity of the complex needs of substance misusers are likely to influence the type and range of interventions

The goals of psychosocial interventions are to improve the psychosocial well-being of alcohol and drug users

The effectiveness of a therapeutic alliance is crucial to the delivery of any treatment intervention and patient outcomes

Brief interventions comprise a single brief advice or several short (15–30 minutes) counselling sessions

There is no evidence for the effectiveness of brief interventions in a variety of settings for alcohol and tobacco

The effectiveness of counselling does not lie with the technique or approach used but with the actual counsellor

Matching counselling techniques to a client's goals is crucial in determining successful outcomes

Motivational interviewing has been found to increase the effectiveness of more extensive psychosocial treatment for substance misusers

There is no evidence that contingency management is a useful treatment for 'non-responsive' clients

In relapse prevention, clients may need support to identify risks associated with their substance misuse

ACTIVITY 26.2

There is only one correct answer to the following multiple-choice questions

The term 'psychosocial' refers to the
a.   Connection of social and family networks
b.   Connections with social and cultural factors
c.   Connections between psychological and medical experience
d.   Connections between psychological and social experience

One of the principles of good practice in psychosocial interventions is based on
a.   The assessment of needs or goals
b.   The assessment of health and social care needs
c.   The enabling of decision-making
d.   The contact between a service provider and the client

Keyworking is a basic
a.   Intervention to reduce alcohol- or drug-related harm
b.   Delivery mechanism for a range of psychosocial components
c.   Provision of alcohol- and drug-misuse-related advice and information
d.   All of the above

The aim of brief intervention is

a. To motivate those at risk to change their substance-use behaviour
b. To help the client understand their substance-misuse problems
c. To encourage clients to reduce or give up their substance use
d. All of the above

Brief interventions are intended to

a. Treat clients with alcohol and drug dependence
b. Treat clients at risk of alcohol problems
c. Treat clients with chronic drug problems
d. Treat clients in primary care only

The motivational enhancing technique originates from

a. Cognitive-behavioural theory
b. Psychodynamic theory
c. Theory of change
d. School of family therapy

Motivational interviewing is employed

a. When clients present are showing no or little commitment to change
b. When clients present are showing readiness to change
c. As a non-directive counselling
d. When pharmacological interventions have failed

Motivational interviewing is a technique that

a. Does not require an in-depth counselling knowledge
b. Involves a judgemental approach
c. Uses closed questioning with the client
d. Expresses sympathy with the client

The principles of motivational interviewing are to

a. Express empathy and develop discrepancy
b. Roll with resistance
c. Support self-efficacy
d. All of the above

Contingency management is the process of

a. Using medical reinforcers to increase desired behaviours
b. Using negative reinforcers to increase desired behaviours
c. Using positive reinforcers to increase desired behaviours
d. Engagement with the service to increase desired behaviours

Cue exposure is aimed at extinguishing conditioned responses

a. Craving and withdrawal-like symptoms
b. Changes in skin temperature
c. In both opiate and cocaine users
d. To increase the desire to use

Relapse prevention is a cognitive-behavioural technique centred on
a.   The teaching of coping skills
b.   The teaching of management skills
c.   A relapse prevention plan
d.   Behavioural rehearsal

The evidence supporting acupuncture's effectiveness in detoxification treatment
a.   Is largely anecdotal
b.   Is evidenced-based
c.   Is gaining increased recognition
d.   Is complementary

The aims of pharmacological interventions are
a.   To reduce harm associated with illicit psychoactive substances
b.   To reduce withdrawal syndromes
c.   To prevent relapse
d.   All of the above

Methadone is
a.   A long-acting opiate
b.   A short-acting opiate
c.   An opiate antagonist
d.   Not effective as a maintenance treatment

Methadone maintenance treatment aims
a.   To relieve withdrawal symptoms
b.   To reduce the opiate craving
c.   To bring a biochemical balance in the body
d.   All of the above

ACTIVITY 26.3

- What does the acronym 'FRAMES' stand for?
- What are the six stages in counselling process?
- What are the advantages in using methadone?
- How would you develop a plan of relapse prevention?

REFERENCES

Addiction-clinics (2007) *Psychosocial Interventions*. www.addiction-clinics.com/substance-misuse/pdf/e5.pdf (accessed 26 November 2007).

Babor, T.F. and Higgins-Biddle, J.C. (2001) *Brief Intervention for Hazardous and Harmful Drinking: A Manual for Use in Primary Care*. Geneva: World Health Organization, Document No. WHO/MSD/MSB/01.6b.

Baker, A. and Reichler, R. (1998) *Motivational Interviewing. Clinical Skills Series: Effective Approaches to Alcohol and Other Drug Problems*. Suffolk: Visual Education.

Baker, A., Lewin, T., Reicher, H., Clancy, R., Carr, V., Garrett, R., Sly, K., Devir, H. and Terry, M. (2002) Motivational interviewing among psychiatric in-patients with substance use disorders. *Acta Psychiatrica Scandinavica*, 106: 233–40.

Barret-Kruse, C. (1994) Brief counselling: a user's guide for traditionally trained counselors. *International Journal for the Advancement of Counselling*, 17: 109–15.

Bien, T.H., Miller, W.R. and Tonigan, J.S. (1993) Brief interventions for alcohol problems: a review. *Addiction*, 88: 315–36.

Childress, A.R., McLellan, A.T., Ehrman, R. and O'Brien, C.P. (1988) Classically conditioned responses in opioid and cocaine dependence: a role in relapse? In B.A. Ray (ed.) *Learning factors in substance abuse*, DHHS Publication no. 88–1576, pp. 25–43. Washington DC: U.S. Government Printing Office.

Conklin, C. and Tiffany, S. (2002) Applying extinction research and theory to cue exposure addiction treatments. *Addiction*, 97: 155–67.

Copello, A.G., Templeton, I. and Velleman, R. (2006) Family interventions for drug and alcohol misuse: is there a best practice? *Current Opinion in Psychiatry*, 19, 3: 271–6.

Department of Health (1999) *Drug Misuse and Dependence – Guidelines on Clinical Management*. London: The Stationery Office.

Department of Health (2007) *Drug Misuse and Dependence: UK Guidelines on Clinical Management*. London: Department of Health.

Gossop, M., Stewart, D., Browne, N. and Marsden, J. (2002). Factors associated with abstinence, lapse or relapse to heroin use after residential treatment: protective effect of coping responses. *Addiction*, 97: 1259–67.

Heather, N. (1998) Using brief opportunities for change in medical settings. In W. Miller and N. Heather (eds) *Treating Addictive Behaviors*. New York: Plenum.

Heather, N., Whitton, B. and Robertson, I. (1986) Evaluation of a self-help manual for media-recruited problem drinkers: six-month follow-up results. *British Journal of Clinical Psychology*, 25: 19–34.

Heather, N. and Kaner, E. (2001) *Brief Interventions: An Opportunity for Reducing Excessive Drinking*. Paper presented to Working Group: Health Systems and Alcohol at Ministerial Conference on Young People and Alcohol, Stockholm, Sweden, 19–21 February.

Institute of Medicine (1990) Gerstein, D. and Harwood, H. (eds) *Treating Drug Problems*. Vol. 1, Washington DC: National Academy Press.

Katims, J.J., Ng, L.K.Y. and Lowinson, J.H. (1992) Acupuncture and transcutaneous electrical nerve stimulation: afferent nerve stimulation (ANS), In K. Lowinson, P. Ruiz, R.B. Millman and J.G. Langrod (eds), *Treatment of Addiction in Substance Abuse: A Comprehensive Textbook*, 2nd edition, pp. 574–83. Baltimore: Williams and Wilkins

Kreek, M.J. and Vocci, F. (2002) History and current status of opioid maintenance treatments. *Journal of Substance Abuse Treatment*, 23: 93–105.

McDonald, L. and Rassool, G. Hussein (1997) Complementary therapies in addiction nursing practice. In G. Hussein Rassool and M. Gafoor (eds) *Addiction Nursing: Perspectives on Professional and Clinical Practice*. Cheltenham: Nelson Thornes.

McLellan, A.T., Wood, G.E., Metzger, D.S., McKay, J. and Altermanv, A.I. (1997) Evaluating the effectiveness of addiction treatments: reasonable expectations, appropriate comparisons. In J.A. Egerton, D.M. Fox and A.I. Leshner (eds) *Treating Drug Abusers Effectively*. Oxford: Blackwell Publications.

Mason, P. (2006) Motivational interviewing. In G. Hussein Rassool (ed.) *Dual Diagnosis Nursing*. Oxford: Blackwell Publications.

Mello, N., Mendelson, J., Kuehnle, J. and Sellers, M. (1981) Operant analysis of human heroin self-administration and the effects of naltrexone. *Journal of Pharmacology and Experimental Therapeutics*, 216: 45–54.

Miller, W.R. and Rollnick, S. (2002) *Motivational Interviewing: Preparing People for Change*, 2nd edition, New York: Guilford Press.

Miller, W.R. and Walker, D.D. (1997) Should there be aromatherapy for addiction? *Addiction*, 92, 4: 486–7.

Monti, P.M., Abrams, D.B., Kadden, R.M. and Cooney, N.L. (1989) *Treating Alcohol Dependence*. New York: Guilford Press.

NICE (2007) *Drug Misuse: Psychosocial Interventions*. NICE Clinical Guideline 51. London: National Institute for Health and Clinical Excellence.

NTA (2006a) *Treating Drug Misuse Problems: Evidence of Effectiveness*. London: National Treatment Agency.

NTA (2006b) *Review of the Effectiveness of Treatment for Alcohol Problems*. London: National Treatment Agency.

Prendergast, M.L., Podus, D., Chang, E. and Urada, D. (2002) The effectiveness of drug abuse treatment: a meta analysis of comparison group studies. *Drug and Alcohol Dependence*, 67: 53–72.

Psychosocial Working Group (2003) *A Framework for Practice*. Edinburgh: Centre for International Health Studies, Queen Margaret University College.

Rollnick, S. and Miller, W.R. (1995) What is motivational interviewing? *Behavioural and Cognitive Psychotherapy*, 23: 325–34.

Roth, A.D. and Pilling, S. (2007) *The Competences Required to Deliver Effective Cognitive and Behavioural Therapy for People with Depression and with Anxiety Disorders*. London: Department of Health.

Sorensen, J.L. and Copeland, A.L. (2000) Drug abuse treatment as an HIV prevention strategy: a review. *Drug Alcohol Dependence*, 59: 17–31.

Spray, J.R. and Jones, S.M. (1995) *The Use of Acupuncture in Drug Addiction Treatment*, News Briefs. http://ndsn.org/SEPT95/GUEST.html (accessed 29 January 2008).

Tonigan, S., Connors, G. and Miller, W.R. (1996) The Alcoholic Anonymous Involvement scale (AAI): reliability and norms. *Psychology of Addictive Behavior*, 10: 75–80.

Trevelyan, T. (1996) A true complement. *Nursing Times*, 92: 5.

Tucker, T., Ritter, A., Maher, C. and Jackson, H. (2004) Naltrexone maintenance for heroin dependence: uptake, attrition and retention. *Drug and Alcohol Review*, 23: 299–309.

Velleman, R. (2001) *Counselling for Alcohol Problems*, 2nd edition. London: Sage Publications.

WHO (1996) Brief Intervention Study Group: a cross-national trial of brief interventions with heavy drinkers. *American Journal of Public Health*, 86: 948–55.

WHO (2005) *Brief Intervention for Substance Use: A Manual for Use in Primary Care Department of Mental Health & Substance Dependence*. Geneva: World Health Organization.

CHAPTER 27

HARM REDUCTION APPROACH

OBJECTIVES

▪ Explain what is meant by harm reduction approach.

▪ Discuss the rationale for harm reduction approach.

▪ Discuss the harm reduction approach to drug, alcohol, tobacco and blood-borne and HIV infections.

▪ Explain what is meant by safer drug use and safer sex practice.

▪ Discuss the advantages and limitations of needle syringe schemes.

▪ Have an awareness of an alternative policy to harm reduction approach.

HARM REDUCTION APPROACH

There is now a broad consensus of opinion that recognises that the misuse of psycho-active substances is, and will continue to be, a part of society. Many individuals are unable or lack the readiness to change to be drug-free but none the less could benefit from intervention. The thinking of the 'unthinkable' approach has brought a sea change in the policy and strategy in tackling alcohol and drug misuse. An open-door policy can result in a harm reduction snowball effect: small improvements can pave the path for further reduction of drug use and an improved lifestyle in other ways. This snowball effect can continue, eventually, to the point of abstinence (Westermeyer 2002).

Since the mid-1980s, the UK government has viewed harm reduction as an integral and important part of the overall HIV prevention strategy and has supported a comprehensive and complementary package of interventions for HIV prevention, treatment and care among drug users. Three phases of the development of harm reduction have been observed (Erickson 1999). The first phase stemmed from a growing concern in the 1960s about the health risks associated with tobacco and alcohol use in the population. The second phase began in 1990 with a sharp focus on AIDS prevention among injecting drug users. Currently there is a third phase in which an integrated public health perspective is being developed for all licit and illicit psychoactive substances. The benefits and limitations of the harm reduction approach are presented in Table 27.1.

Table 27.1 Benefits and limitations of the harm reduction approach

Advantages	Limitations
• Substance-misuse-free society is unrealistic • Is a pragmatic public health approach • Complements approaches that aim for reductions in drug, alcohol and tobacco consumption • Engages people and motivates them to make contact with substance-misuse services • Reduces harm caused by substance misuse • Promotes controlled use of psychoactive substances • Avoids moralistic, stigmatising and judgemental statements about substance misusers • Reduces accidental death and overdose and saves lives • Reduces the transmission of blood-borne infections	• ? Provides a disguise for pro-legalisation efforts • ? Encourages illegal use of psychoactive substances • Encourages drinking behaviour • Discourages substance misusers from attaining abstinence • Undercuts abstinence-oriented treatment programmes

Harm reduction can work alongside approaches that aim for reductions in drug, alcohol and tobacco consumption. Harm reduction means trying to reduce the harm that people do to themselves, or other people, from their substance use. It can be contrasted with primary prevention, which tries to stop people using drugs in the first place or to stop using if they have already started. Harm reduction focuses on 'safer' drug use and has also been developed as a way of educating young people about drug use (Drugscope 2002). Harm reduction has also been described as a set of practical strategies that reduce negative consequences of drug use, incorporating a spectrum of strategies from safer use to managed use to abstinence (Harm Reduction.co.uk 2003). Rosenberg *et al.*'s (2004) study of 436 out of 623 eligible agencies in England, Wales and Scotland provides a valid assessment of the support of harm reduction interventions in British substance-misuse agencies. Harm reduction strategies meet drug users 'where they're at', addressing conditions of use along with the use itself (Harm Reduction.co.uk 2003). The principles of harm reduction (Harm Reduction co.uk 2003) are outlined in Table 27.2.

An important aspect of harm reduction is its focus on public health, which has improved co-operation between health, social, criminal justice system and law enforcement agencies. Harm reduction approaches nudge more substance misusers to engage in prevention and treatment programmes and open the door to helping these individuals to reduce harm in some way that would not otherwise occur. Engagement in treatment can provide a window of opportunity to minimise harms caused by alcohol and drug misuse. It also provides better outcomes for substance misusers as a small reduction in alcohol or drug misuse is better than zero reduction. An important aspect of harm reduction is its focus on public health, which has improved co-operation

Table 27.2 Principles of harm reduction

- Accepts that use of psychoactive substances is a part of our society, and chooses to minimise its harmful effects rather than to ignore or condemn it
- Understands that substance misuse is a complex and multi-faceted phenomenon that encompasses a continuum of behaviours, ranging from dependence to total abstinence, and acknowledges that some ways of using drugs or alcohol are clearly safer than others
- Calls for the non-judgemental, non-coercive provision of services and resources to individuals who use drugs and the communities in which they live in order to assist them in reducing attendant harm
- Ensures that substance misusers and those with a history of substance misuse routinely have a real voice in the creation of programmes and policies designed to serve them
- Affirms substance misusers themselves as the primary agents of reducing the harms of their substance use, and seeks to empower users to share information and support each other in strategies which meet their actual conditions of use
- Recognises that the realities of poverty, class, racism, social isolation, past trauma, sex-based discrimination and other social inequalities affect both people's vulnerability to and capacity for effectively dealing with substance-related harm
- Does not attempt to minimise or ignore the real and tragic harm and danger associated with licit and illicit drug use

---

Source: Harm Reduction co.uk (2003)

between the health, social, criminal justice system and law enforcement agencies. Harm reduction must be carried out in a public health framework and one in which the health, human rights and social needs of drug users, their families and communities are met (Cabinet Office 2005).

HARM REDUCTION: DRUGS

Harm reduction programmes include supervised consumption of methadone or other opiate substitutes, needle exchanges schemes (pharmacy-based needle exchange or other forms of needle exchange), programmes to reduce the risk associated with HIV and hepatitis, health information about safer drug use and safer sex. Information about safer drug use is providing health information for people who choose to use drugs to do so in the safest possible way. The harm reduction advice about safer drug use is presented in Table 27.3.

The first principle of reducing harm involves drawing attention the dangers of specific hazards in the misuse of particular psychoactive substances. In relation to harm reduction for injecting drug users, this may involve drawing attention to technique-specific hazards (related to the technology of injecting and sharing of equipment). For example, one important initiative in harm reduction approach has been the implementation of needle syringe schemes which provide sterile equipment, information on safer injecting and other services to people who usually are using illegal drugs. The procedure of safer injecting and methods of cleaning injecting equipment are presented in Table 27.4.

A hierarchy of goals is provided for those drug misusers in order to reach the abstinence stage. In order to achieve the reduction of harm, measures are used to that include: persuading drug users to stop sharing injecting equipment; moving from injection to oral drug use; decreasing drug use; and ultimately abstaining altogether.

Table 27.3 Safer drug use

Safer places to use drugs	• Taking drugs with friends is safer than doing it alone • Avoid using drugs in isolated places (e.g. toilets, derelict buildings, canal banks, railway lines)
Safer methods of taking drugs	• Swallowing, smoking or inhaling drugs is safer than injecting
Injecting drugs is more risky because of	• Overdose • Infection • Abscesses • Blood clots (thromboses) • Blood poisoning (septicaemia) • Gangrene • Death
If you intend to inject drugs	• Help and advice are available from your local needle and syringe exchange • It is safer *not* to inject • It is more dangerous to inject in big veins like the groin or neck
Sharing needles, syringes, filters, spoons and water should always be avoided to reduce the risk of HIV and hepatitis B and C transmission	• Ask your GP about hepatitis B vaccination • Do not use other people's 'wash outs' • It is not just the needle that's dangerous, it is everything used for injecting that could pass on the virus
Hygiene	• It is very important when injecting drugs to always remember to use clean, preferably new, equipment and make sure your hands and the injection site are clean
Mixing drugs	• Avoid cocktails of drugs – mixing drugs makes it more difficult to predict what will happen and for how long
Combining alcohol and drugs	• Can lead to respiratory depression • May choke on your vomit • Accidental overdoses and deaths

Source: Adapted from *Problem Drug Use: A Guide to Management in General Practice*, Nottingham Alcohol and Drug Team, The Wells Road Centre, Nottingham, NG3 3AA

HARM REDUCTION: ALCOHOL

Moderate or controlled drinking has been the health education message of the past few decades and can be regarded as alcohol harm reduction strategy. Alcohol harm reduction can be broadly defined as measures that aim to reduce the incidence of problem drinking and its negative consequences. Harm reduction offers a pragmatic approach to alcohol consumption and alcohol-related problems based on three core objectives: to reduce harmful consequences associated with alcohol use; to provide an alternative to zero-tolerance approaches by incorporating drinking goals (abstinence or moderation) that are compatible with the needs of the individual; and to promote access to services by offering low-threshold alternatives to traditional alcohol prevention and treatment (Marlatt and Witkiewitz 2002).

Table 27.4 Harm reduction and injecting drug users

Safer injecting use	<ul><li>Always inject with the blood flow</li><li>Rotate injection sites</li><li>Use sterile new injecting equipment, with the smallest-bore needle possible</li><li>Avoid neck, groin, breast, feet and hand veins</li><li>Mix powders with sterile water and filter solution before injecting</li><li>Always dispose of equipment safely (either in a bin provided or by placing the needle inside the syringe and placing both inside a drinks can)</li><li>Avoid injecting into infected areas</li><li>Do not inject into swollen limbs, even if the veins appear to be distended</li><li>Poor veins indicate a poor technique. Try to see what is going wrong</li><li>Do not inject on your own</li><li>Learn basic principles of first aid and cardiopulmonary resuscitation in order that you may help friends at times of crisis</li></ul>
Method of cleaning injecting equipment	1. Pour bleach into one cup (or bottle) and water into another 2. Draw bleach up with the dirty needle and syringe 3. Expel bleach into sink 4. Repeat steps 2 and 3 5. Draw water up through needle and syringe 6. Expel water into sink 7. Repeat steps 5 and 6 at least two or three times

Source: Department of Health (1999) *Drug Misuse and Dependence – Guidelines on Clinical Management.* London: HMSO.

A comprehensive alcohol policy needs population-level interventions, which focus on the availability and accessibility of alcohol (such as taxation and restricted licensing hours) and alcohol harm reduction interventions (International Harm Reduction Association (IHRA 2003). The focus of harm reduction strategies on particular risk behaviours (such as drinking and driving, binge drinking), risk groups, special populations (such as pregnant women, young people) and particular drinking contexts (such as bars and clubs). These approaches have broadened the sphere of interest in alcohol-related harms to include social nuisance and public order problems (IHRA 2003). The examples and benefits of alcohol harm reduction approach are presented in Table 27.5.

Table 27.5 Examples and benefits of alcohol harm reduction approach

Examples	*Benefits*
<ul><li>Promoting safer design of drinking environment</li><li>Campaigns against drinking and driving</li><li>Serving alcohol in shatter-proof glass to prevent injuries</li><li>Training bar staff to serve alcohol responsibly</li><li>Minimising violence and antisocial behaviour by managing drinking context</li><li>Brief interventions</li><li>Health education on controlled drinking in educational institutions</li><li>Providing shelters for homeless drinkers and intoxicated individuals.</li></ul>	<ul><li>Practical approaches</li><li>Realistic approaches</li><li>Not based on national policies, legislation or funding</li><li>Delivered by local communities based on local needs</li><li>Short-term aim is to minimise the impacts of alcohol consumption</li><li>Long-term aim is to change drinking cultures – promoting the benefits of responsible drinking and discouraging harmful drinking</li></ul>

HARM REDUCTION: TOBACCO

The harm reduction approach to tobacco smoking has remained controversial despite the universal use of tobacco smoking. Currently, tobacco harm reduction strategy is based on supply and demand reduction strategies (Esson and Leeder 2005). Thus, in light of (1) the high number of smokers worldwide, (2) the regular failure of smokers to give up their tobacco addiction, (3) the direct role of several smoke components, and, to a much lesser extent, nicotine, in most tobacco-related diseases, and (4) the possible use of much less toxic, but still addictive, tobacco products, evaluation of less harmful products, such as oral tobacco, for the purpose of harm reduction is warranted (Martinet *et al.* 2007). According to the proponents of tobacco harm reduction, this approach to tobacco smoking should also be evaluated and/or promoted within a hierarchy of 'achievable' goals (Martinet *et al.* 2007). Abstinence-oriented treatment such as nicotine replacement therapy may be a viable option for most smokers. Advising cigarette smokers who cannot give up smoking to use oral tobacco could be an efficient way to reduce harm related to nicotine addiction (Fagerström and Schildt (2003).

HARM REDUCTION: HIV AND BLOOD-BORNE INFECTIONS

In the context of HIV and other blood-borne diseases, harm reduction strategies aim to reduce the health and social harms of drug injecting. Prevention of HIV transmission among injecting drug users (IDUs) can best be achieved by implementing a core package of interventions including (Cabinet Office 2005), exchange syringe schemes, methadone maintenance, hepatitis vaccination, safer sexual practice, sexual health, access to drug and HIV treatment and clinical and home-based care. A more comprehensive list is provided in Table 27.6.

Table 27.6 Prevention of HIV among IDUs: core package of interventions

- Availability of and referral to a variety of drug treatment options
- Substitution therapy such as methadone maintenance therapy
- Sterile needle and syringe access and disposal programmes
- Outreach programmes and community-based interventions
- Primary healthcare, such as hepatitis B vaccination, abscess and vein care
- Prevention of sexual transmission among drug users and their partners, including access to condoms
- Prevention and treatment of other sexually transmitted infections (STIs)
- Voluntary confidential counselling and HIV testing (VCT)
- Access to AIDS treatment for injecting drug users
- Provision of information, advice and education about HIV, other diseases, and sexual and reproductive health
- Access to affordable clinical and home-based care, essential legal and social services, psychosocial support and counselling services.

Source: Adapted from Cabinet Office (2005)

NEEDLE EXCHANGE SCHEMES

Syringe exchange schemes provide paraphernalia (syringe, citric and vitamin C sachets, water ampoules, stericups and sterifilts), educational resources (for example, on safer drug use, safer sexual practice, overdose, first aid) and health interventions to enable injecting drug users to protect themselves and their communities through safer injection practices and harm reduction methods. The World Health Organization (2004) report stated there is evidence to suggest that providing access to and encouraging utilisation of sterile needles and syringes for people who inject drugs is now generally considered to be a fundamental component of any comprehensive and effective HIV-prevention programme. There was no evidence that needle exchange programmes increased either the number of people using drugs or the frequency of injecting drug use. However, it is important to tailor harm reduction programmes to meet the specific needs where cocaine injection is prevalent. Cocaine injectors tend to inject much more frequently than heroin injectors, and therefore require much greater quantities of sterile needles and syringes than usually provided by most needle exchange programmes (WHO 2004). Many needle exchanges often target self-identified injecting drug users and miss occasional or recreational drug users, especially among young people. Strategies should be developed to focus on young people who are occasional or recreational users.

In some countries, there is provision of syringe-dispensing machines and mobile vans as part of the needle exchange schemes. Syringe-dispensing machines are automatic commercial dispensing machines that exchange new for used syringes, or provide sterile equipment for a coin or free-of-cost. This scheme is to provide exchange services after closure of the day needle exchange services. The needle exchange scheme-mobile introduced, in 1986, in Amsterdam, the Netherlands, was a methadone-dispensing bus that also offered syringe and needle exchange (Moore *et al.* 2004). The exchange needles and syringes using mobile vans were introduced in both London and Liverpool in the same year (Buning 1993).

The rationale for dispensing machines and mobile vans offers the potential to provide injecting equipment to hard-to-reach and high-risk groups of injecting drug users (Islam and Conigrave 2007). Access to needle syringe schemes is usually limited outside business hours, and many injecting drug users need access to services in the evening, at night or at weekends. Consequently, dispensing machines were introduced to supply sterile needles and syringes together with condoms, health information pamphlets and other minor health supplies (Loxley *et al.* 1991) and provide anonymity. Unlike dispensing machines, mobile vans do not provide completely anonymous access to sterile injecting equipment but can provide outreach services to those high-risk groups such as homeless users, chaotic users, young recreational drug users and drug users from Black and ethnic minority groups. There is evidence to support the notion that dispensing machines and mobile vans can accommodate different patterns of user, diversifying services to meet various needs are crucial elements in continuing efforts in reducing the spread of HIV and other blood-borne viruses among injecting drug users (Islam and Conigrave 2007)

A more recent technological innovation of the harm reduction approach is the introduction of the 'Nevershare syringe' . The Nevershare syringe is the world's first syringe designed for injecting drug users with plungers in a range of colours to reduce accidental sharing (Exchange Supplies 2008). By supplying syringes with coloured plungers, blood-borne virus transmission can be reduced more effectively by:

- reducing the risk of accidental sharing
- reinforcing the importance of having your own equipment, and not sharing
- making the issue of sharing explicit with every syringe
- promoting strategies to prevent accidental sharing. (Exchange Supplies 2008).

ALTERNATIVES TO THE HARM REDUCTION APPROACH

EURAD (Europe against drugs) is a non-voluntary organisation providing drug information network and advocacy that promotes the creation of healthy drug-free cultures in the world and opposes the legalisation of drugs. Its philosophy is based on Article 33 of the UN Convention against Illicit Traffic of Narcotic Drugs and Psychotropic Substances of 1988, which refers to 'publicly inciting or inducing others, by any means, . . . to use narcotic drugs or psychotropic substances illicitly' and requires each party to establish such conduct as a criminal offence under its domestic law.

EURAD states that it is the drug taking in itself and the behaviour drug misuse causes that is the root of the 'harm'. EURAD fears that strategies like harm reduction might well increase and change the nature of the problem in the future. The organisation suggests that methadone programmes have little or no place in communities that run efficient demand restrictive policies of prevention and early intervention with brakes all the way down the slope of drug abuse. EURAD does not support harm reduction policies, recognising that these enable addiction and lead to harm production policies. EURAD believes that the way forward in combating the drugs epidemic is to reduce the demand for drugs while supporting families afflicted by drug misuse.

Even though EURAD is not in favour of methadone programmes, it sets a number of strict criteria if services introduce methadone programmes. It also has objections directed against needle exchange schemes. Its objections are based on the notions that needle exchange schemes reduce the threshold against injecting drug use and thus encourage injecting among those who still take drugs orally or by sniffing. In addition, it believes that focusing on needles or syringes might make society forget that HIV/AIDS is spread to a greater extent by sex than by the sharing of needles or syringes. It emphasises that needle or syringe distribution programmes, as well as poorly controlled methadone programmes, have no place in communities that run efficient demand restrictive policies of early intervention with brakes all the way down the slope of drug misuse.

KEY POINTS

- Harm reduction means trying to reduce the harm that people do to themselves, or other people, from their substance use.
- Harm reduction can work alongside approaches that aim for reductions in drug, alcohol and tobacco consumption.
- Harm reduction focuses on safer drug use and safer sexual practice.
- It provides better outcomes for substance misusers as a small reduction in alcohol or drug misuse is better than zero reduction.

- Harm reduction programmes include supervised consumption of methadone or other opiate substitutes and needle exchanges schemes (pharmacy-based needle exchange or other forms of needle exchange).
- A comprehensive alcohol policy needs population-level interventions, which focus on the availability and accessibility of alcohol and alcohol harm reduction interventions.
- The harm reduction approach to tobacco smoking has remained controversial despite the universal use of tobacco smoking.
- Currently, tobacco harm reduction strategy is based on supply and demand reduction strategies.
- In the context of HIV and other blood-borne diseases, harm reduction strategies aim to reduce the health and social harms of drug injecting.
- There was no evidence that needle exchange programmes increased either the number of people using drugs or the frequency of injecting drug use.
- Many needle-exchanges often target self-identified injecting drug users and miss occasional or recreational drug users, especially among young people.
- EURAD does not support harm reduction policies, recognising that these enable addiction and lead to harm production policies.

ACTIVITY 27.1

Please state whether the following statements are true or false. Reflect on the statements and give reason(s) for choosing a particular option

	True	False
The UK views harm reduction as an integral and important part of the overall HIV prevention strategy		
Harm reduction cannot work alongside approaches that aim for reductions in drug, alcohol and tobacco consumption		
Harm reduction focuses on 'safer' drug use and has also been developed as a way of educating young people about drug use		
Harm reduction approaches nudge more substance misusers to engage in prevention and treatment programmes		
Engagement in treatment can provide a window of opportunity to minimise harm caused by alcohol and drug misuse		
Harm reduction does not provide better outcomes for substance misusers		
A comprehensive alcohol policy needs population-level interventions focusing on the availability and accessibility of alcohol and alcohol harm reduction interventions		
Currently, tobacco harm reduction strategy is based on supply and demand reduction strategies		
Abstinence-oriented treatment such as nicotine replacement therapy may be a viable option for most smokers		
In the context of HIV and other blood-borne diseases, harm reduction strategies aim to reduce the health and social harms of drug injecting		

There is no evidence to suggest that harm reduction is effective in HIV prevention programmes

There is no evidence that needle exchange programmes increased either the number of people using drugs or the frequency of injecting drug use

It is important to tailor harm-reduction programmes to meet the specific needs of cocaine users

Many injecting drug users need access to services in the evening, at night or in weekends

---

ACTIVITY 27.2

There is only one correct answer to the following questions

Harm reduction programmes include
a. Supervised consumption of methadone
b. Needle exchange schemes
c. Ideas to reduce the risk associated with HIV and hepatitis
d. All of the above

The first principle of reducing harm involves drawing attention to
a. The dangers of drugs and technique-specific hazards
b. The dangers of psychoactive drugs
c. The dangers of needle exchange schemes
d. The dangers of not using sterile equipment.

Alcohol harm reduction can be broadly defined as measures that aim
a. To reduce the incidence of problem drinking
b. To reduce controlled drinking
c. To reduce alcohol consumption
d. To promote zero tolerance

Syringe exchange schemes provide
a. Paraphernalia
b. Educational resources
c. Health interventions
d. All of the above

Needle exchanges should target
a. Self-identified injecting drug users
b. Recreational drug users
c. Homeless injecting drug users
d. All of the above

ACTIVITY 27.3

- List the benefits and limitations of a harm reduction approach
- Identify the hierarchy of goals for drug misusers to reach the abstinence stage
- Discuss the harm reduction approach to drug, alcohol, tobacco and blood-borne and HIV infections
- Explain what is meant by safer drug use and safer sex practice
- Discuss the advantages and limitations of needle syringe schemes
- What is the rationale for dispensing machines and mobile vans in the provision of injecting equipment?

REFERENCES

Buning, E. (1993) Outreach work with drug users: an overview. *International Journal of Drug Policy*, 4, 2: 78–82.

Cabinet Office (2005) *Harm Reduction: Tackling Drug Use and HIV in the Developing World*. London: Department for International Development.

Drugscope (2002) *Drug Terms*. London: Drugscope. www.drugscope.org.uk.

Erickson, P.G. (1999) Introduction: the three phases of harm reduction. An examination of emerging concepts, methodologies, and critiques. *Substance Use and Misuse*, 34: 1–7.

Esson, K.M. and Leeder, S. (2005) *The Millennium Development Goals and Tobacco Control: An Opportunity for Global Partnership*. Geneva: World Health Organization.

EURAD www.eurad.net (accessed 25 November 2007).

Exchange Supplies (2008) www.exchangesupplies.org (accessed 25 November 2007).

Fagerström, K.O. and Schildt, E.B. (2003) Should the European union lift the ban on snus? Evidence from the Swedish experience. *Addiction*, 98: 1191–5.

Harm Reduction co.uk (2003) *Harm Reduction*. www.harmreduction.co.uk/index3.html (accessed on 25 November 2007).

International Harm Reduction Association (IHRA) (2003) *What Is Alcohol Harm Reduction*. www.ihra.net/alcohol (accessed 26 November 2007).

Islam, M.M. and Conigrave K.M. (2007) Assessing the role of syringe dispensing machines and mobile van outlets in reaching hard-to-reach and high-risk groups of injecting drug users (IDUs): a review. *Harm Reduction Journal*, 4: 14doi:10.1186/1477-7517-4-14. www.harm reductionjournal.com/content/4/1/14 (accessed 26 November 2007).

Loxley, W., Watt, P., Kosky, M., Westlund, B., Watson, C. and Marsh A. (1991) Western Australian initiatives to prevent the spread of HIV/AIDS amongst injecting drug users. *International Journal on Drug Policy*, 2, 4: 13–16.

Marlatt, G.A. and Witkiewitz, K. (2002) Harm reduction approaches to alcohol use: health promotion, prevention, and treatment. *Addictive Behaviors*, 27, 8: 867–86.

Martinet, Y., Bohadana, A. and Fagerström, K. (2007) Introducing oral tobacco for tobacco harm reduction: what are the main obstacles? *Harm Reduction Journal*, 4: 17doi:10.1186/14 77-7517-4-17. www.harmreductionjournal.com/content/4/1/17 (accessed 26 November 2007).

Moore, G., McCarthy, P., MacNeela, P., MacGabhann, L., Philbin, M. and Proudfoot, D. (2004) *A Review of Harm Reduction Approaches in Ireland and Evidence from the International Literature*. Dublin: National Advisory Committee on Drugs.

Rosenberg, H., Melville, J. and McLean, P.C. (2004) Non pharmacological harm-reduction interventions in British substance-misuse services. *Addictive Behaviours*, 29, 6: 1225–9.

Westermeyer, R. (2002) *Harm Reduction and Illicit Drug Use*. www.habitsmart.com/index.html (accessed 26 November 2007).

WHO (2001) *The World Health Report 2001 – Mental Health: New Understanding, New Hope*. Geneva: World Health Organization.

WHO (2004) *Effectiveness of Sterile Needle and Syringe Programming in Reducing HIV/AIDS among Injecting Drug Users*. Geneva: World Health Organization. www.who.int/hiv/pub/prev_care/en/effectivenesssterileneedle.pdf (accessed 26 November 2007).

CHAPTER 28

INTOXICATION AND OVERDOSE: HEALTH INTERVENTIONS

OBJECTIVES

- Define intoxication and overdose.

- Identify the reasons of the need for emergency medical attention.

- Discuss the effects of acute intoxication.

- Identify the risks associated with alcohol and drug misuse.

- Describe the interventions in acute intoxication.

- Identify the risk factors associated with an increased likelihood of overdose.

- Describe the interventions in overdose.

Intoxication and overdose are the potential consequences of substance misuse whether the psychoactive substance is illicit, prescribed or over-the-counter. Emergency medical attention is often required by those misusing psychoactive substances as a result of:

- toxic or adverse effects of the substance
- the route of administration (injecting may lead to blood poisoning and deep vein thrombosis)
- lifestyle behaviours (poor malnutrition, dehydration)
- risk-taking whilst under the influence of psychoactive substances (accidents, self-harm).

Psychoactive substances taken in combination with alcohol or drugs, even drugs normally considered safe, increase the risk of death by overdose and can have serious long-term consequences. Intoxication is a state when there is an intake of more than the normal amount of a psychoactive substance which produces behavioural or physical changes. An overdose is the accidental or intentional use of a psychoactive substance which exceeds the individual's tolerance. This chapter covers two aspects of substance misuse – intoxication and overdose – and relevant health interventions are outlined.

ACUTE INTOXICATION

Acute intoxication frequently occurs in persons who have more persistent alcohol- or drug-related problems. It is a transient condition following the administration of alcohol or other psychoactive substance, resulting in disturbances in level of consciousness, cognition, perception, affect or behaviour, or other psycho-physiological functions and responses (WHO 2005).

Most psychoactive substances will have an effect upon the central nervous and the cardiopulmonary systems. The type, the dose of drug and the individual's level of tolerance have a significant influence on the state of intoxication. However, it is important to recognise the symptoms of alcohol or drug intoxication not only to confirm the presence and severity of the alcohol effect but also to be able to differentiate the symptoms from other conditions. These conditions may mimic or mask the symptoms of alcohol or drug intoxication. The symptoms of intoxication do not always reflect the desired or expected effects of the psychoactive substance. For instance, depressant drugs (alcohol or GHB) may lead to symptoms of agitation or hyperactivity, and stimulant drugs (amphetamine or cocaine) may lead to socially withdrawn and introverted behaviour. In alcohol intoxication, for example, the level of intoxication will largely be influenced by body weight, tolerance, the volume of alcohol consumption, alcohol percentage in the drinks consumed and the period over which the alcohol was taken. The cultural and personal expectations regarding the effects of the drug will also influence the level of intoxication. The common features of psychoactive intoxication include disinhibition, euphoria, lack of co-ordination and impaired judgement. Alcohol and drug intoxication may influence a person's mental health problem and may imitate or mask symptoms of an underlying mental or physical disorder. The resulting lack of inhibition and the depressant effect on the central nervous system may increase the risk of harm to self and others and exacerbate the risk of suicide.

RISKS OF ALCOHOL AND DRUG INTOXICATION

An individual in an acute stage of intoxication of alcohol is most frequently seen in accident and emergency departments. Alcohol intoxication rarely requires treatment but it may precipitate seizures by lowering the seizure threshold level. Because the symptoms of alcohol withdrawal are related to a relative drop in alcohol levels, seizures may paradoxically occur during intoxication. It is extremely common for an intoxicated individual to vomit once or twice. However, continued vomiting may be a sign of head injury or other serious illness.

Alcohol and drugs affect co-ordination and reactions, so individuals are prone to accidents. Trauma and head injuries, caused by poor co-ordination and judgement when intoxicated, are common. Head injury also increases the risk of seizures. It is possible for an individual who has acute alcohol poisoning to go into respiratory arrest while they are asleep and they can also choke to death on their vomit. Hypothermia is also a high risk factor for homeless problem drinkers. The individual may become belligerent, paranoid and even violent, necessitating the risk of caution and sensitivity when approaching them. The use, desired effects and acute intoxication of psychoactive substances are discussed in Chapters 7 to 12.

INTERVENTIONS IN ACUTE INTOXICATION

Health interventions are based on the urgency and seriousness of the individual with acute intoxication. When an individual is acutely intoxicated, first aid procedures are implemented in relation to:

- *A* – Airway
- *B* – Breathing
- *C* – Circulation / cardiac.

The interventions required for an individual with acute intoxication are presented in Table 28.1.

Additional interventions may be the monitoring of withdrawal syndrome; the screening for drug and alcohol problems (assessment, urine or saliva testing); referral to an appropriate service to meet these needs; contact point for further help (self-help groups); harm-reduction (advice to reduce the harm caused by drug use, such as safer modes of use or how to access sterile injecting equipment); provision of information literature on overdose prevention, viral transmission and local drug services. Developing close liaison with drug treatment providers facilitates better access to treatment.

Table 28.1 Health Interventions: Intoxication

Medical or physical needs	Psychosocial needs
<ul><li>Place in recovery position – if appropriate</li><li>Assessment of airway, breathing and circulation</li><li>Assess level of consciousness (Glasgow coma scale)</li><li>Monitor vital signs</li><li>Implement seizure safety precautions</li><li>Monitor fluid intake and output</li><li>Implement interventions to decrease systemic absorption of drugs (use of absorbents (activated charcoal), induced diarrhoea, induced vomiting, gastric lavage), if appropriate</li><li>Administration of antidote, if appropriate</li></ul>	<ul><li>Orientation</li><li>'Being there'</li><li>Non-judgemental approach in interactions</li><li>Create a supportive environment</li><li>Assess for 'risk behaviours' (self-harm, potential for violence)</li><li>Contact relatives or friends who are best able to support and reassure the patient</li></ul>

OVERDOSE

There has been concern about the high prevalence of mortality amongst substance misusers. Drug-related deaths are defined as 'Deaths where the underlying cause is poisoning, drug abuse, or drug dependence and where any of the substances are controlled under the Misuse of Drugs Act (1971)' (ONS 2003). The report by the Advisory Council on the Misuse of Drugs (ACMD 2000, xi, 6) on *Reducing Drug-related Deaths* highlighted its concern about this issue and acknowledged that the prevention of drug-related deaths is a matter of pressing urgency. The report indicated that the number of such deaths must be substantially reduced. In England and Wales, there were more than 2,300 drug-related deaths due to accidental or intentional overdose during 1998 and the trend is rising (ACMD 2000). Following the recommendations of the ACMD Report (2000), and the *Action Plan to Prevent Drug-related Deaths* (Department of Health 2001), the government's updated drug strategy (Home Office 2002) has given a higher profile to a range of harm reduction measures to reduce premature death amongst drug users associated with fatal and non-fatal overdoses.

An overdose is 'an event in which a person intentionally or accidentally ingests one or more psychoactive substances at unsafe levels, leading to physical trauma, which may require immediate medical care to reverse and manage symptoms and other complications' (National Treatment Agency 2002: 156). Whilst many victims of drug overdose recover without long-term consequences, there can be serious implications for health due to the failure of the respiratory or circulatory systems or major organs like the kidneys or liver. The pattern of the type of drug taken in overdose has changed in recent years, largely with changes in their availability and accessibility. Substance misusers are at higher risk of suicide than the general population, and prescribed drugs, notably antidepressants and methadone, heighten that risk.

Drug overdose is the most common method of suicide amongst substance misusers and the likelihood of overdose is increased when drugs are taken by injection: fatal overdose (immediate death) is particularly associated with injecting opioid users. (Oyefeso *et al*. 1999, NTA 2002). There is evidence to suggest that about 80% of people who present to accident and emergency departments following self-harm will have taken an overdose of prescribed or over-the-counter medication and most will meet criteria for one or more psychiatric diagnosis at the time they are assessed (Haw *et al*. 2001, Horrocks *et al*. 2003).

About one-third of those who self-harm will be misusing drugs or alcohol on a regular basis (Haw *et al*. 2001). The misuse of a combination of psychoactive substances such as benzodiazepines and alcohol with opiates or combining heroin with cocaine as a 'speedball' can increase the chances of an overdose. In a prospective study of mortality among drug misusers, Gossop *et al*. (2002) found that the majority of deaths (68%) were associated with drug overdoses. Opiates were the drugs most commonly detected during post-mortem examinations. In the majority of cases, more than one drug was detected. Polydrug use and, specifically, heavy drinking, and use of benzodiazepines and amphetamines, were identified as risk factors for mortality. The use of antidepressants amongst polysubstance users has also been found to heighten the risk of fatality (Oyefeso *et al*. 2000).

The are several risk factors that are reported to be associated with an increased likelihood of overdose. The multiple risk factors include: administration by injection;

Table 28.2 Predictors of risk associated with overdose

- Injecting drugs (heroin users, high level of dependence)
- Polydrug use (combinations of drugs such as heroin, methadone, alcohol and benzodiazepines)
- High tolerance levels (users who have experienced non-fatal overdoses recently)
- Low tolerance levels (using opiates when tolerance is low particularly after a break in use following imprisonment or detoxification)
- Cocaine and crack (cocaine and crack use among heroin users can play a role in fatal overdoses, as they can temporarily mask the sedative effects of heroin and other depressant-type drugs)
- Poor mental health, depression, hopelessness and suicidal thoughts
- Not being in treatment (heroin injectors not in methadone treatment are around four times more likely to die than those in treatment)
- Premature termination of treatment (loss of tolerance, increased polydrug use after detoxification)
- Solitary alcohol or drug use (using drugs alone, especially injecting, places a person at increased risk)

Source: Adapted from Roberts and McVeigh (2004)

concomitant use of other depressant drugs; loss of tolerance after a period of abstinence; injecting in public places (which may be associated with the use of untested drugs) or solitary drug use; a long history of opiate dependence; older age; and possibly unexpected changes in purity (EMCDDA 2003). A summary of risk factors associated with incidence of overdose is presented in Table 28.2.

INTERVENTIONS WITH OVERDOSE

Drug overdose amongst substance misusers is a relatively common phenomenon and an acute life-threatening emergency. For many substance misusers, the first or only point of contact with health services is the accident and emergency (A&E) departments following overdoses, accidents or psychological crises. There are some general principles that define interventions of individuals with drug overdose, and, in any settings, emergency treatment should begin immediately. The priority is treating life-threatening problems such as respiratory depression, airway obstruction, cardiovascular collapse and convulsions (epileptic-form seizures) alongside specific measures to treat the overdose.

Emergency Interventions include:

- establishment of a patent airway
- provision of ventilation support (artificial respiration, respirator)
- maintenance of adequate circulatory status (chest compressions, defibrillator, intravenous line)
- controlling of seizures (safety measures, intravenous diazepam)
- administration of drug, if appropriate (for example, opiate overdose-naloxone).

After implementing acute interventions to stabilise the individual, a through history and physical examination are completed. Obtain information about the substance: name, route of administration, amount taken, when and period of time taken. If the individual is unable to participate in the assessment process, collateral information should be obtained whenever possible from family members or significant others or past medical notes. Investigations for routine blood count and chemistry,

Table 28.3 Continuing interventions in overdose

• Monitor vital signs including temperature
• Perform electrocardiogram (EEG) and continue to monitor
• Check the level of consciousness continue to be monitored at 15-minute intervals using the Glasgow coma scale (Teasdale and Jennett 1974)
• Maintaining hydration and monitoring fluid intake and output
• Safety precautions must be maintained during acute interventions as the individual may show signs of varying level of consciousness, hallucinations and seizures
• Reassurance and support should be provided
• Measures to decrease systemic absorption of the substance such as gastric lavage, induced emesis (vomiting), absorbents (activated charcoal) or induced diarrhoea (magnesium) should be used as appropriate
• An antidote may be administered depending upon the type of psychoactive substance used

urinalysis and toxicological screens of blood and urine will provide further evidence about the overdose. Monitor vital signs including temperature. Perform electrocardiogram (EEG) and continue to monitor. The level of consciousness should be checked and should continue to be monitored at 15-minute intervals using the Glasgow Coma Scale (Teasdale and Jennett 1974). The continuing interventions of overdose are presented in Table 28.3.

In the case of a loss of consciousness, it is important not to presume that alcohol or drugs are the sole cause. Other possible causes may include trauma, epilepsy, diabetes, hepatic failure, hypercalcaemia, renal failure, cerebral haemorrhage, cerebral thrombosis, abscess, tumour, arrhythmias, myocardial infarction and infections such as meningitis or encephalitis. Once the overdose has been treated it is important to assess for depression or self-harm and explore the withdrawal management and treatment interventions options. It is also a good opportunity for harm reduction interventions and the provisions of health information and information related to specialist alcohol or drug services.

INTERVENTIONS FOR OPIATE OVERDOSE

Opiate users are prone to accidental overdose because they often overestimate their own tolerance or are unaware of the potency of the drug they use. The presenting features of opiate overdose are:

• slow respiration (2–7/minute), usually deep compared with the shallow and more rapid respiration associated with intoxication by barbiturates, etc.
• pinpoint pupils
• cyanosis, weak pulse, bradycardia
• possible pulmonary oedema
• twitching of muscles
• subnormal temperature may occur.

The treatment of overdose from opiates is the antidote naloxone hydrochloride (Naloxone). A dose at 0.8–2 mg by intravenous injection should be administered, repeated at intervals of 2–3 minutes to a maximum of 10 mg. If respiratory function does not improve, other diagnostic options such as other drug intoxication, or other organic causes of loss of consciousness, including hypoglycaemia, should be considered (Department of Health 1999). If an intravenous route is not accessible owing to vein collapse, subcutaneous or intramuscular injection routes should be used. Naloxone is short-acting, and repeated injections or intravenous infusion may be needed if a longer-acting opiate such as methadone has been taken. Naloxone can be given as a continuous intravenous infusion of 2 mg diluted in a 500 ml intravenous solution titrated at a rate determined by the clinical response (Department of Health 1999). In methadone overdose, the effects can persist for up to 72 hours. Even in circumstances where patients have been resuscitated, depending on the magnitude of the overdose, they should be observed as an inpatient for a period of up to 72 hours. For high-dose intoxication, naloxone infusion should be considered.

INTERVENTIONS FOR OTHER DRUG OVERDOSES

No antidote exists for the treatment of overdose from other drugs such as amphetamines, cocaine, cannabis, LSD, ecstasy, barbiturates and alcohol. In such overdoses, respiration must be maintained by artificial means until the drugs are removed from the system. Some drugs may help speed the excretion of the barbiturates. The use of the tricyclic antidepressants is common with substance misusers. Antidepressants in large dosage can cause coma, cardiac arrhythmias and anti-cholinergic effect, and mortality risk is high. Treatment interventions should therefore be aimed at the presenting symptoms and may include:

- management of the unconscious patient
- management of hypothermia
- management of acute psychosis.

Overdose of GHB can be difficult to treat because of its multiple effects on the body. GHB overdose often causes life-threatening respiratory depression, bradycardia and consequent heart failure. GHB tends to cause nausea and vomiting, particularly when combined with alcohol; so a substance misuser may be simultaneously unconscious, vomiting and convulsing (Miotto and Roth 2001). The most likely risk of death from GHB overdose is inhalation of vomit while unconscious. Individuals are most likely to vomit as they become unconscious, and as they wake up. This risk can be partially prevented by laying the patient down in the recovery position.

KEY POINTS

- Intoxication and overdose are the potential consequences of substance misuse whether the psychoactive substance is illicit, prescribed or over-the-counter.
- Psychoactive substances taken in combination with alcohol or drug increase the risk of death by overdose and can have serious long-term consequences.

- Acute intoxication frequently occurs in persons who have more persistent alcohol- or drug-related problems.
- The type and dose of drug and the individual's level of tolerance have a significant influence on the state of intoxication.
- Alcohol and drug intoxication may influence a person's mental health problem and may imitate or mask symptoms of an underlying mental or physical disorder.
- Drug-related deaths are deaths where the underlying cause is poisoning, drug abuse, or drug dependence
- The government's updated drug strategy has given a higher profile to a range of harm reduction measures to reduce premature death amongst drug users associated with fatal and non-fatal overdoses.
- Substance misusers are at higher risk of suicide than the general population, and prescribed drugs, notably antidepressants and methadone, heighten that risk.
- Drug overdose is the most common method of suicide amongst substance misusers, and the likelihood of overdose is increased when drugs are taken by injection.
- Fatal overdose (immediate death) is particularly associated with injecting opioid users.
- Overdose amongst substance misusers is an acute life-threatening emergency.
- The treatment of overdose from opiates is the antidote naloxone hydrochloride (Naloxone).
- No antidote exists for the treatment of overdose from other drugs such as amphetamines, cocaine, cannabis, LSD, ecstasy, barbiturates and alcohol.

ACTIVITY 28.1

Please state whether the following statements are true or false. Reflect on the statements and give reason(s) for choosing a particular option

	True	False
Intoxication and overdose are the potential consequences of substance misuse		
Psychoactive substances, taken in combination with alcohol or drugs, are considered safe		
Intoxication is a state when there is an intake of more than the normal amount of a psychoactive substance		
An overdose is the accidental or intentional use of a psychoactive substance which exceeds the individual's tolerance		
Some medical or psychological conditions may mimic or mask the symptoms of alcohol or drug intoxication		
The cultural and personal expectations regarding the effects of the drug will also influence the level of intoxication		
Trauma and head injuries increase the risk of seizures		
Substance misusers have a lower risk of suicide than the general population		
Drug overdose is the most common method of suicide amongst substance misusers		

Combining heroin with cocaine as a 'speedball' can increase the chances of an overdose

The use of antidepressants amongst polysubstance users has been found to heighten the risk of fatality

The treatment of overdose from opiates is the antidote naloxone hydrochloride

Overdose of GHB can be difficult to treat because of its multiple effects on the body

ACTIVITY 28.2

There is only one correct answer to the following multiple-choice questions

Emergency medical attention is often required by substance misusers because of
a.   Toxic or adverse effects of the substance
b.   The route of administration
c.   Poor malnutrition and dehydration
d.   All of the above

Factors that have a significant influence on the state of intoxication include
a.   The type of psychoactive substance
b.   The dosage of the psychoactive substance
c.   The level of tolerance
d.   All of the above

In alcohol intoxication the level of intoxication will largely be influenced by
a.   Body weight
b.   Tolerance
c.   Volume of alcohol consumption
d.   All of the above

Alcohol intoxication
a.   Rarely requires treatment
b.   May precipitate seizures
c.   May induce vomiting
d.   All of the above

Once emergency care in acute intoxication is given it is important to
a.   Monitor of withdrawal syndrome
b.   Screen for drug and alcohol problems
c.   Refer to a specialist service
d.   All of the above

Types of health information that should be given to substance misusers
a.   A contact point for further help (self-help groups)
b.   Harm reduction

c.   Overdose prevention
d.   All of the above

Overdose can have serious implications such as
a.   Respiratory failure
b.   Circulatory failure
c.   Liver failure
d.   All of the above

The likelihood of overdose is increased when drugs are taken
a.   By injection
b.   Orally
c.   By inhalation
d.   None of the above

The risk factors of fatal overdose include
a.   Administration by injection
b.   Loss of tolerance after a period of abstinence
c.   Unexpected changes in drug purity
d.   All of the above

The emergency interventions in overdose interventions include:
a.   Establishing a patent airway and providing ventilation support
b.   Maintaining adequate circulatory status
c.   Controlling seizures
d.   All of the above

General treatment interventions should include
a.   Management of the unconscious patient
b.   Management of hypothermia
c.   Management of acute psychosis
d.   All of the above

REFERENCES

ACMD (Advisory Council on the Misuse of Drugs) (2000) *Reducing Drug-related Deaths.* A report by the Advisory Council on the Misuse of Drugs. London: The Stationery Office.

Department of Health (1999) *Drug Misuse and Dependence – Guidelines on Clinical Management.* London: The Stationery Office.

Department of Health (2001) *Action Plan to Prevent Drug-related Deaths.* London: Department of Health.

European Monitoring Centre for Drugs and Drug Addiction. (2003) *Annual Report 2003: The State of the Drugs Problem in the European Union and Norway.* Lisbon: EMCCDA.

Gossop, M., Duncan, S., Samantha, T. and Marsden, J. (2002) A prospective study of mortality among drug misusers during a 4-year period after seeking treatment. *Addiction*, 97, 1: 39–47.

Haw, C., Hawton, K., Houston, K. and Townsend, E. (2001) Psychiatric and personality disorders in deliberate self-harm patients. *British Journal of Psychiatry*, 178: 48–54.

Home Office (2002) *Updated Strategy 2002*. London: Home Office. www.drugs.gov.uk.

Horrocks, J., Price, S., House, A. and Owens, D. (2003) Self-injury attendances in the accident and emergency department. *British Journal of Psychiatry*, 183: 34–9.

Merrill, J., Milner, G., Owens, D. and Vale, A. (1992). Alcohol and attempted suicide. *British Journal of Addictions*, 87: 83–9.

Miotto, K. and Roth, B. (2001) Patients with a history of around-the clock use of gamma hydroxybutyrate may present as disturbing and difficult to manage. *UCLA Integrated UTSW Toxicology Substance Abuse Program Training Service*. www.tcada.state.tx.us.

NTA(2002) *Models of Care for Treatment of Adult Drug Misusers*. London: National Treatment Agency .

Office for National Statistics (2003) Deaths related to drug poisoning: results for England and Wales, 1993 to 2001. London: *Health Statistics Quarterly* (Spring).

Oyefeso, A., Ghodse, A.H., Clancy, C. and Corkery, J.M. (1999) Suicide among drug addicts in the UK. *British Journal of Psychiatry*, 175: 277–82.

Oyefeso, A., Valmana, A., Clancy, C., Ghodse, A.H. and Williams, H. (2000) Fatal antidepressant overdose among drug abusers and non-drug abusers. *Acta Psychiatrica Scandinavia*, 102: 295–9.

Roberts, L. and McVeigh, J. (2004) *LIFEGUARD: ACT FAST SAVE A LIFE. An Evaluation of a Multi-component Information Campaign Targeted at Reducing Drug-related Deaths in Cheshire and Merseyside*. Centre for Public Health, Faculty of Health & Applied Social Sciences, Liverpool: Liverpool John Moores University.

Teasdale, G. and Jennett, B. (1974) Assessment of coma and impaired consciousness, a practical scale. *Lancet*, 2: 81–4.

WHO (2005) *The ICD-10 Classification of Mental and Behavioural Disorders: Diagnostic Criteria for Research*. Geneva: World Health Organization.

CHAPTER 29

DRUG MISUSE: PHARMACOLOGICAL AND PSYCHOSOCIAL INTERVENTIONS

OBJECTIVES

■ Define the term detoxification.

■ Describe the management strategies for opioids users.

■ Outline the management strategies for polydrug users.

■ Describe management strategies for stimulant users.

■ Describe the pharmacological interventions in pregnancy.

The aims of this chapter are to outline the specific treatment strategies and phar-macological interventions and the detoxification of psychoactive substances. Specific psychosocial interventions are also included. The *Models of Care* for substance misuse treatment – promoting quality, efficiency and effectiveness in drug misuse treatment services (NTA 2002, 2006) outline how organisations should work together to pro-vide effective drug treatment services, and this includes a national framework for commissioning drug treatment to meet the needs of diverse local populations. There is a range of community-based and residential services which are provided solely for alcohol and drug users in structured programmes of care and interventions. Services include advice and information, needle exchange facilities, day programmes, community drug and alcohol services, community prescribing services, inpatient services and residential rehabilitation. There are a number of different ways in which people can access drug treatment. The majority of people refer themselves into drug treatment services and some are referred by general practitioners, social workers or hospital staff.

Some people enter drug treatment through the criminal justice routes following a court order or through the Drugs Intervention Programme (DIP), administered by the Home Office.

The treatment of drug addiction is focused on three main components: dealing with detoxification and withdrawal effects; maintenance (also known as substitution or harm-reduction therapies); and abstinence. Drug treatment may include drug detoxification, methadone maintenance therapy, motivational interviewing and counselling, other cognitive behaviour therapies, marital and family therapy, relapse prevention and the 12-Step approach. In addition, self-help groups such as Narcotics Anonymous and Cocaine Anonymous are also part of the package of care for the service user's treatment journey. Both pharmacological and psychosocial interventions are used, often complemented by educational and vocational rehabilitation.

DETOXIFICATION

Drug misusers must undergo a detoxification process as part of the initial stage of the treatment plan. This is followed by treatment with psychosocial approaches and/or substitute medication. Detoxification is the process of allowing the body to rid itself of a psychoactive substance while managing the symptoms of withdrawal. The process is gradual and can involve the use of substitute medication to alleviate physical withdrawal symptoms. Some drug users go through a stabilization process where they are prescribed a substitute for the psychoactive substance (such as methadone for heroin users).

OPIOIDS DETOXIFICATION AND PSYCHOSOCIAL INTERVENTIONS

Opioid detoxification refers to the process by which the effects of opioid drugs are eliminated from dependent opioid users in a safe and effective manner, such that withdrawal symptoms are minimised (NICE 2007a). Detoxification should be a readily available treatment option for people who are opioid-dependent and have expressed an informed choice to become abstinent (NICE 2007a). Heroin, morphine, codeine and methadone will produce similar withdrawal signs and symptoms but withdrawal symptoms from shorter-acting opiates will appear and abate sooner. The time of onset and the duration of the withdrawal syndrome will depend on the drug itself, the total intake of the drug, the duration of use and the health of the individual. Withdrawal from heroin or morphine begins 8–12 hours after the last dose of the drug and the effects become less over a period of five to seven days. The signs and symptoms from methadone begin 12 hours after the last dose and the peak intensity occurs on the third day of abstinence. Symptoms usually subside after two to three weeks. The common signs and symptoms of opiate withdrawal syndrome are described in Chapter 8.

Before the implementation of the detoxification process, there is a need to provide information, advice and support. Service users should be informed about detoxification and the associated risks (NICE 2007a), including:

- the physical and psychological aspects of opioid withdrawal, including the duration and intensity of symptoms, and how these may be managed
- the use of non-pharmacological approaches to manage or cope with opioid withdrawal symptoms
- the loss of opioid tolerance following detoxification, and the ensuing increased risk of overdose and death from illicit drug use that may be potentiated by the use of alcohol or benzodiazepines
- the importance of continued support, as well as psychosocial and appropriate pharmacological interventions, to maintain abstinence, treat co-morbid mental health problems and reduce the risk of adverse outcomes (including death).

The detoxification process should be carried out under healthcare personnel supervision as part of hospital or community-based programme. However, it is recommended that service users who have not benefited from previous formal community-based detoxification; who need medical and/or nursing care because of significant co-morbid physical or mental health problems; who require complex polydrug detoxification (for example concurrent detoxification from alcohol or benzodiazepines); and who are experiencing significant social problems should not undertake community-based detoxification (NICE 2007a).

Once the presence and severity of opioid dependence is established, the process of detoxification can take place. Methadone or buprenorphine should be offered as the first-line treatment in opioid detoxification (NICE 2007a). The baseline dose of methadone aims to minimise the severity of the withdrawal, produce a degree of comfort and lessen the risk of overdose. Dose reduction of methadone can be undertaken depending on the results of the assessment and treatment plan. The most rapid regime can be carried out by incremental cuts in dose over seven to 21 days and slower regimes may take several months to complete. When there are complex social or other needs, slow reductions of methadone are prescribed, the general principle being that at higher dose levels the greater the reduction possible, as it represents a smaller percentage of the total. As the dose falls, reduction should be more gradual (Department of Health 1999). This gradual reduction of methadone can occur at any time interval, for instance, daily, alternate days, weekly. In order to decrease the individual's anxiety and increase their sense of control, it may be necessary to hold the reduction steady at a given dose over a few days. Delays in the rate of reduction should be accompanied by psychological support. Progress should be monitored at intervals and the individual's progress should be discussed with the multidisciplinary team. All detoxification programmes require relapse-prevention strategies and psychological support after detoxification because relapse rates are high.

Some clients can rapidly achieve total abstinence from opioids through detoxification and psychosocial interventions. However, others may require a methadone maintenance approach for longer than a few months. The aims of the methadone maintenance approach are to:

- reduce illicit heroin use
- reduce reducing craving
- preventing withdrawal
- eliminating the hazards of injecting
- reduce criminal behaviour
- enhance stability to prevent clients returning to previous patterns of drug use.

It is necessary to provide psychosocial interventions during and after pharmacological interventions for the opioid users to achieve full benefits of the overall treatment package. A range of psychosocial interventions are effective in the treatment of drug misuse; these include contingency management and behavioural couples therapy for drug-specific problems and a range of evidence-based psychological interventions, such as cognitive behavioural therapy, for common co-morbid mental health problems (NICE 2007b). Counselling and support are important both during and after withdrawal from medication. Counselling sessions can be used to explore underlying emotional conflicts and to provide an opportunity to set mutually agreed goals that will help the client to stay off drugs and improve their self-esteem. NICE (2007b) recommended that contingency management aimed at reducing illicit drug use should be considered both during detoxification and for up to 3–6 months after completion of detoxification.

Behavioural couples therapy should be considered for people who are in close contact with a non-drug-misusing partner and who present for treatment of opioid misuse (including those who continue to use illicit drugs while receiving opioid maintenance treatment or after completing opioid detoxification (NICE 2007b)). Individual and group-based psycho-educational interventions should be provided to give information about lifestyle changes, about reducing exposure to blood-borne viruses and/or about reducing sexual and injection risk behaviours for people who misuse drugs. In relapse-prevention programmes, client should be able to identify high risk situations or 'cues' and develop coping skills to prevent relapse. Some clients may require help to deal with problems such as anxiety and sleeplessness, while others need more practical help to deal with issues such as accommodation, homelessness and unemployment. Assistance with housing and benefit issues as well as practical help in finding suitable employment is sometimes necessary. Attendance at self-help groups such as Narcotics Anonymous and Cocaine Anonymous should be facilitated for clients who show an interest. For a few clients a period of stay in a residential rehabilitation facility might be the only way in which they are able to achieve abstinence. For clients with co-existing substance misuse and psychiatric disorders (for example, depression and anxiety), cognitive behavioural therapy is recommended (NICE 2007b).

POLYDRUG USERS

Multiple drug taking or polydrug use has become a common feature with opiate users. Drugs such as benzodiazepines, amphetamines, cocaine and alcohol are frequently used in various combinations either to complement the effects of opiates or to alleviate withdrawal symptoms. Alcohol detoxification in most cases (except for clients with a history of seizures or serious physical or psychiatric conditions) can be carried out at community-structured services using a benzodiazepine drug such as Valium or Librium (see Chapter 30). Benzodiazepine withdrawal is usually achieved by converting to a long-acting drug like valium and reducing every two to three weeks. It is recommended to withdraw the client from any hypno-sedative drugs first before attempting to reduce the methadone. For some polydrug users, admission to hospital may be necessary to stabilise their medication needs or for safer detoxification, particularly if there is a risk of withdrawal seizures. Healthcare professionals should be aware that medications used in opioid detoxification are open to risks of misuse and diversion in all settings (including prisons), and should consider monitoring of medication concordance and methods of limiting the risk of diversion where necessary, including supervised consumption (NICE 2007a). The drug naltrexone which blocks the effects of opiates may be used to prevent relapse in patients who are opiate-free.

A small minority of opiate users are prescribed injectable methadone and pharmaceutical injectable heroin (diamorphine) for the management of their addiction. For guidance on the principles guiding injectable maintenance prescribing see *Injectable Heroin (and Injectable Methadone): Potential Roles in Drug Treatment* (NTA 2003).

BENZODIAZEPINES

Benzodiazepines have their own addictive potential and are often taken in combination with opiates. Sudden cessation in the use of benzodiazepines can lead to a recognised withdrawal state. Many opiate users use benzodiazepines as part of polydrug use. The withdrawal states associated with benzodiazepines use include anxiety, panic attacks, insomnia, perceptual disturbances, fits, aches and pain, poor memory and concentration, difficulty in thinking and confusion. The discontinuation of benzodiazepine dependence should be done under nursing and medical supervision. The two essential pillars of a successful benzodiazepine withdrawal strategy are: gradual dosage reduction and anxiety management. Of these, dosage reduction is by far the easier but psychological support is equally important for successful outcome, particularly for reducing the incidence and severity of post-withdrawal syndromes (Aston 1994). An alternative strategy is the substitution of a long-acting benzodiazepine.

For clients on therapeutic doses of benzodiazepines, withdrawal is best completed in a community-based service. For high-dose and chronic benzodiazepine users, admission to a hospital may be indicated where drug reduction can be initiated at a faster rate. Withdrawal prescribing should be initiated only where there is clear evidence that the individual is dependent on benzodiazepine(s). The management of withdrawal from benzodiazepines involves the gradual tapering of the dose, and this may be extended over the course of several weeks depending on the length of use and severity of symptoms. The rate of withdrawal should be individually tailored to the patient's lifestyle, personality, environmental stresses and reasons for taking benzodiazepines and amount of support available (Aston 1994).

The use of a long-acting benzodiazepine such as diazepam is widely accepted as the most effective way of withdrawing patients because it leaves the system gradually and therefore slows down the onset of withdrawal symptoms. Short-acting benzo-diazepines on the other hand may cause more abrupt and severe withdrawal reactions. The duration of a typical withdrawal period is six to eight weeks but this can be extended for a few months for patients experiencing severe symptoms. However, too prolonged a withdrawal programme can be counterproductive for some patients who might become unduly preoccupied with their symptoms. If the client is also receiving a long-term prescription of methadone for concomitant opiate dependence, the methadone dose should be kept stable throughout the benzodiazepine reduction period (Department of Health 1999). Concurrent detoxification of both drugs is not recommended in a community setting.

Many clients will experience anxiety symptoms and difficulties in sleeping regardless of the rate of reduction. These can be helped with the provision of counselling and psychological support as well as practical advice such as the use of relaxation tapes and anxiety and sleep management. The degree of support and intervention will vary with different patients, and other approaches such as yoga, massage, aromatherapy and physical exercises can also help to reduce symptoms (Gafoor 1998). Those clients who are experiencing more severe withdrawal symptoms, for example, panic attacks, agoraphobia or depression, may require more intensive cognitive behavioural treatment.

STIMULANTS

Amphetamine, cocaine and ecstasy are the most commonly abused stimulants and they do not produce a major physiological withdrawal syndrome. There is a lack of consensus over the existence of a stimulant withdrawal syndrome and no specific detoxification protocol for stimulant withdrawal (Feigenbaun and Allen 1996). Regular users of stimulants may experience exhaustion, insomnia, intense dreaming and depressed mood. These symptoms tend to subside over a period of two to four days of abstinence from the drug. However, the withdrawal symptoms differ between intermittent binge users and chronic users of stimulants. The aim of treatment interventions is to address the complexity of biochemical, psychological and social factors which perpetuate stimulant use.

There is no indication for the prescription of cocaine or methylamphetamine in the treatment of stimulant withdrawal, and it is not recommended that other stimulants, such as methylphenidate or phentermine, be prescribed (Department of Health 1999). But there may be a limited place for the prescription of dexamphetamine sulphate 5 mg in the treatment of amphetamine misuse. After cessation of stimulant use, antidepressants drugs are sometimes prescribed. Antidepressants, such as fluoxetine, can be effective in the management of major depressive episodes associated with stimulant use, but occasional toxic reactions have been described when selective serotonin re-uptake inhibitors (SSRIs) are prescribed and stimulants continue to be taken (Barrett et al. 1996). Ghodse (1995) outlines a treatment plan advocating oral or intravenous diazepam to settle agitation. In some individuals with a dual diagnosis, abrupt cessation of stimulants may trigger a profound transient depression with suicidal thoughts necessitating hospitalisation or close monitoring (Banerjee et al. 2002).

Studies have found that an abstinence-based psychosocial treatment approach, linking counselling and social support, had the greatest impact on cocaine misuse (Donmall et al. 1995). Complementary therapies, such as acupuncture, are being more widely used for crack cocaine detoxification (Lipton et al. 1994) although there is only limited evidence to support their effectiveness. This alternative treatment may be one of the ways to appeal to those who have limited contact with drug specialist services. General principles of management, such as harm reduction approach about safer injecting practice and safer sex, should be part of the psychosocial and educational programme.

GHB

A GHB withdrawal syndrome that has aspects of alcohol and benzodiazepine withdrawal has been reported. The syndrome appears to manifest itself in individuals who have self-administered GHB every two to three hours and are at increased risk for the emergence of severe symptoms. GHB withdrawal can occur after several months of regular use. Management of the withdrawal syndrome has necessitated the use of high dosages of hypno-sedative and physical restraints to control the confusion, delirium, psychosis and resultant agitation.

CANNABIS, HALLUCINOGENS AND PHENCYCLIDINE

There is no acute abstinence syndrome associated with withdrawal from cannabis. Some individuals are irritable and have difficulty sleeping for a few days after chronic use. Where agitation and severe insomnia are prominent, short-term low doses of anti-psychotics are sometimes the appropriate measures. There are also no acute withdrawal syndrome with hallucinogens and phencyclidine (PCP), although chronic use of PCP may lead to a toxic psychosis. Pharmacological treatments for cannabis and stimulant misuse are not well developed, and therefore psychosocial interventions are the mainstay of effective treatment.

PHARMACOLOGICAL TREATMENT FOR DRUG MISUSERS IN PREGNANCY

The use of psychoactive substances such as cocaine and heroin during pregnancy is common. A study of a UK inner-city clinic demonstrated that approximately 16% of the women had taken one or more illicit substances (Sherwood *et al.* 1999). The overall aim of antenatal treatment varies according to the type of drug being misused. Methadone remains the drug of choice for opiate or opioid substitution, with proven medical and social benefits due to stabilisation of drug use and lifestyle and contact with services. Methadone maintenance, when compared with the illicit use of heroin, is associated with greater access of antenatal care and hence better maternal and infant outcomes, including a reduced risk of preterm delivery and low birth weight (Jarvis and Schnoll 1995). Neonatal abstinence syndrome, however, may be more common in infants whose mothers took methadone rather than heroin (Chasnoff *et al.* 1990).

Detoxification can therefore be carried out at any stage of pregnancy and at any speed but should be undertaken only if appropriate and if there is a reasonable prospect of success (Hepburn 2004). Antenatal detoxification from benzodiazepines, to reduce risk of maternal convulsion, should therefore be carried out under cover of a short reducing course of diazepam and an initial dose of 10 mg three times daily reducing by 5 mg each day (rotating the dose to be reduced) has proved safe in practice (Hepburn 2004). Withdrawal from alcohol can be safely managed with the same regime as used for benzodiazepine withdrawal. There is no evidence to support substitution therapy during pregnancy for any other type of drug.

KEY POINTS

- The *Models of Care* for substance misuse treatment outline how organisations should work together to provide effective drug treatment services.
- Services include advice and information, needle exchange facilities, day programmes, community drug and alcohol services, community prescribing services, inpatient services and residential rehabilitation.
- The treatment of drug addiction is focused on three main components: dealing with detoxification and withdrawal effects; maintenance (also known as 'substitution' or 'harm reduction' therapies) and abstinence.
- Drug misusers must undergo a detoxification process as part of the initial stage of the treatment plan.
- The detoxification is followed by treatment with psychosocial approaches and/or substitute medication.
- Opioid detoxification refers to the process by which the effects of opioid drugs are eliminated from dependent opioid users in a safe and effective manner, such that withdrawal symptoms are minimised.
- Service users should be informed about detoxification and the associated risks.
- Methadone or buprenorphine should be offered as the first-line treatment in opioid detoxification.
- All detoxification programmes require relapse-prevention strategies and psychological support after detoxification because relapse rates are high.
- The aims of the methadone maintenance approach are to: reduce illicit heroin use; reduce reducing craving and prevent withdrawal; eliminate the hazards of injecting; reduce criminal behaviour; and enhance stability to prevent clients returning to previous patterns of drug use.
- A range of psychosocial interventions is effective in the treatment of drug misuse; these include contingency management and behavioural couple's therapy for drug-specific problems.
- Cognitive behavioural therapy is effective for common co-morbid mental health problems.
- Many opiate users use benzodiazepines as part of polydrug use.
- Concurrent detoxification of both heroin and benzodiazepines is not recommended in a community setting.
- There is no specific detoxification protocol for stimulant withdrawal.
- After cessation of stimulant use, antidepressants drugs are sometimes prescribed.
- A GHB withdrawal syndrome that has aspects of alcohol and benzodiazepine withdrawal has been reported.
- There is no acute abstinence syndrome associated with withdrawal from cannabis.
- The overall aim of antenatal treatment varies according to the type of drug being misused.
- Methadone remains the drug of choice for opiate or opioid substitution with proven medical and social benefits.

ACTIVITY 29.1

Please state whether the following statements are true or false. Reflect on the statements and give reason(s) for choosing a particular option

	True	False
The Models of Care for substance-misuse treatment outlines how organisations should provide effective drug treatment services		
Intervention strategies include pharmacological and psychosocial interventions and educational and vocational rehabilitation		
Drug misusers must undergo a detoxification process as part of initial stage of the treatment plan		
Detoxification should be a readily available treatment option for people who are opioid-dependent and have expressed an informed choice to become abstinent		
Heroin, morphine, codeine and methadone will not produce similar withdrawal signs and symptoms		
Withdrawal from heroin or morphine begins 8–12 hours after the last dose of the drug		
Service users with significant comorbid physical or mental health problems are able to undertake community-based detoxification		
The most rapid methadone regime can be carried out by incremental cuts in dose over 7–21 days		
Contingency management and behavioural couples therapy are effective in the treatment of drug misuse		
Multiple drug taking or polydrug use has become a common feature with opiate users		
The drug naltrexone may not be used to prevent relapse in patients who are opiate-free		
For clients on therapeutic doses of benzodiazepines, withdrawal is best completed in community-based services		
Amphetamine, cocaine and ecstasy are the most commonly abused stimulants and they produce a major physiological withdrawal syndrome		

ACTIVITY 29.2

There is only one correct answer to the following multiple-choice questions

The ways people can access drug treatment are
a.   Self-referral
b.   Primary health care

c.   Criminal justice system
d.   All of the above

The treatment of drug addiction is focused on
a.   Dealing with detoxification and withdrawal effects
b.   Maintenance 'substitution'
c.   'Harm reduction' therapies)
d.   All of the above

Detoxification is the process of
a.   Treatment for drug users
b.   Rapid cessation to reduce withdrawal effects
c.   Allowing the body to rid itself of a psychoactive substance
d.   Prescribing a substitute psychoactive substance

Opioid detoxification refers to the process by which
a.   The effects of opioid drugs are eliminated
b.   Withdrawal symptoms are minimized
c.   A safe and effective procedure is carried out
d.   All of the above

The time of onset and the duration of the withdrawal syndrome will depend on
a.   The drug itself
b.   The total intake of the drug
c.   The duration of use
d.   All of the above

The following substance should be offered as the first-line treatment in opioid detoxification
a.   Methadone or buprenorphine
b.   Methadone or benzodiazepines
c.   Heroin and methadone
d.   None of the above

The baseline dose of methadone aims to
a.   Reduce the severity of the withdrawal
b.   Produce a degree of comfort
c.   Lessen the risk of overdose
d.   All of the above

This gradual reduction of methadone can occur at
a.   Daily intervals
b.   Alternate days intervals
c.   Weekly intervals
d.   All of the above

All detoxification programmes require
a.   Relapse prevention strategies
b.   Psychological support

   c.   Medical prescribing
   d.   All of the above

The aims of the methadone maintenance approach include
   a.   The reduction of illicit heroin use
   b.   The reduction of craving
   c.   The prevention of withdrawal
   d.   All of the above

Behavioural couples therapy should be considered for people
   a.   Who are in close contact with a non-drug-misusing partner
   b.   Who present for treatment opioid misuse
   c.   After completing opioid detoxification
   d.   All of the above

Relapse prevention programme includes
   a.   Identification of high-risk situations
   b.   Identification of high-risk 'cues'
   c.   Development of coping skills
   d.   All of the above

For some polydrug users, admission to hospital may be necessary in order
   a.   To stabilise their medication needs
   b.   To provide safer detoxification
   c.   To deal with the risk of withdrawal seizures
   d.   All of the above

Sudden cessation in the use of benzodiazepines can lead to
   a.   A recognised withdrawal state
   b.   Psychological dependence
   c.   Physical dependence
   d.   Tolerance

The essential pillars of a successful benzodiazepine withdrawal strategy are
   a.   Gradual dosage reduction
   b.   Anxiety management
   c.   Psychological support
   d.   All of the above

There is no acute abstinence syndrome associated
   a.   With withdrawal from cannabis
   b.   With withdrawal from hallucinogens
   c.   With withdrawal from phencyclidine
   d.   All of the above

Methadone maintenance when compared with the illicit use of heroin is associated
   a.   With greater access of antenatal care
   b.   With better maternal and infant outcomes

c.   With reduced risk of preterm delivery and low birth weight
d.   All of the above

REFERENCES

Aston, H. (1994) The treatment of benzodiazepine dependence. *Addiction*, 89: 1535–41.

Banerjee, S., Clancy, C. and Crome, I. (2002) *Co-existing Problems of Mental Disorder and Substance Misuse (Dual Diagnosis)*. London: Royal College of Psychiatrists Research Unit.

Barrett, J., Meehan, O. and Fahy, T. (1996) SSRI and sympathominetic interaction. *British Journal of Psychiatry*, 168: 253.

Chasnoff, I.J., Landress, H.J. and Barrett, M.E. (1990) The prevalence of illicit-drug use during pregnancy and discrepancies in mandatory reporting in Pinellas County, Florida. *New England Journal of Medicine*, 322: 1202–6.

Department of Health (1999) *Drug Misuse and Dependence – Guidelines on Clinical Management*. London: The Stationery Office.

Donmall, M., Seivewright, N., Douglas, J., Draycott, T. and Millar, T. (1995) *National Cocaine Treatment Study: The Effectiveness of Treatments Offered to Cocaine/Crack Users*. A report to the Task Force. London: Department of Health.

Feigenbaum, J.C. and Allen, K.M. (1996) Detoxification. In K.M.Allen (ed.) *Nursing Care of the Addicted Client*, pp. 139–75. Philadelphia: Lippincott.

Gafoor, M. (1998) Benzodiazepines: clinical care and nursing interventions. In G. Hussein Rassool (ed.) *Substance Use and Misuse: Nature, Context and Clinical Interventions*. Oxford: Blackwell Science.

Ghodse, H. (1995) *Drugs and Addictive Behaviour: A Guide to Treatment*, 2nd edition. Oxford: Blackwell Scientific Publications.

Hepburn, M. (2004) Substance abuse in pregnancy. *Current Obstetrics and Gynaecology*, 14: 419–25.

Jarvis, M.A.E. and Schnoll, S.H. (1995) Methadone use in pregnancy. *NIDA Research Monograph*, 149: 58–77.

Lipton, D.S., Brewington, V. and Smith, M. (1994) Acupuncture for crack-cocaine detoxification: experimental evaluation of efficacy. *Journal of Substance Abuse Treatment*, 11, 3: 205–15.

NTA (2002) *Models of Care for Adult Drug Misusers. Parts 1 and 2*. London: National Treatment Agency.

NTA (2003) *Injectable Heroin (and Injectable Methadone): Potential Roles in Drug Treatment*. London: National Treatment Agency.

NTA (2006) Models of Care for adult drug misusers Updated, London: NTA.

NICE (2007a) *Drug Misuse: Opioid Detoxification*, NICE clinical guideline 52. London: National Institute for Clinical Excellence. www.nice.org.uk/CG52 (accessed January 2008).

NICE (2007b) *Drug Misuse: Psychosocial Interventions*, NICE clinical guideline 51. London: National Institute for Clinical Excellence. www.nice.org.uk/CG51 (accessed January 2008).

Sherwood, R.A., Keating, J., Kavvadia, V. Greenough, A. and Peters, T.J. (1999) Substance misuse in early pregnancy and relationship to fetal outcome. *European Journal of Pediatrics*, 158: 488–92.

CHAPTER 30

ALCOHOL MISUSE: PHARMACOLOGICAL AND PSYCHOSOCIAL INTERVENTIONS

OBJECTIVES

▪ List the screening instruments for identifying alcohol problems.

▪ Describe the management and treatment of harmful and hazardous drinkers.

▪ Describe the management and treatment of moderate and severe dependent drinkers.

▪ Discuss the advantages and limitations of community detoxification.

▪ Discuss the pharmacological management of withdrawal.

▪ Discuss the psychosocial interventions in management and treatment of alcohol problems.

The *Models of Care for Alcohol Misusers* (MoCAM) (NTA 2007) provide best practice guidance for local health organisations and their partners in delivering a planned and integrated local treatment system for adult alcohol misusers. The *Review of the Effectiveness of Treatment for Alcohol Problems* (Heather *et al*. 2006) suggests that provision of alcohol treatment to 10% of the dependent drinking population within the UK would significantly reduce public sector resource costs. MoCAM identifies four main categories of alcohol misusers who may benefit from some kind of intervention or treatment: hazardous drinkers; harmful drinkers; moderately dependent drinkers and severely dependent drinkers.

Hazardous drinkers are drinking at levels over the sensible drinking limits, either in terms of regular excessive consumption or less frequent sessions of heavy drinking, and they have so far avoided significant alcohol-related problems. Harmful drinkers are usually drinking at levels above those recommended for sensible drinking and show clear evidence of some alcohol-related harm. Both groups may benefit from advice, health information and brief interventions. The main groups of alcohol users who clearly may benefit from specialist alcohol treatment are those who are moderately and severely dependent. The effectiveness review (Heather *et al.* 2006) suggests that, for treatment planning purposes, the most useful categorisation is into 'moderate dependence', 'severe dependence' and 'dependence with complex needs'. This is because the latter 'severe and complex' group is likely to require a higher level of intervention at the outset than those with moderate dependence. Moderately dependent drinkers' treatment can often be managed effectively in home or community settings. However, many severely dependent drinkers, those with complex needs such as polydrug misusers and those with alcohol and psychiatric problems, may need inpatient-assisted alcohol withdrawal, multiple agency services and residential rehabilitation.

MoCAM advocates a stepped model of care for alcohol misusers:

- provision of brief interventions for those drinking excessively but not requiring treatment for alcohol dependence
- provision of treatment interventions for those with moderate or severe dependence and related problems.

Alcohol misusers require specialist treatment from community alcohol teams, inpatient detoxification units and structured day or residential programmes. Self-help groups such as Alcoholics Anonymous (AA) and other voluntary agencies may also play an important role in the management of care and treatment interventions. The choice of setting in each individual circumstance will depend on the range of accompanying physical, psychological or social problems, including risks posed to the drinker and risks to others from the drinker's behaviour (NTA 2007). Problem drinkers making contact with healthcare professionals either in primary care or at specialist units are usually offered a detoxification programme as a prelude to further psychosocial interventions.

SCREENING FOR ALCOHOL PROBLEMS

A number of screening tools are available to identify current or potential alcohol problems among service users (see Chapter 24). In a review of the effectiveness of treatment for alcohol problems, Heather *et al.* (2006) recommended the following: The AUDIT (Alcohol Use Disorders Identification Test) can be embedded in a general health questionnaire and is an efficient tool for the detection of hazardous drinking; the FAST is a rapid and efficient screening tool for detecting alcohol misuse in the A&E settings; and clinical history and physical examination can be used to detect harmful drinking. Laboratory tests, such as the test for the liver enzyme gamma-glutamyltransferase (GGT), may also reveal the presence of unsuspected alcohol problems. It is important to carry out an initial or comprehensive assessment to determine the nature and severity of the drinking problems, and this would determine the selection of a problem drinker to have detoxification at home, in the community or at an inpatient detoxification unit.

WORKING WITH HARMFUL AND HAZARDOUS DRINKERS

Any encounter with a service user attending primary healthcare and hospitals settings provides an occasion for opportunistic triage screening, health information, advice and brief interventions. As standard practice, hazardous and harmful drinkers without complex needs should be offered simple, structured advice to promote reduced consumption of alcohol to less risky levels. Brief interventions may be offered to those who do not respond effectively to advice and health information. Brief interventions are effective in a variety of settings, including medical settings, such as primary care and A&E, and in generic non-specialist services (Heather *et al.* 2006).

Those who need further interventions as a result of their high level of alcohol consumption should be referred to specialist alcohol agencies. Interventions can often be completed in one session using a minimal intervention such as ensuring that patients have access to the health information they need to make informed choices: sensible drinking limits, clear and safe advice on alcohol reduction and completion of simple alcohol diaries (Moore 2006). A follow-up appointment is useful but not essential. In some circumstances, hazardous and harmful drinkers with complex needs including people with psychiatric problems, people with learning disabilities, some older people, and some with social and housing problems may require more intensive or prolonged multiple-agency interventions (see Moore 2006). The Department of Health (2002) recommends that dual diagnosis issues at this level require care co-ordination in order to manage integrated treatment across multiple agencies.

WORKING WITH MODERATE TO SEVERE DEPENDENT DRINKERS

Community or home detoxification can be offered to moderately dependent drinkers depending on the nature and associated physical, psychological or social problems, including risks posed to the drinker and risks to others. However, severely dependent drinkers may have serious and long-standing problems including significant alcohol withdrawal. Given adequate risk assessment and a comprehensive and intensive care plan, medically assisted alcohol withdrawal can safely be provided to many severely dependent drinkers in the home or in community settings (NTA 2007). But more severely dependent drinkers require inpatient-assisted detoxification and residential rehabilitation. Severe dependent drinkers have complex needs including multiple substance misuse, complicated alcohol withdrawal, co-existing psychiatric disorders or social problems

The comprehensive alcohol assessment builds on the initial alcohol assessment, and includes patterns of use, withdrawal symptoms, psychological history, physical problems, self-harm, levels of risk for both mental health and alcohol use and history of trauma. Others areas that need to be assessed are social issues related to childcare, relationships, domestic violence, housing, employment and financial standing. A history of contact with forensic services, legal problems, arrests, fines, charges or any outstanding warrants should be explored. In relation to mental health needs, key cues for targeted questioning would relate to presentations that include stress, tension, anxiety, low mood and psychological distress (Royal College of Psychiatrists 2005). For dependent drinkers with psychiatric problems, the degree of immediate risk is used to determine how, when and where psychiatric services intervene. Based on assessment, individualised care plans reflecting mental health and alcohol use are developed covering the initial presentation, with a stepwise approach to individualised treatment, considering risk, and strategies that address psychosocial functioning (Moore 2006). Key areas of a care plan are presented in Table 30.1.

Table 30.1 Alcohol: key areas of care plan

Needs or problems	Expected outcome	Interventions
Poor physical health	• Improvements in daily intake of nutrition	• Assessment of daily intake of nutrients • Vitamin supplements
Fear of withdrawal symptoms	• Prevention of withdrawal symptoms	• Health information and advice
Risk behaviour	• Elimination or reduction of risk behaviour	• Assessment and monitoring
Low self-esteem	• Adoption of more positive attitude	• Counselling
Lack of assertive skills	• Development of assertive skills	• Counselling and cognitive behavioural techniques
Anxiety	• Control of anxiety	• Anxiety or stress management
Boredom	• Reduction boredom	• Encourage participation in alternative leisure activities
Detoxification	• Client will not experience any physical distress and discomfort while undergoing detoxification	• Explain the role of medication in facilitating detoxification and overcoming withdrawal
Dealing with loss or grief reactions	• Facilitating the grieving process • Resolution of grieving process	• Counselling
Relapse	• Prevention of relapse	• Relapse prevention

Source: Adapted from Gafoor and Rassool (1998)

DETOXIFICATION

Where alcohol causes physical withdrawal syndromes, detoxification is a treatment intervention. Medically assisted detoxification can be delivered both in the community and in inpatient settings. Community detoxification is based on the principle that the service users remain in their own natural environment, and this approach is rooted in social learning theory (Gafoor and Rassool 1998). This is based on the premise that drinking is a learned behaviour in response to environmental and social cues. Detoxification can be regarded as a prelude to further social and psychological interventions aimed at influencing and motivating the service users to change their behaviours (Gafoor and Rassool 1998). The potential benefits of community detoxification are presented in Table 30.2.

There is evidence to suggest that home detoxification can be as safe and effective as hospital-based care as long as standards and policies are adhered to (Stockwell *et al.* 1991). Finally and most importantly, there must be no previous history of alcohol withdrawal fits or delirium tremens. Clients with moderate or severe withdrawal may require inpatient detoxification. The indications for inpatient detoxification are presented in Table 30.3.

Table 30.2 Potential benefits and limitations of community detoxification

Benefits	Limitations
• Interventions in a familiar environment • Support of family network and significant others • Client able to resist environmental cues to drinking and develop new coping strategies • Stigma of admission to hospital or specialist unit is disengaged • A more accessible and flexible service • Enabling service user to seek help at an early stage of their drinking career • Client remains at work during treatment interventions • More dependent drinkers can be recruited for detoxification rather than being on a waiting list for inpatient detoxification • Cost-effective	• Clients remain in an environment which might be perpetuating alcohol misuse • Family or carer do not have any respite • Some clients may not view their problems as severe • Not suitable for those with complex needs or history of mental health problems and severe withdrawal

Source: Adapted from Gafoor and Rassool (1998)

Table 30.3 Indications for inpatient detoxification

- Alcohol delirium or seizures present at the time of assessment
- A history of seizures or alcoholic delirium and high alcohol consumption
- A history of high-dose polydrug use
- Pyrexia greater than 38.5°C
- A history of recent head injury with loss of consciousness
- Illnesses requiring medical or surgical treatment
- Wernicke's encephalopathy
- Conditions requiring psychiatric admission (self-harm, severe anxiety or depression, psychotic disorders)

MANAGEMENT OF WITHDRAWAL

The main objectives of pharmacological interventions in alcohol withdrawal are the relief of subjective withdrawal symptoms, the prevention and management of more serious complications and preparation for more structured psychosocial and educational interventions.

The alcohol withdrawal syndrome lasts for about five days, with the greatest risk of severe withdrawal in the first 24 to 48 hours. Chlordiazepoxide or diazepam loading shortens the detoxification period, is safer and avoids the indiscriminate use of medication (Wasilewski *et al.* 1996). In addition, diazepam has an anti-convulsant effect which helps to safeguard against seizures. A typical specimen prescribing regime is presented in Table 30.4.

The principles of management in alcohol detoxification include monitoring of dehydration, blood pressure, dietary intake, orientation to time, place and person, and sleep. A framework for the management of alcohol withdrawal (Shaw *et al.* 1981) is presented in Table 30.5.

Preparation is important to build the service user's confidence and maximise the benefits from the detoxification episode (Heather *et al.* 2006). Clients need a non-stimulating and non-threatening environment, and low lighting at night will help reduce perceptual disturbances. Whilst detoxification can be a very physical process, there are a number of psychological elements that nurses are skilled at observing and managing,

Table 30.4 Specimen prescribing regime for diazepam

Dosage	Duration
10 mg tds	1 day
5 mg qds	1 day
5 mg tds	1 day
5 mg bd	1 day
5 mg nocte	1 day

Table 30.5 A framework for supportive care for alcohol withdrawal

Needs	Interventions
Environmental stimuli	Nursing in quiet area with only one staff in contact
Body temperature	Control body temperature: apply or remove bed clothing when necessary
Blood pressure	Monitor blood pressure
Foods and fluids	Offer fluids every 60 minutes and record fluid intake
Rest and sleep	Allow rest or sleep between monitoring of vital signs
Elimination	Assist to bathroom and record output
Epigastric distress	Deep breathing and relaxation
Physical comfort	Change position if necessary
Reality orientation	Time, place and person
Providing positive reinforcement	Reinforce positive elements of the intervention
Visitors	No visitors during supportive care

Source: Adapted from Shaw *et al.* (1981)

including hallucinations, delirium, altered mental states, hyper-vigilance, anxiety, paranoia, depression, tactile hallucinations and levels of risk (Moore *et al*. 2006). There is evidence that therapeutic interventions combined with carefully monitored medication are an important factor in the treatment of alcohol withdrawal syndrome (Bennie 1998).

PSYCHOSOCIAL INTERVENTIONS

The goals of psychosocial interventions are to complement pharmacological interventions (for example, in detoxification or relapse prevention) and to enable clients to regain stability and a healthier lifestyle. The use of brief interventions has been described in Chapter 26. In summary, brief interventions have been found effective for helping harmful or hazardous drinkers to reduce or stop drinking and for motivating moderate or severe alcohol-dependent users to enter long-term alcohol treatment. Motivational interviewing is the preliminary psychological intervention in specialist settings for those clients with moderate or severe dependence who are not willing to change their risk behaviour. Motivational interviewing increases the effectiveness of more extensive psychological treatment (Heather *et al*. 2006). In Table 30.6 the Stage of Change Model and interviewing strategies provide examples of motivational interviewing questions that correspond to the various stages of readiness to change (Burge and Schneider 1999, Rollnick *et al*. 1992).

The use of cognitive-behavioural approaches has been found to be effective in reducing or stopping alcohol use. One example is the community reinforcement approach (CRA). It consists of a broad range of treatment with the aim of engineering the service user's social environment (including the family and vocational environment)

Table 30.6 Stage of change model and interviewing strategies

Stage of change	Strategies	Description
Pre-contemplation	Lifestyle, stresses and alcohol use	Discuss lifestyle and life stresses. 'Where does your use of alcohol fit in?'
Pre-contemplation	Health and alcohol use	Ask about health in general. 'What part does your drinking play in your health?'
Pre-contemplation	A typical day	'Describe a typical day, from beginning to end. How does alcohol fit in?'
Contemplation	'Good' things and 'less good' things	'What are some good things about your use of alcohol?' 'What are some less good things?'
Contemplation	Providing information	Ask permission to provide information. Deliver information in a non-personal manner. 'What do you make of all this?'
Contemplation	The future and the present	'How would you like things to be different in the future?'
Preparation or action	Exploring concerns	Elicit the patient's reasons for concern about alcohol use. List concerns about changing behaviour
Preparation or action	Helping with decision-making	'Given your concerns about drinking, where does this leave you now?'

Source: Adapted from Burge and Schneider (1999) and Rollnick, Heather and Bell (1992)

so that abstinence is rewarded and intoxication unrewarded (Heather *et al.* 2006). There is evidence to suggest that CRA is an effective treatment intervention with those with severe alcohol dependence. However, pharmacological treatment in the form of prescribing Disulfiram is an essential component of the CRA (Heather *et al.* 2006).

Social behaviour and network therapy can also be used with service users in modifying and maintaining changes in alcohol consumption. The basic premise is to enable clients to develop positive social networks. The components of social behaviour and network therapy are described in Copello *et al.* (2002). Other interventions such as coping and social skills training are effective with service users with moderate dependent alcohol use (Heather *et al.* 2006). There are significant numbers of alcohol misusers who have marital problems. Marital therapy, based on the cognitive-behavioural approach, has been found to be effective in improving interpersonal relationships and in the reduction of drinking problem (Heather *et al.* 2006).

For service users with co-existing alcohol and anxiety problems, several psychological therapies, such as relaxation training, stress management and skills training, may be employed in the treatment of both anxiety and alcohol disorders. Cognitive-behavioural therapy, pharmacological treatments, social skills and assertiveness training, self-control training and stress management have been found to be effective (Oei and Loveday 1997). Techniques to identify and manage anxiety may also prevent relapse to alcohol use among co-morbid patients (Petrakis *et al.* 2002). Service users with anxiety and alcohol misuse have difficulty in engaging in treatment interventions. For example, patients with anxiety symptoms such as panic attacks or social phobia may have difficulty attending group meetings (Modesto-Lowe and Kranzler 1999). After treatment has been initiated, clinicians must monitor both drinking behaviour and psychiatric symptoms, since alcohol dependence and anxiety disorders both tend to have a relapsing course (Modesto-Lowe and Kranzler 1999).

However, there is no fully validated treatment package for the treatment of co-existent anxiety disorders and alcohol misuse (Oei and Loveday 1997) and no compelling evidence to support any one psychosocial treatment over another to reduce substance use (or improve mental state) by individuals with serious mental illnesses (Cleary *et al.* 1999). Short- or long-term psychosocial interventions for service users with alcohol and psychiatric disorders require clear and consistent approaches, across multiple agencies, with realistic time-frames for interventions to work.

One of the key components of psychosocial interventions is the prevention of relapse and the promoting and the maintenance of abstinence. Relapse prevention should be incorporated in all specialist treatment for alcohol problems, and there is good evidence of its effectiveness (Heather *et al.* 2006). The programme on relapse prevention enables the service user to identify high-risk situations or triggers which can lead to problem drinking, and to manage these by developing alternative coping skills and strategies (Gafoor and Rassool 1998). Pharmacotherapy is also used in relapse prevention. Dusulfiram taken under supervision is an effective component of relapse prevention strategies (Heather *et al.* 2006). Anti-craving medications such as naltrexone and acamprosate may also be used as part of psychosocial interventions, including relapse prevention.

Vitamin deficiency in alcoholism is common and causes Wernicke's encephalopathy and is most commonly seen in heavy drinkers with a poor diet. The Royal College of Physicians (2001) has recommended that for service users undergoing alcohol detoxification in the community 200 mg four times a day of oral thiamine and vitamin

B strong tablets (30 mg/day) is the treatment of choice for the duration of the detoxification. Both supplements could be continued if there is evidence of cognitive impairment (thiamine 50 mg four times a day) or poor diet (vitamin B strong 30 mg/day).

Ito and Donovan (1986) suggested that a well-planned programme for continued assistance will increase the service user's chances of a successful long-term outcome. The after-care programme may include further psychological interventions such as counselling or marital therapy in combination to attendance at self-help groups such as Alcoholics Anonymous. There is evidence to suggest that planned and structured after-care is effective in improving outcome following the initial treatment of service users with severe alcohol problems (Heather *et al.* 2006). Multidimensional pharmacological and psychosocial interventions and a multi-professional approach are required to provide better and more effective outcomes for those with alcohol-related problems.

KEY POINTS

- Four main categories of alcohol misusers may benefit from some kind of intervention or treatment: hazardous drinkers; harmful drinkers; moderately dependent drinkers; and severely dependent drinkers.
- Both hazardous and harmful drinkers may benefit from advice, health information and brief interventions.
- The main groups of alcohol users who clearly may benefit from specialist alcohol treatment are those who are moderately and severely dependent.
- Alcohol misusers require specialist treatment from community alcohol teams, inpatient detoxification units and structured day or residential programmes.
- A number of screening tools are available to identify current or potential alcohol problems among service users.
- Community or home detoxification can be offered to moderately dependent drinkers.
- Severely dependent drinkers have complex needs including multiple substance misuse, complicated alcohol withdrawal, co-existing psychiatric disorders or social problems.
- Where alcohol causes physical withdrawal syndromes, detoxification is a treatment intervention.
- There is evidence that therapeutic interventions combined with carefully monitored medication are an important factor in the treatment of alcohol withdrawal syndrome.
- Motivational interviewing increases the effectiveness of more extensive psychological treatment.
- Social behaviour and network therapy can also be used with service users in modifying and maintaining changes in alcohol consumption.
- Other intervention such as coping and social skills training is effective with service users with moderately dependent alcohol use.
- Psychosocial interventions for service users with alcohol and psychiatric disorders require clear and consistent approaches, across multiple agencies, with realistic time-frames for interventions to work.

- Relapse prevention should be incorporated in all specialist treatment for alcohol problems and there is good evidence of its effectiveness.
- There is evidence that planned and structured after-care is effective in improving outcome following the initial treatment of service users with severe alcohol problems.

ACTIVITY 30.1

Please state whether the following statements are true or false. Reflect on the statements and give reason(s) for choosing a particular option

	True	False
Provision of alcohol treatment would not significantly reduce public sector resource costs		
Hazardous drinkers may benefit from advice, health information and brief interventions		
Harmful drinkers may benefit from advice, health information and brief interventions		
The main groups of alcohol users who clearly may benefit from specialist alcohol treatment are those who are moderately and severely dependent		
The AUDIT (Alcohol Use Disorders Identification Test) is an efficient tool for the detection of hazardous drinking		
The FAST is a rapid and efficient screening tool for detecting alcohol misuse in all settings		
Brief interventions are effective in a variety of settings, including medical settings, such as primary care and A&E, and in generic non-specialist services		
Where alcohol causes physical withdrawal syndromes, detoxification is a treatment intervention		
There is no evidence to suggest that home detoxification can be as safe and effective as hospital-based care		
There is evidence that therapeutic interventions combined with carefully monitored medication are an important factor in the treatment of alcohol withdrawal syndrome		
There is evidence to suggest that the Community Reinforcement Approach is an effective treatment intervention with those with severe alcohol dependence		
Cognitive-behavioural therapy, pharmacological treatments, social skills and assertiveness training, self-control training and stress management have been found to be effective		
There is a validated treatment package for the treatment of co-existent anxiety disorders and alcohol misuse		

ACTIVITY 30.2

There is only one correct answer to the following multiple choice questions

Hazardous drinkers
a.   Are drinking at levels over the sensible limits
b.   Have less frequent sessions of heavy drinking
c.   Have avoided significant alcohol-related problems
d.   All of the above

Harmful drinkers
a.   Are usually drinking at levels above sensible limits
b.   Show clear evidence of some alcohol-related harm
c.   Have more frequent sessions of heavy drinking
d.   All of the above

A stepped model of care for alcohol misusers comprises
a.   Provision of brief interventions for those drinking excessively
b.   Provision of treatment interventions for moderate drinkers
c.   Provision of treatment interventions for severe drinkers
d.   All of the above

The choice of setting in each individual circumstance will depend
a.   On the range of accompanying physical problems
b.   On the range of accompanying social problems
c.   On the range of accompanying psychological problems
d.   All of the above

Hazardous and harmful drinkers without complex needs should be offered
a.   Simple, structured advice
b.   Brief intervention
c.   Harm reduction
d.   All of the above

Community or home detoxification can be offered to
a.   Moderately dependent drinkers
b.   Severe dependent drinkers
c.   Those with complex needs
d.   Those who have risky behaviours

Severely dependent drinkers have
a.   Complex needs
b.   Multiple substance misuse
c.   Complicated alcohol withdrawal
d.   All of the above

Community detoxification is based on the principle that
a.   The service users remain in their own natural environment
b.   Drinking is a learned behaviour

c. Service users respond to environmental and social cues
d. All of the above

The main objectives of pharmacological interventions in alcohol withdrawal are
a. The relief of subjective withdrawal symptoms
b. The prevention and management of more serious complications
c. The preparation for more structured psychosocial interventions
d. All of the above

Chlordiazepoxide or diazepam is the main choice of detoxification because
a. It shortens the detoxification period
b. It is safer than other drugs
c. It has an anti-convulsant effect
d. All of the above

The principles of management in alcohol detoxification include
a. Monitoring of dehydration
b. Monitoring dietary intake
c. Orientation to time, place and person
d. All of the above

The goals of the psychosocial interventions are
a. To complement pharmacological interventions
b. To enable clients to regain stability and a healthier lifestyle
c. To provide family and social network support
d. All of the above

Relapse prevention
a. Is a key components of psychosocial interventions
b. Promotes and maintains abstinence
c. Enables the service user to identify high risk situations
d. All of the above

ACTIVITY 30.3

- What are the potential benefits and limitations of community or home detoxification?
- What are the pharmacological management problems of withdrawal?
- What are the psychosocial interventions in management and treatment of alcohol problems?
- What are the indications for inpatient detoxification?
- Why is it important to have planned follow-up or after-care for service users with alcohol problems?

REFERENCES

Bennie, C. (1998) A comparison of home detoxification and minimal intervention strategies for problem drinkers. *Alcohol and Alcoholism*, 33, 2: 157–63.

Burge, S. and Schneider, F.D. (1999) Alcohol-related problems: recognition and intervention. *American Academy of Family Physician*, 59 2: 361–72.

Cleary, M., Hunt, G., Matheson, S., Siegfried, N. and Walter, G. (1999) *Psychosocial Interventions for People with Both Severe Mental Illness and Substance Misuse.* Cochrane Database of Systematic Reviews 1999, Issue 2. Art. no.: CD001088. DOI: 10.1002/14651858.CD001088.pub2 (accessed 10 December 2007).

Copello, A., Orford, J., Hodgson, R., Tober, G. and Barrett, C. (2002) Social behaviour and network therapy: basic principles and early experiences. *Addictive Behaviours*, 27: 354–6.

Department of Health (2002) *Dual Diagnosis Good Practice Guide Mental Health Implementation Policy Guide.* London: Department of Health.

Gafoor, M. and Rassool, G. Hussein (1998) Alcohol: community detoxification and clinical care. In G. Hussein Rassool (ed.) *Substance Use and Misuse: Nature, Context and Clinical Interventions.* Oxford: Blackwell Science.

Heather, N., Raistrick, D. and Godfrey, C. (2006) *A Review of the Effectiveness of Treatment for Alcohol Problems.* London: National Treatment Agency.

Ito, J.R. and Donovan, D.M. (1986) Aftercare in alcoholism treatment: a review. In W.R. Miller and N. Heather (eds) *Treating Addictive Behaviours: Processes of Change.* New York: Plenum Press.

Modesto-Lowe, V. and Kranzler, H.R. (1999) Diagnosis and treatment of alcohol-dependent patients with comorbid psychiatric disorders. *Alcohol Research & Health*, 23, 2: 144–9.

Moore, K. (2006) Alcohol & dual diagnosis. In G. Hussein Rassool (ed.) *Dual Diagnosis Nursing.* Oxford: Blackwell Publications.

National Treatment Agency (2007) *Models of Care for Alcohol Misusers.* London: NTA Publications.

Oei, T.P.S. and Loveday, W.A.L. (1997) Management of comorbid anxiety and alcohol disorders: parallel treatment of disorders. *Drug and Alcohol Review*, 16: 261–74.

Petrakis, I.L., Gonzalez-Haddad, G., Rosenheck, R. and Krystal, J.H. (2002) Comorbidity of alcoholism and psychiatric disorders. *Alcohol Research and Health*, 26: 81–9.

Rollnick, S., Heather, N. and Bell A. (1992) Negotiating behaviour change in medical settings: the development of brief motivational interviewing. *Journal of Mental Health*, 1: 25–37.

Royal College of Physicians (2001) *Report on Alcohol: Guidelines for Managing Wernicke's Encephalopathy in the Accident and Emergency Department.* London: The Royal College of Physicians.

Royal College of Psychiatrists (2005) *Alcohol: Our Favourite Drug. Fact Sheet.* London: RCP.

Shaw, J.M., Kolesar, G.S., Sellers, E.M., Kaplan, H.L. and Sandor, P. (1981) Development of optimal treatment tactics for alcohol withdrawal, assessment and effectiveness of supportive care. *Journal of Clinical Psychopharmacology*, 1, 6: 382–8.

Stockwell, T., Bolt, L. and Russel, G. (1991) Home detoxification from alcohol: its safety and efficacy in comparison to inpatient care. *Alcohol and Alcoholism*, 26: 645–50.

Wasilewski, D., Matsumoto, H., Kur, E., Dziklinska, A., Wozny, E., Stencka, K., Chaba, P. and Szelenberger, W. (1996) Assessment of diazepam loading dose therapy of delirium tremens. *Alcohol and Alcoholism*, 31, 3: 273–8.

CHAPTER 31

SMOKING CESSATION: HEALTHCARE INTERVENTIONS

OBJECTIVES

- Describe the feature of a smoking cessation service.

- Discuss the benefits of smoking cessation.

- Identify the psychological interventions used in smoking cessation.

- Identify the nicotine and non-nicotine replacement therapy used in smoking cessation.

- Discuss the assessment and interventions to enable smokers to quit.

The dependence of nicotine is classified as a psychiatric disorder in ICD-10 and DSM-IV. Nicotine-dependence defining features include failed attempts to abstain, powerful urges to use nicotine and withdrawal symptoms on cessation. The World Health Organization (2008) report on status of global efforts against tobacco indicates that only 5% of the global population is protected by comprehensive national smoke-free legislation; 40% of countries still allow smoking in hospitals and schools; and services to treat tobacco dependence are fully available in only nine countries, covering 5% of the world's people.

An important element of the UK strategy on smoking (Department of Health 1998) is the establishment of smoking cessation services in the NHS, in recognition that many smokers want to stop, but find it hard to do so. The government in England has set up a comprehensive NHS Stop Smoking Service which is now available across the NHS in England. This provides counselling and support to smokers wanting to quit, complementing the use of stop-smoking aids, nicotine replacement therapy (NRT) and

Bupropion (Zyban). The NHS Stop Smoking Service has successfully helped many people to quit smoking, but quit rates are still lower among people in routine, casual and manual work than among those in higher socio-economic groups (Willis 2007).

An evaluation of the NHS Stop Smoking Service (Information Centre 2008) shows that the majority of those setting a quit date for smoking cessation received NRT (74%), 10% received Champix (Varenicline), 4% received Bupropion (Zyban) and fewer than 1% received both NRT and Bupropion. Champix was the most successful smoking cessation aid in helping people quit. The findings from an evaluation of the NHS Stop Smoking Services programme funded by the Department of Health (Bauld *et al.* 2005) showed that it can contribute to a (modest) reduction in health inequalities: long-term quit rates show about 15% of people continue not to smoke at 52 weeks; and that it is cost-effective in helping smokers quit. This shows that a smoker who tries to quit with the NHS Stop Smoking Service, using NRT or Zyban is up to four times as likely to succeed than by willpower alone. A Cochrane review (Stead *et al.* 1996) of the evidence on NRT found that it roughly doubles the chances of a smoker successfully quitting compared to someone using no therapy.

SMOKING CESSATION SERVICE

A smoking cessation service should include both psychological (motivational) and pharmacological treatment interventions. The NHS Stop Smoking Service typically combines behavioural support, delivered in a group or individual setting, with pharmacotherapy (NRT or Bupropion). The aims of the service are to provide an accessible, effective smoking cessation counselling service for staff, clients and the local community and to deliver training on smoking cessation to health professionals (Mills 1998)

Referrals to the clinics are usually from general practitioners, health professionals or smokers who have contacted the service via free-phone helplines. Once contact is made with the smoking cessation service, an information session can be used to provide details of the services, brief intervention advice and information on treatments and interventions to aid smoking cessation. Service users attending smoking clinics are offered help and advice in preparation for their quit date as well as motivational support and encouragement through their first month. All service users are required to attend an assessment interview, followed by joining either group therapy sessions or a 'one to one' therapy. The duration of 'one to one' therapy sessions may depend on the clients' needs and progress made. The duration of group sessions is variable and depends on local services and needs of service users. In some services, specialist smoking courses for heavily addicted smokers who wish to quit are provided. Drop-in services are available without the need to make an appointment. To encourage pregnant women to access the service, partnerships with the maternity services have been set up in some smoking cessation schemes. Using modern technology, the service can now measure the carbon monoxide levels and chronological age of the lungs. The feedback provided and the benefits identified can be a motivating factor in nudging pre-contemplators to contemplation or action.

Psychological interventions play an integral role in smoking cessation treatment, either in conjunction with medication or alone. A variety of methods to assist smokers in quitting include coaching individuals to recognise high-risk smoking situations, develop alternative coping strategies, manage stress and improve problem-solving skills, as well as increase social support. Self-help materials are also provided to complement the psychological interventions.

HEALTH GAINS AND BENEFITS OF SMOKING CESSATION

Improvement in overall health and health gains will be gained through smoking cessation. The risk of death of former smokers compared to that for continuing smokers begins to decline shortly after giving up until after some 15 years of abstinence. Smoking cessation substantially reduces the risk of coronary heart disease among men and women, and reduces the risk of stroke. A reduction of risk between 30% and 50% for lung cancer has been reported after ten years' abstinence. Bladder cancer and cervical cancer risks are also substantially lower after a few years of abstinence. Women who stop smoking before becoming pregnant have infants of the same birth weight as those born to women who have never smoked. A summary of the key benefits of quitting smoking is presented in Table 31.1.

Table 31.1 Benefits of quitting smoking (time lapse)

Time	Changes
20 minutes	• Blood pressure drops to normal • Pulse rate drops to normal • Temperature of hands and feet increases to normal
8 hours	• Carbon monoxide level in blood returns to normal • Oxygen level in blood returns to normal
24 hours	• Immediate risk of heart attack starts to fall
48 hours	• Nerve endings start to regrow • Ability to taste and smell enhanced
14 days	• Circulation improves • Walking becomes easier • Lung function increases up to 30%
1 month	• Most nicotine withdrawal symptoms disappear
3 months	• Lung function improves • Nagging cough disappears • Cilia regrow in the lungs, increasing their ability to handle mucus, clean themselves and reduce infection
9 months	• Risk of pregnancy complications and foetal death reduced to level of non-smoker
1 year	• Excess risk of coronary heart disease half that of a smoker • There is no safe point beyond which relapse will not occur
5 years	• Risk of lung cancer decreases by half • Stroke risk same as non-smoker • Risk of mouth, throat and oesophageal cancer half that of a smoker
10 years	• Lung cancer death rate same as non-smoker • Pre-cancerous cells replaced
15 years	• Risk of coronary heart disease same as a non-smoker

Source: Adapted from www.quitsmokingsupport.com/benefits.htm (accessed 15 December 2007)

ASSESSMENT AND INTERVENTIONS

The assessment of nicotine dependence and motivation to quit is based on the Fagerström test for nicotine dependence (Heatherton *et al.* 1991). The taking of a smoking history is presented in Table 31.2. The assessment interview may last for 20–30 minutes and is common to all potential quitters. It is during the assessment interview that the client may decide not to join the next group but prefer 'one to one' counselling. On admission to the clinic, a contract or ground rules are discussed with the service user and a setting and a 'quit date' are agreed. It is valuable at this stage to allow service users to express any anxieties regarding the quit attempt and to examine previous failed attempts. The type of NRT should be decided (patches or gum) and its use and limitations explained to the client.

The ECO level (measuring carbon monoxide) is taken, as carbon monoxide levels are an indicator of the amount of tobacco smoke inhaled by an individual smoker (Foulds 1996). ECO measurement is a quick, simple, non-invasive test but the levels of carbon monoxide can be affected by the time elapsed since the last cigarette. Readings taken in the afternoon give a more accurate indication than morning readings and it is important to point this out to the client (Mills 1998). ECO levels can also be affected by recent exercise, and the depth and frequency of inhalation. Carbon monoxide is excreted by the body quite rapidly and will reduce considerably within hours of giving up smoking. Using an ECO monitor where clients can see one of the positive effects of not smoking can add a major incentive towards quitting (Mills 1998).

A second appointment should be made for the quit date and the service user should be encouraged to make immediate preparations to quit. This involve making changes such as disposing of smoking equipment as well as changes in daily routine at work or at home. The client needs also to be prepared to deal with stress without nicotine and socialisation with partner or friends who are smokers. During this session, for those who have quit smoking prior to the appointment, it is important to explore their feelings and the coping strategies they have used during this period. Clients often describe the first week as 'not too bad', appearing to be almost euphoric and confident, while others describe cravings and physical discomforts such as sleeplessness, anxiety and difficulty concentrating (Foulds *et al.* 1993). It is important to caution the over-confident that the euphoria may lessen somewhat, while pointing out the positive results of quitting to those who are perhaps viewing the prospect of being a non-smoker as less attractive as a result of their present discomfort (Mills 1998).

Further sessions can be arranged for the provision of support and counselling and for ECO measurements. Telephone contact and support may be a suitable alternative

Table 31.2 Taking a smoking history

- Number of years as a smoker?
- How soon after waking is the first cigarette?
- Does the client crave a cigarette when in a no-smoking area or situation?
- Examine any previous attempts to quit
- Assess suitability for nicotine replacement therapy (NRT), for example, no contraindications (in certain cases written permission from the client's GP may need to be obtained)
- Ensure the client has realistic expectations of the efficacy of the treatment
- Discuss concerns, for example, withdrawal discomfort
- Measure expired carbon monoxide levels (ECO)

for clients unable to attend the clinic on a regular basis. The measurement of ECO level of carbon monoxide should be undertaken at four weeks from the quit date for most quitters. Many smokers will need to make multiple attempts to quit before achieving long-term success and it is therefore important that services remain committed to providing repeat interventions for those who are motivated to make a new quit attempt following a relapse.

BRIEF INTERVENTIONS FOR SMOKERS

The psychological technique of brief interventions involves opportunistic advice, discussion, negotiation or encouragement (see Chapter 26) and is delivered in a range of primary and community service provisions. For smoking cessation, brief interventions (NICE 2006) typically take between five and ten minutes and may include one or more of the following:

- simple opportunistic advice to stop
- assessment of the patient's commitment to quit
- pharmacotherapy and/or behavioural support
- provision of self-help material and referral to more intensive support such as the NHS Stop Smoking Service.

NICE (2006) has recommended that everyone who smokes should be advised to quit and that, for a service user who presents with a smoking-related disease, the cessation advice may be linked to their medical condition. Advice to stop smoking should be sensitive to the individual's preferences, needs and circumstances. General practitioners and nurses in primary and community care should advise all patients who smoke to quit and offer a referral to an NHS Stop Smoking Service. All other health professionals, such as hospital clinicians, pharmacists and dentists and community workers, should refer people who smoke to an intensive support service (for example, NHS Stop Smoking Service). Figure 31.1 shows the intervention strategies for smokers.

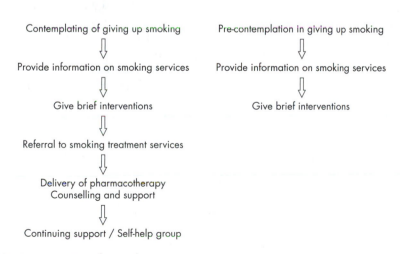

FIGURE 31.1 Interventions for smokers

PHARMACOLOGICAL INTERVENTIONS

The main forms of pharmacological treatment covered are nicotine replacement therapy (NRT) and the antidepressant Bupropion. Nice (2002) has recommended that, in deciding which therapies to use and in which order they should be prescribed, practitioners should take into account:

- intention and motivation to quit, and likelihood of compliance
- the availability of counselling or support
- previous usage of smoking cessation aids
- contraindications and potential for adverse effects
- personal preferences of the smoker

NICOTINE REPLACEMENT THERAPY

The aims of NRT are to reduce withdrawal symptoms associated with stopping smoking by replacing the nicotine from tobacco smoking. NRT is available as skin patches that deliver nicotine slowly, and chewing gum, nasal spray, inhalers, and lozenges or tablets, all of which deliver nicotine to the brain more quickly than skin patches, but less rapidly than smoking cigarettes (Stead *et al.* 1996). NRT is currently produced as:

- transdermal patch (varying doses, 16 hours and 24 hours duration)
- gum (2 mg and 4 mg)
- sublingual tablet (2 mg)
- nasal spray (0.5 mg per dose, usually administered two doses at a time)
- inhalator or inhaler
- lozenge (1, 2 and 4 mg)

NRT substitutes produce less severe physiological alterations than tobacco-based systems, do not contain the carcinogens and gases associated with tobacco smoke and have little abuse potential since they do not produce the pleasurable effects of tobacco products (NIDA 2006). A Cochrane review (Stead *et al.* 1996) found evidence that all forms of NRT made it more likely that a person's attempt to quit smoking would succeed. The chances of stopping smoking were increased by 50% to 70%. The review also indicated that heavier smokers may need higher doses and works with or without additional counselling.

NON-NICOTINE-BASED PHARMACOLOGICAL MEDICATION

Some smokers may prefer a treatment that is not nicotine-based: the atypical antidepressant Bupropion has been well studied and is the only non-nicotine medication licensed as an aid to smoking cessation (Hughes *et al.* 2004). Bupropion is an effective intervention and should be offered as a treatment option for patients requesting help with smoking cessation, unless any of the contraindications apply. However, Bupropion is unsuitable for some patient groups (for example, pregnant women, people with a history of seizures or eating disorders) for which nicotine replacement may be considered (Lingford-Hughes *et al.* 2004). Bupropion is not recommended for smokers under the age of 18 years, as its safety and efficacy have not been evaluated for this group. Bupropion should normally be prescribed only as part of an abstinent-contingent treatment (ACT), in which the smoker makes a commitment to stop smoking on or before a particular date (target stop date) (NICE 2002). There is currently insufficient evidence to recommend the use of NRT and Bupropion in combination.

Varenicline (Champix, Pfizer) has also been recommended as an option for smokers who have expressed a desire to quit smoking (NICE 2007). The summary of product characteristics states that smokers should set a date to stop smoking, that treatment with Varenicline should start one to two weeks before this date and that smoking cessation therapies are more likely to succeed for patients who are provided with additional advice and support. However, Varenicline may be associated with nausea and other gastrointestinal disorders such as vomiting.

Several other non-nicotine medications are being investigated for the treatment of tobacco addiction, including other antidepressants and an anti-hypertensive medication, among others. Scientists are also investigating the potential of a vaccine that targets nicotine for use in relapse prevention. The nicotine vaccine is designed to stimulate the production of antibodies that would block access of nicotine to the brain and prevent nicotine's reinforcing effects (NIDA 2006).

KEY POINTS

- The NHS Stop Smoking Service provides counselling and support to smokers wanting to quit, complementing the use of stop smoking aids, nicotine replacement therapy (NRT) and Bupropion (Zyban).
- An evaluation of the NHS Stop Smoking Service shows that the majority of those setting a quit date for smoking cessation received NRT.
- A smoking cessation service should include both psychological (motivational) and pharmacological treatment interventions.
- Brief intervention advice and information on treatment interventions to aid smoking cessation are provided.
- The assessment of nicotine dependence and motivation to quit is based on the Fagerström test for nicotine dependence
- NICE has provided a care pathway for smokers who wish to quit tobacco smoking.
- NICE has recommended that everyone who smokes should be advised to quit.
- The aims of NRT are to reduce withdrawal symptoms associated with stopping smoking by replacing the nicotine from tobacco smoking.
- Some smokers may prefer a treatment that is not nicotine-based.
- The atypical antidepressant Bupropion has been well studied and is the only non-nicotine medication licensed as an aid to smoking cessation.
- Bupropion is unsuitable for some patient groups (e.g. pregnant women or people with a history of seizures or eating disorders) for which nicotine replacement may be considered.

- Varenicline (Champix, Pfizer) has also been recommended as an option for smokers who have expressed a desire to quit smoking.
- Varenicline may be associated with nausea and other gastrointestinal disorders such as vomiting.
- Several other non-nicotine medications are being investigated for the treatment of tobacco addiction, including other antidepressants and an anti-hypertensive medication.
- Scientists are also investigating the potential of a vaccine that targets nicotine for use in relapse prevention.

ACTIVITY 31.1

Please state whether the following statements are true or false. Reflect on the statements and give reason(s) for choosing a particular option

	True	False
Dependence on nicotine is classified as a psychiatric disorder in ICD-10 and DSM-IV		
Smokers' quit rates are still higher among people in routine, casual and manual work		
An evaluation of the NHS Stop Smoking Service shows that the majority of those setting a quit date for smoking cessation received both NRT and bupropion		
There is evidence that NRT doubles the chances of a smoker successfully quitting compared to someone using no therapy		
Using modern technology the service can now measure the carbon monoxide levels and the chronological age of the lungs		
Many smokers will need to make multiple attempts to quit before achieving long-term success		
The aim of NRT is to reduce withdrawal symptoms associated with stopping smoking		
Some smokers may prefer a treatment that is not nicotine-based		
Bupropion is recommended for smokers under the age of 18 years		
There is current evidence to recommend the use of NRT and bupropion in combination		
Varenicline (Champix, Pfizer) has been recommended as an option for smokers		

ACTIVITY 31.2

There is only one correct answer to the following multiple choice questions

Features defining nicotine dependence include
a. Failed attempts to abstain
b. Powerful urges to use nicotine
c. Withdrawal symptoms on cessation
d. All of the above

The NHS Stop Smoking Service provides
a. Counselling and support to smokers wanting to quit
b. Behavioural interventions and social support
c. Nicotine replacement therapy and bupropion
d. All of the above

Referrals to the clinics are usually from
a. General practitioners
b. Health professionals
c. Smokers who have contacted the service
d. All of the above

A variety of methods to assist smokers in quitting include
a. Identifying high-risk smoking situations
b. Developing alternative coping strategies
c. Managing stress
d. All of the above

The assessment of nicotine dependence and motivation to quit is based on the
a. Model of change
b. Fagerström test
c. Assessment interview
d. Counselling

The ECO level is taken to measure
a. Carbon dioxide levels
b. Carbon monoxide levels
c. Smoke inhalation
d. Inhaled nicotine

ECO levels can also be affected by
a. Recent exercise
b. Depth of inhalation
c. Frequency of inhalation
d. All of the above

The psychological techniques of brief interventions involve
a.   Opportunistic advice
b.   Negotiation
c.   Encouragement
d.   All of the above

NRT is available as
a.   Skin patches
b.   Chewing gum
c.   Nasal spray
d.   All of the above

Bupropion is an effective intervention and should be offered
a.   As a treatment option
b.   To clients who are pregnant
c.   To clients with history of seizures
d.   To clients with eating disorders

ACTIVITY 31.3

- Describe the feature of a smoking cessation service
- Discuss the benefits of smoking cessation
- Identify the psychological interventions used in smoking cessation
- Identify the nicotine and non-nicotine replacement therapy used in smoking cessation
- Discuss the assessment and interventions to enable smokers to quit

REFERENCES

Bauld, L., Coleman, T., Adams, C., Pound, E. and Ferguson, J. (2005) Delivering the English smoking treatment services. *Addiction*, 100: 19–27. doi:10.1111/j.1360-0443.2005.01024.x (accessed 12 December 2007).

Department of Health (1998) *Smoking Kills*. London: Department of Health.

Foulds, J. (1993) Does nicotine replacement therapy work? *Addiction*, 88: 1473–78.

Foulds, J. (1996) Strategies for smoking cessation. *British Medical Bulletin*, 52, 1: 157–73.

Foulds, J., Stapleton, J., Hayward, M., Russell, M.A., Feyerabend, C., Fleming, T. and Costello, J. (1993) Transdermal nicotine patches with low-intensity support to aid smoking cessation in outpatients in a general hospital. A placebo-controlled trial. *Arch. Fam. Med.*, 2, 4: 417–23.

Heatherton, T.F., Kozlowski, L.T., Frecker, R.C. and Fagerström, K.O. (1991) The Fagerström Tolerance Questionnaire. *British Journal of Addiction*, 86: 1119–27.

Hughes, J., Stead, L. and Lancaster, T. (2004) Antidepressants for smoking cessation (Cochrane Review). In *The Cochrane Library*. Chichester: John Wiley & Sons, Ltd.

Information Centre (2008) *Statistics on NHS Stop Smoking Services in England, April to September 2007*. www.ic.nhs.uk (accessed 12 December 2007).

Lingford-Hughes, A.R., Welch, S. and Nutt, D.J. (2004) Evidence-based guidelines for the pharmacological management of substance misuse. *Journal of Psychopharmacology*, 18, 3: 293–335.

Mills, C. (1998) Nicotine addiction: health care interventions. In G. Hussein Rassool (ed.) *Substance Use and Misuse: Nature, Context and Clinical Interventions*. Oxford: Blackwell Publications.

National Institute of Drug Abuse (2006) *Research Report Series. Tobacco Addiction*. NIDA, NIH Publication Number 06-4342. Bethesda, MD: NIDA.

NICE (2002) *Guidance in the Use of Nicotine Replacement Therapy (NRT) and Bupropion for Smoking Cessation*, Summary, TA39. London: National Institute for Clinical Excellence.

NICE (2006) *Brief Interventions and Referral for Smoking Cessation in Primary Care and Other Settings*, Public Health Guidance No. 1. London: National Institute for Clinical Excellence.

NICE (2007) *Varenicline: Guidance for Smoking Cessation*, TA123. London: National Institute for Clinical Excellence.

Stead, L.F., Perera, R., Bullen, C., Mant, D. and Lancaster, T. (1996) *Nicotine Replacement Therapy for Smoking Cessation*. Cochrane Database of Systematic Reviews 1996, Issue 3. Art. No.: CD000146. DOI: 10.1002/14651858.CD000146.pub3 (accessed 12 December 2007).

Willis, N. (2007) *NHS Stop Smoking Services – Service and Monitoring Guidance 2007/08*. London: Department of Health.

WHO (2008) *Global Efforts Against Tobacco*. Geneva, World Health Organization.

CHAPTER 32

COMPETENCE AND PROFESSIONAL DEVELOPMENT

OBJECTIVES

▪ Provide an awareness of current policies regarding the integration of alcohol and drug in professional education.

▪ Provide an awareness of the integration of substance misuse in the curriculum.

▪ Identify the barriers in health professionals' reluctance to work with substance misusers.

▪ Outline the knowledge and skills required for staff working in the substance misuse field.

There is an increasingly acknowledgement that drug and alcohol misuse is a major public health problem, and the previous chapters have reinforced this notion. The argument for raising the profile of alcohol and drug misuse problems is challenging in the realisation that substance misuse is more likely to be the norm than the exception among the population. The recognition, screening, and brief psychosocial interventions with alcohol and drug misusers are very much 'core business' for primary and community health services.

There is a pressing need for health and social care professionals to develop their knowledge and clinical expertise in substance misuse in order to respond effectively to potential misusers and to those with severe substance misuse problems. However, education and training in alcohol and drug use and misuse have been largely patchy and limited, and have lagged behind the growth in service provision. Many reports have recommended that professional bodies in health and social work should continue to design training in the early identification of drug and alcohol misuse and appropriate referral skills for professionals working in health, social care and the criminal justice system. The goal of education and training in substance use would be to: provide an increased awareness and recognition of the needs of the patients, enhance the sharecared and collaborative approaches between the different disciplines, improve the evidenced-based intervention strategies required and provide high-quality care (Rassool 2002).

REVIEW OF RECOMMENDATIONS: INTEGRATION OF SUBSTANCE MISUSE IN THE CURRICULUM

Several governmental reports have identified the importance and the need for the educational preparation of health and social care professional and allied disciplines in working with substance misusers. The reports mentioned in this section are presented in the context of education and training of health and social care professionals. Governmental strategies have focused on the importance of staff working in different agencies, including primary healthcare workers and staff in the prison health system, to receive adequate training in substance-use education strategy for tackling drug misuse. The Advisory Council on the Misuse of Drugs (ACMD 1988, 1989, 1990, 1991) reports recommended that information on the recognition and management of drug misusers should be part of the basic training of all professionals who are likely to have contact with them. The reports further recommended that relevant training bodies should take steps to ensure that appropriate arrangements for training are instituted as a matter of urgency.

The ACMD report (1990) *Problem Drug Use: A Review of Training* recommended the integration of substance use and misuse as part of the core curriculum should be at both undergraduate and postgraduate levels. The report made further recommendation that specialist training should equip those who are directly involved in the management of drug-related problems to embrace a whole range of knowledge and skills, including interventions, counselling, knowledge of drink/drugs interaction, research and evaluation. The National Alcohol Training Strategy report (Alcohol Concern 1994), recommended that the basic training which is provided for professionals staff such as doctors, nurses, social workers and probation officers should ensure that they are competent in the performance of their professional role. It does not, however, always include the competences required for the early identification of alcohol misuse, for offering appropriate response and for making appropriate referrals where indicated. Professional staff also need opportunities for post-basic training to enable them to specialise in work with alcohol misusers. The All-Party Parliamentary Drug Misuse Groups' report (2000) recommended that better training in substance misuse and dual diagnosis for doctors, nurses, social workers, probation officers, police and prison officers and voluntary sector personnel would assist in the early recognition of the condition and better accessibility to appropriate treatment provision.

ALCOHOL AND DRUGS IN THE EDUCATIONAL PROGRAMME

Despite the recommendations at national and international levels (WHO 1993), the substance-misuse component in the undergraduate medical, nursing, social work, pharmacy and psychology curriculum lags behind current awareness of substance misuse as a major national health problem. Education about drugs and alcohol and their impact on health still find insufficient space within the medical curriculum (Glass 1990). In England, a review on the preparation of nurses for both pre-registration and post-registration in substance misuse by the English National Board reaffirms the lack of adequate preparation of nurses, midwives and health visitors, the low priority accorded to the substance-misuse component and the incongruity of curricular content (ENB 1995). The ENB recommends that substance use and misuse should be included in all pre-registration and post-registration nursing, midwifery and health visiting curricular guidelines.

In a survey of substance-misuse education in British medical schools, Crome (1999) found that medical students are receiving six hours of formal training and stated that the amount of input had halved in the last ten years. However, she found that only one department, within a medical school, delivers 30 hours of substance misuse education and co-ordinates another 30 hours throughout the undergraduate medical education. Day *et al.* (1999) found that fewer than half of the respondents of 143 psychiatrists surveyed in the UK had received formal training in the management of substance misuse in the previous five years. In social work and probation qualifying training, Harrison (1993) suggested that there has been some improvement in integrating alcohol-related knowledge and skills in the curriculum. It seems that several social work courses are providing students with an extensive educational programme on substance use problems, in one case amounting to eight weeks of full-time formal education (Harrison 1993). In nursing, there is little evidence to suggest that the integration of the substance-misuse component in the undergraduate and postgraduate curriculum has been implemented in educational institutions (Murphy-Parker and Rassool 2000, Rassool 2000). However, it is acknowledged that in the UK and the USA the integration of substance use and misuse components in the undergraduate and postgraduate nursing curriculum is still restricted to a few centres of excellence.

ATTITUDINAL BARRIERS

Health and social care professionals may be reluctant to respond appropriately because of the lack of adequate preparation and negative attitudes towards substance misusers. Social prejudice, negative attitudes and stereotyped perceptions of substance misusers (Rassool 1998, Selleck and Redding 1998) and dual diagnosis patients (Williams 1999) are held widely amongst healthcare professionals, and this may lead to minimal care being given to this population. Studies support the idea that the development of a more positive and non-judgemental attitude and confidence and skills in identifying and working with substance misuse and related problems may be partly related to the provision of education and training. However, much professional education and training reinforces the view that dealing with substance misuse is the job of a specialist

(Rassool 1993, 2000). In the case of dual diagnosis patients, the responsibility for health and social care provisions can be shifted from one discipline to another and this 'diffusion of responsibility' is all too apparent (Rassool 2006).

TRAINING NEEDS AND GOOD PRACTICE

Education and training in alcohol and drug misuse, at a local level, should not be ad hoc but be based upon a systematic planning. Initially, purchasers should develop an educational strategy with local authorities, educationalists and providers of services to identify the target needs and the planning of an educational programme. It is acknowledged that, although this process is complex and time-consuming, it is invaluable in the delivering of high-quality training and is service-driven. A training needs analysis is of paramount importance and should be part of a coherent strategy. The targeted audience for training should be mental health and addiction nurses, psychiatrists, social workers, prison healthcare staff, probation officers and others in the criminal justice system and primary health care teams and staff in the non-statutory organisations – in effect, all those who come in contact with service users, generic and specialist staff, in both hospital and community settings. This question here is not who needs training in dual diagnosis but what kind and levels of training are required.

The principles of good practice in education and training and the design and delivery of training require the setting of clear aims, learning outcomes, content, teaching methodologies and evaluation. The teaching and learning strategies used should be innovative and these should be directed and guided by the learning outcomes. Visits and structured clinical placements should be incorporated into the educational plan. An important component in the design of the curriculum is the selection of tools and procedures to be used in the assessment of learning and the evaluation of the course. The challenge for educators and trainers in professional education is to change from a traditional method of course development by adopting a framework based on the learning or occupational needs and curriculum model.

KNOWLEDGE AND SKILLS FOR TACKLING SUBSTANCE MISUSE

The knowledge and skills specification below outlines the key areas of knowledge and skills from Skills for Health (2007) that members of staff are likely to need in their first six months in post. The knowledge and skills areas can be used as a framework as a basis for learning outcomes and training courses. This could include all the areas in the specification, or be tailored for participants from particular professional backgrounds. To perform competently in the substance-misuse field, you need to know and understand the following.

substances and their effects
- the difference between legal and illegal drugs, the reasons for the different classifications under law and the social construction of the law in relation to substance use

- the range of different substances, their appearance, methods of taking them, their effects, the risks they pose and their implications for the delivery of services
- the interactions between different drugs
- substance-misuse jargon and commonly used terminology
- the impact of the language used to describe substance use and users upon the development and maintenance of therapeutic relationships

substance use and dependence
- the underlying issues that may lead to substance misuse
- the continuum of substance use from recreational to problematic
- the relationship between the settings in which substances are used and the activities of the individuals using substances
- the interrelationship between the background of individuals and the effect of substances on them: experience and expectations, mental and psychological state (including dual diagnosis), physical health problems (including related diseases), energy levels at the time of consumption, body weight
- the prevalence of substance use, age of use and relationship to substance type, relationship between (problematic) substance use and economic disadvantage and/or emotional deprivation
- issues of diversity including differing patterns of use in groups, such as Black and ethnic minority groups and women, and responses to use with these groups
- the nature of poly-substance use
- the nature of dependence (psychological and physical) on substances
- the reasons why individuals decide to reduce or cease substance use

substance misuse specific legislation, strategies and policies
- relevant and specific legislation, e.g. the Misuse of Drugs Act (1971) and the Medicines Act (1968)
- national strategies, frameworks and standards, e.g. *Tackling Drugs to Build a Better Britain* and the *Alcohol Harm Reduction Strategy for England, Tackling Substance Misuse in Wales: A Partnership Approach, Models of Care Framework for Developing Local Systems of Effective Drug Misuse Treatment in England, Drug Misuse and Dependence – Guidelines on Clinical Management*, DANOS, QuADS etc.
- local and organisational policies and protocols which support the delivery of services to substance misusers, e.g. confidentiality, information sharing, joint working, health and safety regulations, etc.

substance-misuse harm minimisation strategies and interventions
- the risks substance misuse may pose to individuals (both in the short and the long term), and how to recognise, assess and minimise these risks and the effects of these risks
- the range of actions to take appropriate to your assessment of risk
- the range of harms associated with different methods of drug use, including blood-borne viruses
- interventions commonly used to minimise the harms of substance misuse
- sources of substance-misuse harm minimisation advice
- the reasons why it is important to supervise methadone consumption
- how and when to conduct relapse prevention interventions

recognising substance misuse
- the range of behaviours that can be expected from substance users, and how to deal with these
- the range of different indications of substance-misuse-related problems including drug use, alcohol use, psychological problems, physical problems, social problems and legal problems
- how to investigate situations sufficiently to allow you to make a reasonable judgement about whether individuals are misusing substances
- other factors which can produce indications that may be interpreted as caused by substance misuse
- the range of actions that can be taken when individuals may be misusing substances, and how to decide what action is appropriate

dealing with overdose situations
- the signs and behaviours associated with overdose of a range of substances, and how to deal with these
- the reasons for obtaining personal details from the individual or any person near the individual who has used the substance, and how to do so
- the importance of obtaining information on the substance used from the individual or any person near the individual who has used the substance, and how to do so
- how to encourage substance users suspected of overdose to describe any pain or discomfort they may be experiencing
- how to administer first aid, and assess if safe to do so

screening, assessment and referral of substance users
- the importance of responding promptly to individuals presenting for substance-misuse services in order to maintain their motivation and seize the opportunity for intervention
- the range of needs relating to their substance use individuals may have, and ways of assessing and meeting these needs
- the range of co-existing needs (e.g. physical health, mental health, legal, social and economic) that substance users may have, and ways of assessing and meeting these needs
- the levels of screening and assessment used in substance-misuse services
- the risks to children of substance users, and ways of assessing and addressing these risks
- ways of addressing substance misuse during screening and/or assessment processes
- how to elicit the patient's own views of their substance misuse
- how to respond to clients expressing concern about their substance misuse
- screening and or assessment documentation (paper and electronic), and how to complete it
- the national drug treatment monitoring form, and how to complete it
- policies and protocols for referring individuals to other services
- how to respond to individuals who do not want to be referred to other services

care planning
- how and where to access information and support that can inform your practice when assessing individual needs and preferences, and contributing to the development, implementation and review of care plans

- government reports, inquiries and research reports relevant to the assessment of individual needs and the development, implementation and review of care plans

theories and best practice relevant to:
- the assessment of the holistic needs and circumstances of individuals
- care planning, implementation and review generally, and specifically to the individuals with whom you work
- methods of monitoring, reviewing and evaluating care plans

methods of supporting individuals to:
- contribute to assessments and reviews
- express their needs and preferences
- understand and take responsibility for promoting their own health and care
- identify how their care needs should be met
- assess and manage risks to their health and well-being

role of relationships and support networks in:
- the assessment of individual needs
- care planning, implementation and review
- factors that affect the health, well-being, behaviour, skills, abilities and development of individuals and key people
- the significant changes that are likely to affect needs and circumstances of individuals with whom you work and how these will impact on care needs assessment and the development, implementation and review of care plans
- reasons for revising care plans and how to deal with the affect this may have on individuals

substance-misuse services and other services
- forms of service provision commonly found in the substance misuse sector, e.g. shared care, inpatient prescribing, community prescribing, needle exchange, residential rehabilitation, structured day programmes, Drug Treatment and Testing Orders, arrest referral
- the range of interventions commonly used with substance users and their underpinning theoretical models, e.g. the cycle of change, basic counselling skills, solution-focused therapy, prescribing substitute medication
- the range of substance-misuse services, specialist advice or therapy agencies and support groups *in* the local area, the services they provide, and how to access them
- the range of substance-misuse services, specialist advice or therapy agencies and support groups *outside* the local area, the services they provide, and how to access them
- methods for engaging with hard-to-reach individuals and communities
- the range of services available for substance users who also have housing and social needs, and how to access them
- the range of services available for substance users who also have mental health needs, and how to access them
- the range of services available for substance users who also have criminal justice needs, and how to access them

professional practice and development

- ways of keeping your own knowledge about substances and indications of substance misuse up to date
- ways of keeping up to date with, and adding to, the evidence base for substance misuse interventions
- the limits of your own responsibility and competence and whom to refer to for assistance or advice.

CONCLUSIONS

In this chapter the emphasis has been on the importance of professional education and development on aspects of alcohol and drug misuse. Professional development will always be most effective when it is part of a strategic plan to create an organisational learning culture (Rassool 1997). There are challenges and barriers that need to be overcome if we are to provide high-quality care to alcohol and drug misusers. The denial of healthcare workers and the general public alike of the existence of substance misuse continues to present an obstacle to the provision of early recognition, health education initiatives and effective care. Furthermore, health and social care professionals have a dissonance between their personal belief-therapeutic pessimism – that is there is nothing that can be done or should be done – and their professional roles (de-skilled, lacking in confidence, etc.) (Rassool 2000). Another challenge is to overcome the marginalisation of the importance of the substance-misuse component in health and social care sciences curricula and clinical practice, at undergraduate and postgraduate levels.

The consequences of lack of adequate education and training at all levels are a self-perpetuating cycle. Where a low priority is accorded to both policy and educational development in this area, there is no opportunity for health and social care professionals to develop role adequacy. This results in reinforcing the negative attitudes and the reluctance of healthcare professionals to respond effectively to substance misusers (Rassool 1993, 2000). Owing to the nature and extent of substance misuse as a major public health problem, a cultural shift is required in many of the paradigms that have traditionally guided the work of generic and specialist health and social care professionals. One of the most important aspects of an educational programme is not only knowledge acquisition, changes in attitudes and skills development but also the transfer of 'learning' in clinical practice for the delivery of high-quality care to those with substance-misuse problems. The attainment of positive educational outcomes is only part of the solution, but how to maintain the 'new' experiences' and behaviours in clinical practice is the critical predicament (Rassool and Rawaf 2007).

KEY POINTS

- There is a pressing need for health and social care professionals to develop their knowledge and clinical expertise in substance misuse.
- Many reports have recommended that professional bodies in health and social work should continue to design training in the early identification of drug and

alcohol misuse and appropriate referral skills for professionals working in health, social care and the criminal justice system.

- Several governmental reports have identified the importance and the need for the educational preparation of health and social care professional and allied disciplines in working with substance misusers.

- The substance-misuse component in the undergraduate medical, nursing, social work, pharmacy and psychology curriculum lags behind current awareness of substance misuse as a major national health problem.

- Health and social care professionals may be reluctant to respond appropriately owing to the lack of adequate preparation and negative attitudes towards substance misusers.

REFERENCES

Advisory Council on the Misuse of Drugs (1988) *Aids and Drug Misuse. Part 1*. London: HMSO.

Advisory Council for the Misuse of Drugs (1989) *Aids and Drug Misuse. Part 2*. London: HMSO.

Advisory Council on the Misuse of Drugs (1990) *Problem Drug Use: A Review of Training*. London: HMSO.

Advisory Council on the Misuse of Drugs (1991) *Drug Misusers and the Criminal Justice System*. London: HMSO.

Alcohol Concern (1994) *A National Alcohol Training Strategy*. London: Alcohol Concern.

All-Party Parliamentary Drugs Misuse Group (2000) *Report on Drug Misuse and Mental Health: Learning Lessons on Dual Diagnosis*.

Crome, I.B. (1999) The trouble with training: substance misuse training in British medical schools revisited. What are the issues? *Drugs: Education, Prevention and Policy*, 6, 1: 111–23.

Day, E., Arcelus, J. and Kahn, A. (1999) Perceived role of psychiatrists in the management of substance misuse: a questionnaire survey. *Psychiatric Bulletin*, 23, 11: 667–70.

English National Board for Nursing, Midwifery and Health Visiting (1995) *Press Release*, July. London: ENB.

English National Board for Nursing, Midwifery and Health Visiting (1996) *Substance Use and Misuse: Guidelines for Good Practice in Education and Training of Nurses, Midwives and Health Visitors*. London: ENB.

Glass, I. (1990) Alcohol misuse as a challenge to medical education: a belated remedy. *British Medical Bulletin*, 50, 1: 164–70.

Harrison, L. (1993) *Substance Misuse: Designing Social Work Training*. London: Central Council for Education and Training in Social Work.

Murphy-Parker, D. and Rassool, G. Hussein (2000) *Education of Addictions in Nursing School Curriculum in the United States and the United Kingdom: The Urgent Need to Stir the Waters, Turn the Tide, Steer the Course and Effect a Change*. Paper presented at the 25th National Nurses Society on Addictions Education Conference, Chicago, 29 March – 2 April.

Rassool, G. Hussein (1993) Substance misuse: responding to the challenge. *Journal of Advanced Nursing* 18: 9.

Rassool, G. Hussein (1997) Professional education and training. In G. Hussein Rassool and M. Gafoor (eds) *Addiction Nursing: Perspectives on Professional and Clinical Practice*. Cheltenham: Stanley Thornes.

Rassool, G. Hussein (1998) Contemporary issues in addiction nursing. In G. Hussein Rassool (ed.) *Substance Use and Misuse: Nature, Context and Clinical Interventions*. Oxford: Blackwell Science.

Rassool, G. Hussein (2000) Addiction: global problem and global response complacency or commitment? *Journal of Advanced Nursing*, 32, 3: 505–8.

Rassool, G. Hussein (2002) Substance misuse and mental health: an overview. *Nursing Standard*, 16, 50: 47–53.

Rassool, G. Hussein (2006) Educational development & clinical supervision. In G. Hussein Rassool (ed.) *Dual Diagnosis Nursing*. Oxford: Blackwell Publications.

Rassool, G. Hussein and Rawaf S. (2007) Predictors of educational outcomes of undergraduate nursing students in alcohol and drug education. *Nurse Education Today*, 28: 691–701, doi:10.1016/j.nedt.2007.11.005.

Selleck, C.S. and Redding, B.A. (1998) Knowledge and attitudes of registered nurses towards perinatal substance abuse. *Journal of Obstetric, Gynaecologic and Neonatal Nursing*, 27: 70–8.

Skills for Health (2007) *Guidance on Competence and Qualifications: Drugs and Alcohol National Occupational Standards*. http://www.skillsforhealth.org.uk/page/competences/completed-competences-projects/list/drugs-alcohol-danos (accessed 15 December 2007).

WHO (1993) *WHO Expert Committee on Drug Dependence*, 28th Report Geneva: World Health Organization.

Williams, K. (1999) Attitudes of mental health professionals to co-morbidity between mental health problems and substance misuse. *Journal of Mental Health*, 8, 6: 606–13.

INDEX

Alcohol and Drug Misuse
Companion Website

Visit the website at
http://www.routledge.com/textbooks/9780415409674
and discover a range of online resources designed to
enhance your learning experience.

The website includes:

Interactive online questions
Test your understanding of alcohol and drug misuse with a variety of
interactive questions, with multiple choice and true or false answers.

Activities
Gain valuable insight and understanding through printable activities, for
independent or group study and available for all of the chapters.